Septic Shock - From Pathophysiology to Patient Care

Edited by Nissar Shaikh

Published in London, United Kingdom

Septic Shock - From Pathophysiology to Patient Care
http://dx.doi.org/10.5772/intechopen.1004967
Edited by Nissar Shaikh

Contributors
Abdelrahman Balal, AbdulHadi Hassan Mallick, Abdullah Raheem, Ahmad M. Obeidat, Alper B. Iskit, Anil Kumar Agarwal, Ashish Kumar, Azha Fatima, Ebtihal Mahmoud, Eduardo Almeida de Souza Minuzzo, Erum Saboohi, Eynas Abdalla, Fateen Shareef, Gamal Alameri, Girish Kumthekar, Hilal Üstündağ, Hossam Algallie, Jawdat Alali, Jonathan Eaton, Khalid Y. Fadul, Louie Keith Scott, Malek Abusannuga, Manan Doshi, Matias Nunes Frizzo, Mirna Stela Ludwig, Mohamed Elgassim, Mohammad Ataur Rahman, Nissar Shaikh, Nissar Sheikh, Pauline Brendler Goettems Fiorin, Philip Keith, Rajasekara Chakravarthi, Roshan Afsha, Sanghamitra Padhy, Sara M.I. Ahmed, Seema Nahid, Seema Nahid, Semin Turhan, Siddhartha Banerjee, Sohel Mohamed Gamal Ahmed, Songul Doganay, Taylor Conrad, Tetsuya Yumoto, Um I. Rubab, Umm E. Amara, Vítor Antunes de Oliveira, Wala Sati, Xiaxia Yu, Yong Liu, Yusra Shahid, Zakaria Attique

First published in London, United Kingdom, 2025 by IntechOpen
IntechOpen is the global imprint of INTECHOPEN LIMITED, registered in England and Wales, registration number: 11086078, 167-169 Great Portland Street, London, W1W 5PF, United Kingdom

For EU product safety concerns: IN TECH d.o.o., Prolaz Marije Krucifikse Kozulić 3, 51000 Rijeka, Croatia, info@intechopen.com or visit our website at intechopen.com.

British Library Cataloguing-in-Publication Data
A catalogue record for this book is available from the British Library

Septic Shock - From Pathophysiology to Patient Care
Edited by Nissar Shaikh
p. cm.
Print ISBN 978-0-85014-709-4
Online ISBN 978-0-85014-708-7
eBook (PDF) ISBN 978-0-85014-710-0

Meet the editor

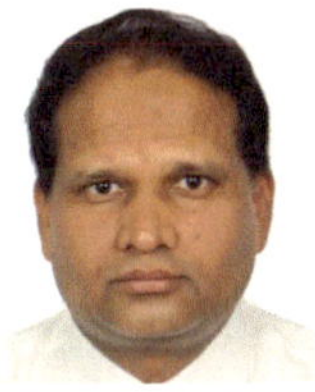

Dr. Nissar Shaikh is a surgical intensive care expert. He is a fellow of the American College of Critical Care Medicine. He has published and presented more than 200 peer-reviewed publications and national and international presentations, and he is actively involved in teaching and clinical care. Dr. Nissar has edited seven books and 41 book chapters. He is a senior consultant in critical care, assistant professor at Weill Cornell Medical College in Doha-Qatar and associate professor at Qatar University. He is the director of the surgical intensive care fellowship at Hamad Medical Corporation in Qatar. He is involved in the fellowship's academic, examination, and administrative activities. He has won three prestigious awards for distinguished services from Hamad Medical Corporation.

Contents

Preface

Sepsis is a worldwide emergency; every 2.8 seconds, one death occurs due to sepsis and septic shock. A delay in diagnosis and management of sepsis by an hour increases the mortality by 8%. In this book, we have tried to simplify the detection and management of sepsis and septic shock so that this clinical emergency will be diagnosed and managed earlier. This book comprises chapters related to the diagnosis, effects on various organs, and management of sepsis and septic shock. It is well-written by experts from their respective fields and different clinical settings. The chapters are written in simple and understandable language. We are sure that this book will not only help and update critical care physicians about sepsis and septic shock but will also be equally helpful for acute care physicians and surgeons, general practitioners, and paramedical critical, intensive care, and acute care staff and technicians in daily medical practice. Editor and authors thank Elvira Baumgartner for her timely, meticulous coordination in bringing up this valuable book. I am thankful to all authors for their writing and patience. I am indebted to my wife, Dr. Firdous and daughters, Dr. Amara and Dr. Jaza, for their unending support and encouragement.

Nissar Shaikh
Surgical Intensive Care,
Hamad Medical Corporation,
Doha, Qatar

Chapter 1

Have You Seen CINMA in Sepsis? An Update on Critical Illness Neuromuscular Abnormalities

Nissar Shaikh, Ashish Kumar, Sanghamitra Padhy and Gamal Alameri

Abstract

Critically ill neuromuscular abnormalities (CINMA) refer to the emergence of new neuromuscular weaknesses in patients receiving intensive care. This condition affects as many as 50% of critically ill individuals in intensive care setting. There are risk factors for CINMA ranging from immobility, sepsis, MODS, hyperglycemia, hypoalbuminemia, use of muscle relaxants, and steroids. The diagnosis is often delayed due to deep sedation of critically ill patients. CINMA can be diagnosed by clinical neuromuscular examination, use of hand grip strength, and MRC sum score. Electrophysiological studies (electromyography and nerve conduction study) are commonly used to diagnose the CINMA. Imaging studies such as ultrasonography, CT (computer tomography), MRI (magnetic resonance tomography), bioimpedance, and dual X-ray absorbometry are being utilized more frequently to diagnose CINMA. There is no definitive treatment of CINMA. Early mobilization, early physical therapy, and adequate nutrition support the corner stone of CINMA therapy. Timely diagnosis and intervention for sepsis are crucial in managing the condition and preventing the onset of CINMA. Additionally, controlling and preventing hyperglycemia are essential to reduce the risk of developing CINMA. Early adequate enteral nutrition support will avoid the total parenteral nutrition and help in muscular mass built up, thus preventing occurrence of CINMA. Careful and judicious use of muscle relaxants and steroids will minimize the chance of CINMA. The presence of CINMA is associated with extended ICU and hospital stays, increased ventilator days, and higher mortality rates at 1- and 5 years post-discharge. Therefore, early diagnosis and prompt management of risk factors are essential to prevent the onset of CINMA.

Keywords: CINMA, myopathy, neuropathy, immobility, nutrition, steroid, muscle relaxants, sepsis, systemic inflammatory syndrome, hyperglycemia, hyperlactatemia, muscle strength, MRC sum score, EMG, nerve conduction study

1. Introduction

In the early nineteenth century, the medical community began to recognize that patients suffering from infections experienced significant muscle mass loss, resulting in weakness. However, over the century, reports increasingly documented this association between acute illness and muscular weakness. However, in late 80s, it was found that these ICU patients exhibited variable degrees of muscle weakness, leading to difficulty and increased efforts to wean them off from ventilatory support. In the early 1980s, a study conducted by Boston described five patients with septic shock and adult respiratory distress syndrome who developed polyneuropathy, leading to prolonged muscle weakness and difficulties in weaning from ventilator [1].

Initially for *Boston et al*; it took years to described five patients of muscular weakness and polyneuropathy; leading to the perception that this condition was a rare clinical occurrence. However, with advancements in medical technologies and therapies along with increased awareness, muscular weakness is now more frequently diagnosed and managed. Although various terminologies are described to define the muscular weakness in critically ill intensive care patients such as critical illness polyneuropathy (CRP), critical illness myopathy, ICU acquired weakness (ICU AW), acute quadriplegic myopathy (AQM), cachectic myopathy, necrotizing myopathy, and thick filament myopathy, often, these terms and their associated causes overlap, prompting the recommendation to use the term critical illness neuromuscular abnormalities (CINMA) to encompass the myopathies and neuropathies observed in patients undergoing intensive care therapy. As in majority of patients, there is coexistence of CIM and CIP with inability to differentiate between the two, it is appropriate to use the term "CINMA" to describe the neuromuscular weakness in the ICU patients.

CINMA is increasingly reported due to clinical awareness, use of ultrashort acting sedation and analgesia in ICU patient, as well as increasing use electrophysiological studies, POCUS (point of care ultrasound). With the recent advancements in the management of ICU patients, the critically ill patients have an improved outcome, but complications such as CINMA increase the financial burden due to extended hospital and ICU stay, as well as increased morbidity.

2. Epidemiology

The CINMA is still underreported and undervalued in critically ill patients, and almost often the loss of muscles and muscular strength is often inaccurately and blindly labeled as ICU acquired weakness without proper investigations and diagnosis, which is not correct. Initially, only four cases were documented over a span of 4 years. By 90s, it became evident that the CINMA occurs more frequently affecting up to 70% of patients with sepsis and multiple organ dysfunction syndrome (MODS) at varying levels of severity [2]. *Steven et al.,* in their systematic review of 24 publications with more than 1000 patients, reported a prevalence of CINMA to be 46%, within 7 days of sepsis and multiple organ dysfunction [3]. More recently, *Fazzini et al.,* in their metanalysis of 3251 patients, reported the overall prevalence of critical illness neuromuscular abnormalities (CINMA) at 48%. They also reported that critically ill patients can lose more than 15% of muscle mass in their first weeks of intensive care stay, equating to a daily loss of approximately 2% of muscle mass. The majority of CINMA occurs in septic shock with MODS other medical conditions such as status asthmatics, 36%, and up to 35% severe acute exacerbation of COPD patients suffer from CINMA [4]. More than 50% of patients who are mechanically ventilated for more than 7 days will develop electrophysiological abnormities and up to 33% develop overt weakness.

CINMA has been observed and reported to occur in higher percentage (up to 67%) in patients with sepsis and septic shock with multiple organ dysfunction and persist in 36% of these patients even after discharge [5].

2.1 Risk factors

The central risk factors for the development of CINMA are sepsis and MODS (multiple organ dysfunction syndrome), along with factors such as muscle inactivity, hyperglycemia, use of steroids, and muscle relaxant [6].

Other risk factors mentioned are higher severity score, use of aminoglycosides, female gender, systemic inflammatory response syndrome (SIRS), hypoalbuminemia, high lactate, parental nutrition, and prolonged use of vasopressors.

These risk factors for CINMA are divided into two: the modifiable and non-modifiable risk factors, as described in **Table 1**.

The longer duration of bed rest was constantly associated with muscle weakness over 24 months of follow up. Increased sedation levels, along with prolonged use of steroids and muscle relaxants, were negatively associated with the development of CINMA [7]. Hyperglycemia and hypoalbuminemia were identified as modifiable risk factors contributing to the complications associated with CINMA.

The elderly patients and female gender were found to have a higher risk for the development of CINMA, along with other non-modifiable risk factors [7].

Non modifiable	Modifiable
1. Higher severity of the disease	1. Prolonged immobilization
2. SIRS and sepsis	2. Hyperglycemia
3. High serum lactate	3. Combine or prolonged use of steroids and muscle relaxant
4. MODS	4. Parental nutrition
5. ARDS and prolonged ventilation	5. Aminoglycosides
6. Female gender	6. Deep and prolonged sedation
7. Elderly patient	7. Prolong vasoactive medications use
	8. Hypoalbuminemia

Table 1.
Risk factors for CINMA.

2.2 Pathophysiology

Due to stress and decrease in protein anabolism and at the same time increase demand, it leads to muscle loss and sarcopenia in critically ill patients. The activation of sympathetic nervous system increases catabolic hormones and generation of proinflammatory cytokines which in turn triggers extensive proteolysis and impairs anabolic processes. Additionally, there is a notable decline in the levels of insulin-like growth factor 1 (IGF-1) in muscle tissue, which is closely linked to the reduction in muscle mass [8].

The mitochondrial function is essential for the life, serving as the energy powerhouse of the human body and providing the necessary energy for muscle contractions. In critically ill patients, particularly in sepsis, the mitochondrial dysfunction leads to accumulation of oxygen free radicals and a decrease in both mitochondrial expression and respiratory chain activity. The mitochondrial mitophagy (cleaves the damaged organelles) is inhibited, thus increasing the risk of death. This accumulation of damaged mitochondria causes degeneration of the muscle fibers and motor neurons leading to sarcopenia and CINMA [9].

Sepsis has a significant negative effect on calcium hemostasis, leading to a decrease in calcium release from the sarcoplasmic reticulum and an increased sensitivity of contractile proteins to calcium. These changes impair membrane excitation in skeletal muscle, ultimately resulting in diminished muscular strength [10].

The normal cell membrane permeability to Na+, K+, and Ca + ions is necessary for action potential generation. In sepsis, the activation and generation of action potential is disturbed due to reduction in membrane Na pumps. The proinflammatory cytokines has a neuro toxic effect and causes depolarization and denervation. Thus, the Na pump inactivation along with the neurotoxic effects of proinflammatory mediators leads to reduced activity in neurons and membranes, which subsequently impacts both muscles and nerves.

The occurrence of polyneuropathy in CINMA is not clear. There is a direct toxic effect of hyperglycemia and mitochondrial dysfunction on neuro-ending and neurons coupled with increased vascular permeability and microvascular alterations within the endoneurium, facilitating the infiltration of neurotoxic substances into nerve endings, leading to axonal degeneration and eventual axonal death [11].

Other mechanism for CINMA in critically ill patients includes destruction of the myofilaments by destruction of regulatory action potential and the concurrent regulation of muscle contraction, an impaired regulation of muscle function by satellite cells [11].

The pathophysiology of CINMA is summarized in **Figure 1**.

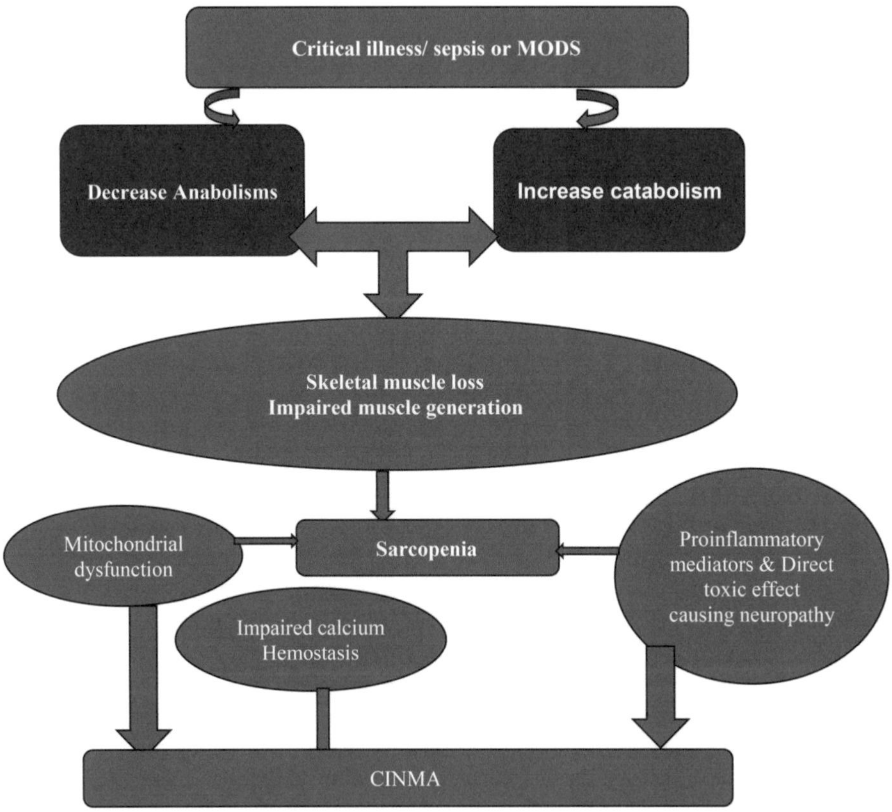

Figure 1.
Pathophysiology of CINMA.

2.3 Diagnosis

Clinical presentation starts within a week of critical illness with variable motor weakness, generally with preservation of sensation. There is a preservation of cranial nerves. There is symmetrical limb weakness, starting from the proximal to the distal muscle involvement. Facial grimacing to pain stimulation without withdrawal or motor response. In CINMA, autonomic dysfunction can occur, leading to fluctuations in heart rate ranging from tachycardia to bradycardia [12].

Early diagnosis of CINMA is essential for reducing associated morbidity and mortality rate. Currently, the diagnosis of CINMA still remains insufficient, often being suspected and confirmed at later stages. This delay can be attributed to staffing challenges and their limited understanding of CINMA, a low prioritization of the condition, and the absence of established guidelines [13].

Most of these ICU patients are sedated and ventilated with disturbed level of consciousness, hemodynamic instability, and complicated early diagnosis.

Manual assessment of hand grip and quadricep strength either through direct measurement or with a handheld dynamometer is a standard method for evaluating neuromuscular weakness in clinical practice. The hand grip strength of less than 11 and 7 kgs in male and female, respectively, may indicate the potential for critical illness neuromuscular weakness (CINMA).

Most used tools to evaluate these patients are manual muscle test scale (in up to 73%) and electrophysiological testing in up to 70%. The most frequently applied method for diagnosing CINMA is the MRC sum score, as described in **Table 2**. A score of less than 48 indicates muscular weakness, and a score of below 36 indicates sever muscle weakness [14].

The MRC sum score is derived from assessments of six upper limb muscles and six lower limb muscles. A higher MRC sum score can also complicate the diagnosis of CINMA, and a notable limitation of this scoring system is that it requires active patient participation.

The advantages of electrophysiological studies offer the benefit of distinguishing between polyneuropathy and myopathies in unconscious patients by direct stimulations and nerve conduction study. The notable drawback of electrophysiological studies is the requirement of expert consultant, along with the time-intensive nature of these studies. Various imaging studies are being increasingly utilized depending on availability and expertise to diagnosed CINMA, although CINMA should be diagnosed on high index of suspicion, thorough patient history, clinical examination,

MRC score	Score	The six muscles to evaluate
1. No contraction	1	Shoulder abduction left and right.
2. Flicker or trace of contraction	2	Elbow flexion left and right
3. Active movement without gravity	3	Wrist extension left and right
4. Active movement against gravity	4	Hip flexion left and right
5. Active movement against gravity with resistance	5	Knee extension left and right
6. Normal movement	6	Ankle dorsiflexion left and right
Normal score: 60		Quadriplegia score:0

Table 2.
The MRC score.

and the exclusion of common neuromuscular disorders. Apart from ultrasonography, the MRI (magnetic resonance imaging), CT (computerized tomography), and dual energy X-ray absorptomography (DXA) are imaging technologies in measuring and quantifying muscle size and thickness. Apart from radiation exposure, these imaging studies are expensive, requires extensive measurement, and are not accurate in larger individuals. Among all these CT and MRI are the gold standard for evaluating muscle

Electrophysiological studies	Advantages	Disadvantages
1. Nerve conduction and needle electromyography (EMG)	Differentiate neuropathy and myopathy	Invasive, expertise required, relatively contraindication in coagulopathy
2. Single nerve conduction study	Less time Less invasive	Required expert to review
3. Direct muscle stimulation	Helps in differentiating myopathies from neuropathies	Not easily available Required experts
Ultrasonography	Bed-side	Not measures muscle mass
	Non-invasive	Operator-dependent
	No radiation	Exact same person and location evaluation
	Abnormal muscle echogenicity is a good test	Not useful in severe body edema and very obese patients Low accuracy No prognostic value
Dual X-ray absorptiometry	Quick diagnosis	Radiation exposure
	Whole body scan	Expensive Experts required Inaccurate with hydration abnormalities
MRI (magnetic resonance Imaging)	Accurate	High cost
	Reliable	Time-consuming
	Valid result in very obese and edematous patients	Patient transport availability
CT (Computerized Tomography)	Accurate	Radiation
	Reliable	Patient transport availability
	Deep muscle evaluation Valid in obese and edematous patients	
Bioelectric impedance	Non-invasive	Not suitable in obese and edematous patients
	Portable Inexpensive	Affected by body position and temperature
Muscle and nerve biopsy	Gives direct and accurate changes in muscles and nerves	Invasive Experts required No prognostic value

Table 3.
Diagnostic modality and their advantages and disadvantages.

quality. DXA is a fast and simple way of measuring body skeletal and non-skeletal mass. The disadvantage is high cost, exposure to radiation, equipment availability is limited, and challenges related to patient mobility. On the other hand, USG (ultrasonography) can evaluate the muscle quality, but the result remains subjective.

Table 3 describes diagnostic modality and their use in the diagnosis of CINMA.

Muscle biopsy can give the accurate idea about muscle mass and its quality; however, it is not commonly conducted due to its invasive nature [15].

3. Differential diagnosis

Before considering a suspicion or diagnosis of CINMA, it is essential to exclude common neuromuscular disorders, including Guillain-Barre syndrome, myasthenia gravis, and high spinal injury, through appropriate diagnostic tests, serological investigations, and a thorough clinical examination.

3.1 Treatment and prevention

As there is no definitive curative treatment for the CINMA currently; the management of these patients focuses on preventive strategies, early detection, and therapeutic interventions.

3.1.1 Preventive measures

1. Timely and early diagnosis of sepsis and septic shock with clinical, serological, diagnostic intervention and administration of appropriate antibiotic along with other therapeutic approaches will prevent further deterioration and complications, particularly, the MODS and preventing proinflammatory storm and thus reducing the likelihood of CINMA [16].

2. The prolonged ICU stay with extended periods of immobilization should be avoided or minimized whenever possible. Early mobilization is essential, as it not only helps prevent but also maintains muscular strength and functionality. Additionally, by giving daily SAT and SBT (spontaneous awakening and spontaneous breathing trail) whenever possible shortens the duration of mechanical ventilation and helps mitigate diaphragmatic and respiratory muscle atrophy and dysfunction, thereby lowering the risk of critical illness neuromuscular abnormalities (CINMA) [16]. Managing hyperglycemia in critically ill patients can help to decrease the incidence of neuromuscular dysfunction and the occurrence of CINMA. Instead of tight control of blood sugar, it is beneficial to have a liberal blood sugar control (between 6 to 8 mmol/L), thus avoiding the hypoglycemia and hyperglycemia and mitigating associated risks and preventing the occurrence [17].

3. In the management of chronically ill patients receiving intensive care therapy, it is essential to administer medications with great caution and under the guidance and supervision of a clinical pharmacist, as few medications may contribute to the development of CINMA. While the existing literature presents inconsistencies, it suggests that neuromuscular blocking agent and steroids should be avoided due to their potential risk in developing CINMA. Prolonged use and

higher dosages of these agents have been shown to adversely affect muscular and neurological function [18].

4. Early initiation of parenteral nutrition is an independent risk factor for the development of CINMA, and hence, it becomes essential to commence enteral nutrition promptly and escalate it rapidly to meet daily energy needs in order to avert malnutrition and the development of CINMA [19].

5. Hypoalbuminemia also described as a potential risk factor for the development of CINMA, and hence, in critical ill patients, hypoalbuminemia should be correct or built up with enteral nutrition [20].

3.2 Early recognition

The early diagnosis of CINMA helps to improve its outcome, thereby decreasing both morbidity and mortality. The early neuromuscular examination and high index of suspicion followed by the use of MRC sum score and followed by confirmation through electrophysiological studies—specifically needle muscle stimulation and peroneal nerve conduction tests—will facilitate the diagnosis of CINMA. Additionally, imaging studies may be utilized based on their availability and the expertise of the medical team.

3.3 Treatment

The early mobilization along with adequate nutritional support are the corner stone for CINMA therapy [21]. The early mobilization or prompt initiation of physical therapy and encouraging patient movement as soon as possible is essential for preserving muscular strength and function in acutely ill individuals. This approach not only helps to prevent muscular atrophy but also enhances metabolic compensation and glycemic control, improving the strength of respiratory muscles. As a result, it contributes to an increase in ventilator-free days, ultimately aiding in the management of CINMA [22].

Nutritional support is very essential to prevent muscle wasting and dysfunction, especially for critically ill patients. It is important to ensure that their diet provides adequate protein and sufficient caloric intake.

The management of CINMA should involve a multidisciplinary team that includes intensivist, physiotherapy, dietitian, clinical pharmacist, and nursing staff.

The application of neuromuscular electric stimulation did not reveal any significant improvement in muscle strength or ventilation-free days when compared to those receiving standard care [23].

4. Morbidity and mortality

CINMA is generally reversible, however, it is associated with increased morbidity and mortality rates. CINMA is an independent risk factor for ICU and in hospital mortility [23]. CINMA is associated with increase ventilator days and length of ICU and hospital stay [23], resulting in higher healthcare-related cost.

CINMA and persistent weakness further increase the mortality in critically ill discharge patients at 1 and 5 years [24].

Most of the patients who survive the CINMA experience prolonged impairment of cognitive, mural, and functional impairment. Most of these patients will have various degree of muscle disability that affect their daily movements [25].

5. Conclusion

The CINMA is more prevalent in critically ill patients than is generally recognized. This condition is multifactorial influenced by the severity of disease, systemic inflammatory response syndrome, use of steroid and muscle relaxant, use of certain antibiotics, or extended periods of immobility.

Diagnosis of CINMA can be achieved through the MRC sum score, while electrophysiological and imaging studies are increasingly utilized for this purpose. Early mobilization, timely weaning from ventilator, and quicker diagnosis of sepsis and immediate treatment not only can help to prevent the progression to more severe illness and multiple organ dysfunction syndrome (MODS), overall reducing the risk of CINMA. Effective management of blood sugar levels is crucial to prevent both hyperglycemia and hypoglycemia. Additionally, addressing hypoalbuminemia, minimizing the prolonged use of steroids and muscle relaxants, ensuring proper nutrition, and promoting early mobilization are essential strategies for preventing and improving outcomes in CINMA patients. It is important to note that CINMA contributes to increased morbidity and mortality among critically ill individuals.

Author details

Nissar Shaikh[1*], Ashish Kumar[1], Sanghamitra Padhy[2] and Gamal Alameri[1]

1 Surgical Intensive Care, Hamad Medical Corporation, Doha, Qatar

2 Department of Anesthesia/ICU and Perioperative Medicine, Hamad Medical Corporation, Doha, Qatar

*Address all correspondence to: nissatfirdous99@gmail.com

References

[1] Bolton CF, Gilbert JJ, Hahn AF, Sibbald WJ. Polyneuropathy in critically ill patients. Journal of Neurology, Neurosurgery, and Psychiatry. 1984;**47**(11):1223-1231

[2] Leijten FS, De Weerd AW, Poortvliet DC, De Ridder VA, Ulrich C, Harink-De Weerd JE. Critical illness polyneuropathy in multiple organ dysfunction syndrome and weaning from the ventilator. Intensive Care Medicine. 1996;**22**(9):856-861

[3] Stevens RD, Dowdy DW, Michaels RK, Mendez-Tellez PA, Pronovost PJ, Needham DM. Neuromuscular dysfunction acquired in critical illness: A systematic review. Intensive Care Medicine. 2007;**33**(11):1876-1891

[4] Appleton R, Kinsella J. Intensive care unit-acquired weakness. Continuing Education in Anesthesia Critical Care & Pain. 2012;**12**(2):62-66

[5] Fan E, Check F, Chlan L, et al. An official thoracic society practice guideline. The diagnosis of intensive care unit acquired weakness in adults. American Journal of Respiratory and Critical Care Medicine. 2014;**190**:1437-1446

[6] Yang T, Li Z, Jiang L, Wang Y, Xi X. Risk factors for intensive care unit-acquired weakness: A systematic review and meta-analysis. Acta Neurologica Scandinavica. 2018;**138**(2):104-114

[7] Vanhorebeek I, Latronico N, Van den Berghe G. ICU-acquired weakness. Intensive Care Medicine. 2020;**46**(4):637-653

[8] Lang CH, Frost RA. Role of growth hormone, insulin-like growth factor-I, and insulin-like growth factor binding proteins in the catabolic response to injury and infection. Current Opinion in Clinical Nutrition and Metabolic Care. 2002;**5**(3):271-279

[9] Kanova M, Kohout P. Molecular mechanisms underlying intensive care unit-acquired weakness and sarcopenia. International Journal of Molecular Sciences. 2022;**23**(15):8396

[10] Zink W, Kaess M, Hofer S, Plachky J, Zausig YA, Sinner B, et al. Alterations in intracellular Ca2+–homeostasis of skeletal muscle fibers during sepsis. Critical Care Medicine. 2008;**36**(5):1559-1563

[11] Bolton CF. Neuromuscular manifestations of critical illness. Muscle & Nerve. 2005;**32**(2):140-163

[12] Shaikh N, Nasser SH, Kettern M. Critical illness polyneuropathy in an obstetric patient: A case report and review. Qatar Medical Journal. 2007;**16**(1):65-67

[13] Yuchen W, Zhang Z, Jiang B, Wang G, Wei H, Li B, et al. Current practice and barriers to ICU-acquired weakness assessment: A cross-sectional survey. Physiotherapy. 2021;**112**:135-142

[14] Hermans G, Clerckx B, Vanhullebusch T. Interobserver agreement of medical research council sum-score and handgrip strength in the intensive care unit. Muscle & Nerve. 2012;**45**(1):18-25

[15] Elkalawy H, Sekhar P, Abosena W. Early detection and assessment of intensive care unit-acquired weakness: A comprehensive review. Acute and Critical Care. 2023;**38**(4):409-424

[16] Petrucci M, Gemmas CL. ICU-acquired weakness: From pathophysiology to management in critical care. Emergency Care and Medicine. 2025;**2**(1):4

[17] Van den Berghe G, Schoonheydt K, Becx P, Bruyninckx F, Wouters PJ. Insulin therapy protects the central and peripheral nervous system of intensive care patients. Neurology. 2005;**64**(8):1348-1353

[18] Yang T, Li Z, Jiang L, Xi X. Corticosteroid use and intensive care unit-acquired weakness: A systematic review and meta-analysis. Critical Care. 2018;**22**(1):187

[19] Chen J, Huang M. Intensive care unit-acquired weakness: Recent insights. Journal of Intensive Medicine. 2023;**4**(1):73-80

[20] Nakano H, Hashimoto H, Mochizuki M, Naraba H, Takahashi Y, Sonoo T, et al. Hypoalbuminemia on admission as an independent risk factor for acute functional decline after infection. Nutrients. 2020;**13**(1):26

[21] Anekwe DE, Biswas S, Bussières A, Spahija J. Early rehabilitation reduces the likelihood of developing intensive care unit-acquired weakness: A systematic review and meta-analysis. Physiotherapy. 2020;**107**:1-10

[22] Kayambu G, Boots R, Paratz J. Physical therapy for the critically ill in the ICU: A systematic review and meta-analysis. Critical Care Medicine. 2013;**41**(6):1543-1554

[23] Zayed Y, Kheiri B, Barbarawi M. Effects of neuromuscular electrical stimulation in critically ill patients: A systematic review and meta-analysis of randomised controlled trials. Australian Critical Care. 2020;**33**(2):203-210

[24] van Wagenberg L, Witteveen E. Causes of mortality in ICU-acquired weakness. Journal of Intensive Care Medicine. 2017;**35**(3):293-296

[25] Wieske L, Dettling-Ihnenfeldt DS, Verhamme C. Impact of ICU-acquired weakness on post-ICU physical functioning: A follow-up study. Critical Care. 2015;**19**(1):196

Chapter 2

Anesthesia and Septic Shock: Pharmacological Approaches and Applications

Semin Turhan

Abstract

Septic shock is a life-threatening complication of sepsis characterized by persistent hypotension, hypoperfusion, and organ dysfunction despite adequate fluid resuscitation. This condition poses significant challenges to anesthesia management and requires a multidisciplinary approach to ensure patient stability during surgery. Key aspects include hemodynamic monitoring, fluid resuscitation, and careful selection of anesthetic agents such as ketamine and etomidate that support cardiovascular function without exacerbating hypotension. Volatile anesthetics such as isoflurane and sevoflurane may provide anti-inflammatory benefits but must be used with caution due to their vasodilatory effects. Postoperative care emphasizes infection control, immune modulation, and prevention of complications such as septic encephalopathy and multiorgan dysfunction. Looking ahead, advances in immune modulation and personalized therapies offer promising avenues for improving outcomes in septic shock patients. These innovations could increase survival rates and minimize the long-term effects of septic shock.

Keywords: septic shock, anesthesia management, pharmacological approaches, drug selection, hemodynamic stability

1. Introduction: Relation of sepsis and septic shock to anesthesiology

Sepsis is a serious infectious condition triggered by a widespread inflammatory response in the body, and septic shock is defined as the most severe form of sepsis. Septic shock is characterized by persistent hypotension, hypoperfusion, and organ dysfunction despite adequate fluid resuscitation [1]. Worldwide, sepsis is a common clinical condition in intensive care units and has a high mortality rate. Septic shock develops in up to 50% of sepsis cases, and the mortality rate for patients with this condition ranges from 40 to 60% [1]. The pathophysiology of septic shock is the result of an abnormal immune response to infection. This response results in a cytokine storm, increased vascular permeability, diffuse vasodilation, and myocardial depression [2].

Septic shock is a major challenge for anesthesia practice. In particular, septic shock patients requiring surgical intervention require a multidisciplinary approach for the safe administration of anesthesia. Cardiovascular and metabolic disturbances caused by septic shock require critical decisions in anesthesia management. Anesthesiologists should develop strategies to ensure hemodynamic stability of these patients before, during, and after surgery [3].

The pathophysiology of sepsis and septic shock is complex and involves the inflammatory response. Sepsis causes systemic inflammatory response syndrome (SIRS) as a result of the body's excessive inflammatory response to infection. In this process, endotoxins from Gram-negative bacteria and exotoxins from Gram-positive bacteria trigger the overproduction of cytokines, reactive oxygen species, and nitrogen species [4]. Cytokines such as TNF-alpha, IL-1, and IL-6 are the major mediators of the inflammatory response, and overproduction of these molecules causes widespread vasodilation and increased vascular permeability, leading to systemic hypotension and organ failure [4]. Myocardial depression is also frequently observed in this process, and the function of the cardiovascular system is severely compromised [1].

Anesthetic management of septic shock requires extremely careful preoperative assessment and intraoperative monitoring. Maintaining blood pressure and tissue perfusion during surgery in these patients is one of the greatest challenges for the anesthesiologist. A cautious pharmacologic approach is required in patients with septic shock because anesthetic agents often have suppressive effects on the cardiovascular system. For example, drugs such as propofol can cause hypotension and should be used with caution in patients with septic shock [5]. Instead, agents with a more stable hemodynamic profile, such as ketamine or etomidate, are recommended [2].

Fluid resuscitation in the preoperative period is critical to ensure hemodynamic stability in patients with septic shock. Adequate fluid therapy should aim to increase intravascular volume and control hypotension. However, vasopressors and inotropic agents should also be used as needed. Norepinephrine is one of the most commonly used vasopressors in these patients and helps to maintain blood pressure by increasing systemic vascular resistance.

In anesthesia practice, the management of sepsis and septic shock should be a multidisciplinary approach, and the perioperative care of these patients requires close collaboration between the surgical and critical care teams. Ensuring cardiovascular stability, preserving organ perfusion, and managing the inflammatory response during anesthesia practice can improve patient survival.

2. Pharmacologic basis: Anesthetic agents used in septic shock

2.1 Volatile anesthetics

Volatile anesthetics should be used with caution in patients with septic shock, as the vasodilating effects of these agents may further decrease blood pressure in septic patients. When using volatile anesthetics such as isoflurane and sevoflurane, dose adjustments are necessary to maintain hemodynamic stability. Isoflurane may preserve cardiac function by reducing myocardial depression, while its general vasodilatory effects may lower blood pressure. Careful hemodynamic monitoring is required when using these agents in septic shock [6].

Volatile anesthetics also have anti-inflammatory effects. Agents such as isoflurane and sevoflurane may reduce the inflammatory response during sepsis by suppressing the production of inflammatory cytokines. These effects of volatile anesthetics on the immune system in sepsis patients may be important for treatment strategies, but careful monitoring is required in clinical practice [5].

2.2 Intravenous anesthetics

Propofol: Propofol should be used with caution in patients with septic shock. The vasodilating and myocardial depressant effects of propofol may exacerbate hypotension in septic patients. When using propofol, especially in patients with septic shock, the lowest effective dose should be preferred, and the patient's hemodynamic status should be carefully monitored. Propofol may increase the inflammatory cytokine response, a factor to be considered in septic patients [6, 7].

Ketamine: Ketamine is an agent that increases cardiovascular support and can be safely used in septic shock patients. The sympathomimetic effects of ketamine can increase blood pressure and stabilize myocardial depression during septic shock. In addition, ketamine has anti-inflammatory effects; it can reduce the inflammatory response by suppressing cytokine production. These properties make ketamine an important option for achieving hemodynamic stability and controlling inflammation in patients with septic shock [8, 9].

Etomidate: Etomidate may be preferred in septic patients because it is a more hemodynamically stable agent. However, etomidate has adrenal suppressive effects, which may be detrimental to septic patients in long-term use. Although a single dose of etomidate is considered safe in septic shock patients, the dose should be carefully adjusted to minimize the effects of adrenal suppression (**Table 1**) [7, 9].

2.3 Role of opioids

Opioids play an important role in the management of analgesia in patients with septic shock. Short-acting opioids (fentanyl, alfentanil, and remifentanil) can be used safely in patients with septic shock and are preferred because they have less effect on blood pressure. These agents can help maintain hemodynamic stability. However, the immunosuppressive effects of opioids should be considered. High doses of opioids may suppress the infection response in septic patients and this should be carefully monitored [7, 8].

Agent	Hemodynamic effects	Inflammatory effects	Adverse effects
Ketamine	Increases BP, supports cardiovascular function	Anti-inflammatory, reduces cytokine production	Increases ICP, sympathomimetic effects
Etomidate	Maintains BP, hemodynamically stable	Minimal inflammatory impact	Adrenal suppression with prolonged use
Propofol	Decreases BP, myocardial depressant	Increases cytokine response	Severe hypotension, cardiovascular depression
Isoflurane	Vasodilation, may reduce BP	Anti-inflammatory effects, reduces cytokine production	Excessive vasodilation, myocardial depression
Sevoflurane	Vasodilation, may reduce BP	Anti-inflammatory effects, reduces cytokine production	Excessive vasodilation, myocardial depression

The "Sedative and Anesthetic Agents in Septic Patients" table should ideally be placed in Section 2: Pharmacologic Basis: Anesthetic Agents Used in Septic Shock, specifically after the detailed discussion of each agent (e.g., Ketamine, Etomidate, Propofol) in Subsection 2.2: Intravenous Anesthetics.

Table 1.
Sedative and anesthetic agents in septic patients.

3. Cardiovascular support and anesthesia practices in septic shock

3.1 Vasopressor and inotropic support

In patients with septic shock, vasopressors and inotropes are often used to maintain hemodynamic stability. The most commonly used vasopressors are norepinephrine and epinephrine. Norepinephrine is the first-line vasopressor for septic shock and increases systemic vascular resistance and blood pressure by peripheral vasoconstriction [10]. Adrenaline may be preferred, especially in refractory septic shock, because of both its vasopressor and inotropic effects. Adrenaline is characterized by its effects of increasing cardiac output and increasing systemic vascular resistance (**Figure 1**) [11].

Dobutamine is used to increase cardiac contractility in septic patients with low cardiac output. Especially when combined with norepinephrine, this agent can improve organ perfusion by increasing hemodynamic support [10]. Vasopressin is rarely used as third-line therapy and is preferred in cases of septic shock refractory to vasopressors. Vasopressin is often given in low doses (0.01–0.04 units/min) in addition to norepinephrine, and this combination provides better blood pressure control [11].

3.2 Fluid resuscitation

Fluid resuscitation in septic shock is the first step in achieving hemodynamic stability. The goal is to improve cardiac output and tissue oxygenation by increasing effective intravascular volume. Crystalloids (e.g., isotonic saline) are usually the first

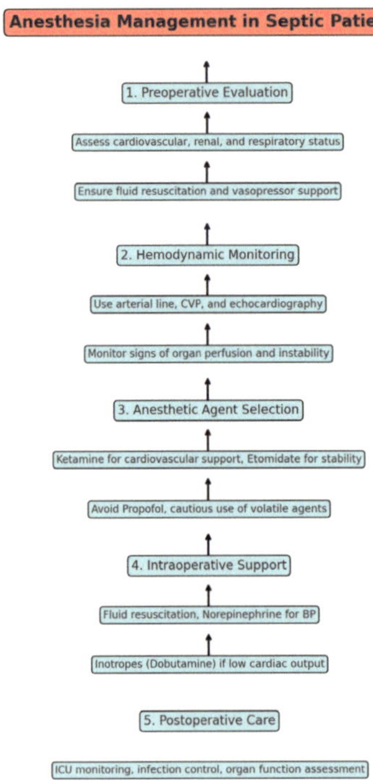

Figure 1.
Anesthesia management in septic patients.

choice of fluid because large studies have shown a favorable effect of crystalloids on mortality [6]. Colloids, on the other hand, can be used especially in patients with hypoalbuminemia, but their cost is higher and some studies have reported adverse effects on renal function [9].

Another important issue to consider in fluid therapy is the appropriate titration of fluid volume. Fluid overload can lead to pulmonary edema and other complications. Therefore, patients' hemodynamic responses should be closely monitored, and fluid therapy should be adjusted according to clinical needs [11.pdf]. Optimal fluid management is a balanced approach in which crystalloids are the first choice to ensure adequate organ perfusion, but colloids can also be used when necessary [9].

4. Special strategies for anesthesia management in septic shock

4.1 Preoperative evaluation

Preoperative evaluation of patients with septic shock is one of the most critical steps in anesthesia management. The presence of organ dysfunction in these patients and the effects of sepsis on the cardiovascular, renal, and respiratory systems are critical to the surgical and anesthetic process. Careful assessment of the hemodynamic status provides information about the patient's fluid balance, blood pressure, and perfusion status. Adequate fluid resuscitation and vasopressor support should be provided. As septic shock leads to hypotension and hypoperfusion, patients should be brought to preoperative cardiovascular stability [11].

Respiratory status is a critical parameter in septic shock. Complications such as acute respiratory distress syndrome (ARDS) may occur in these patients, and respiratory support should be planned. Renal function is often compromised in sepsis and acute kidney injury is common. Preoperative assessment of renal function, diuresis monitoring, and renal replacement therapy, if indicated, play an important role in the planning of anesthetic management [10].

4.2 Anesthesia planning

Anesthetic planning should focus on achieving and maintaining hemodynamic stability in patients with septic shock. These patients are usually hemodynamically unstable, and drug selection should be based on the effects of anesthetic agents on the cardiovascular system. Ketamine is the agent of choice in patients with septic shock because of its effects on cardiovascular support. Etomidate provides hemodynamic stability despite the risk of adrenal suppression when used in a single dose and is considered safe in septic patients [9].

Agents such as propofol should be used with caution in septic shock patients due to its cardiovascular depressant effects. Propofol may worsen hypotension, so careful dose adjustment and continuous hemodynamic monitoring should be used. Vasopressors and inotropic agents are commonly used during anesthesia in patients with septic shock and may be given as continuous infusions to support blood pressure. Norepinephrine is the preferred first-line vasopressor in septic shock and plays an important role in blood pressure stabilization [6].

Invasive hemodynamic monitoring is of great importance in the perioperative period. Continuous blood pressure monitoring by arterial catheterization, fluid balance monitoring by central venous catheterization, and more detailed hemodynamic monitoring by pulmonary artery catheterization should be performed as needed. Echocardiography is also an important tool that can be used to assess cardiac function, especially in patients with septic shock [11].

4.3 Postoperative care

Postoperative care of patients with septic shock requires a multidisciplinary approach in the ICU. In the postoperative period, maintenance of hemodynamic stability, infection control, and monitoring of organ function are critical. Most patients require continuous monitoring in the ICU due to sepsis-related organ dysfunction. Optimal management of therapies such as fluid balance, maintenance of vasopressor and inotrope support, and ventilatory support is essential [9].

In the postoperative period, it is necessary to monitor renal function and assess the need for dialysis, as acute kidney injury due to sepsis may adversely affect the recovery process. Neurological monitoring is also important, and particular attention should be paid to neurological complications that may develop after prolonged hypotension and hypoperfusion [11.pdf]. In addition, long-term effects of anesthesia in septic patients may include cognitive dysfunction and post-sepsis syndrome; therefore, early mobilization and rehabilitation planning is an integral part of postoperative care [11].

5. Postoperative complications and rehabilitation strategies

5.1 Organ dysfunction and supportive therapy

Postoperative multiple organ dysfunction (MODS) is a common and serious complication in patients with septic shock. Acute renal failure and respiratory failure are more common due to the inflammatory response that develops during sepsis. Monitoring of renal function and initiation of renal replacement therapy when necessary plays an important role in postoperative management [5.pdf]. Pulmonary complications may require ventilatory support in patients with sepsis, and lung protective strategies (such as low tidal volume ventilation) should be used [7].

5.2 Septic encephalopathy and neurologic monitoring

Septic encephalopathy is a common neurologic complication in patients with septic shock and requires careful neurologic monitoring in the postoperative period. Hypoperfusion and inflammation during sepsis can lead to impaired brain function. Cognitive impairment and delirium are common long-term sequelae in these patients [8]. Neurological monitoring and cognitive rehabilitation strategies play a critical role in the management of these complications [6].

5.3 Post-sepsis syndrome and rehabilitation

Post sepsis syndrome can have long-term physical, cognitive, and psychological effects in patients with septic shock. This syndrome is more common in elderly patients. Early mobilization of patients in the postoperative period and physical therapy can reduce the effects of post-sepsis syndrome [9.pdf]. In addition, cognitive rehabilitation may be beneficial in reducing the neurological effects of septic shock [10].

5.4 Nutritional support and metabolic management

Nutritional management is critical to support the postoperative recovery of patients with sepsis. Optimal enteral and parenteral nutrition strategies should be implemented in these hypercatabolic patients. Nutritional support is essential to support the immune system and accelerate the healing process [5].

5.5 Long-term cardiac follow-up

The cardiac function of septic shock patients should be monitored for a long time in the postoperative period. Regular assessment of cardiac output and ventricular function by non-invasive methods such as echocardiography is recommended [7]. Cardiac rehabilitation programs should also be planned to minimize the long-term effects of cardiovascular dysfunction in septic shock [11].

6. Immune response and infection control: Immune modulation strategies in septic shock patients

6.1 Sepsis and suppression of immune response

Septic shock leads to an excessive inflammatory response in the body, resulting in significant suppression of the immune system. This leads to impaired immune cell function and an imbalance in cytokine production in patients. In particular, the excessive release of pro-inflammatory cytokines triggers an anti-inflammatory response that suppresses the immune system, leaving patients vulnerable to infection [5]. Immunosuppression after sepsis can lead to an easier spread of infections and therefore regulation of the immune response in patients with sepsis is of vital importance.

6.2 Immune modulatory therapies

Immunomodulatory strategies are treatments used to regulate the immune system in patients with septic shock. These strategies aim to suppress the cytokine response in combination with drugs that regulate the immune response, such as glucocorticoids. However, the effect of these therapies on survival after sepsis is controversial. In some studies, short-term use of glucocorticoids has been shown to accelerate the recovery process in septic shock patients, but these agents may further suppress the immune system when used long-term [7].

IVIG (intravenous immunoglobulin) is another immunomodulatory strategy used to support the immune system during sepsis. By increasing antibody levels, IVIG can strengthen the body's defenses against infection and stabilize the inflammatory response [12]. In patients with septic shock, this treatment may be effective in restoring immune function.

6.3 Infection control

Control of infections in patients with septic shock should be a multidisciplinary approach in the intensive care unit. Antibiotic treatment should be initiated early to rapidly control infections. Empiric antibiotic therapy should be performed with broad-spectrum antibiotics in particular and should be limited according to culture results [11].

However, implementation of aseptic techniques and strict infection control measures in the ICU is critical to minimize the risk of recurrent infection. It should be noted that catheters and invasive monitoring devices can be a source of infection and regular replacement of these devices should be ensured [13].

6.4 Immune system restoration and rehabilitation

In patients recovering from septic shock, it may take time for the immune system to fully recover. Restoring immune system function in these patients requires a multidisciplinary approach, including nutritional supplementation, physical rehabilitation, and mental health support. Micronutrient supplements should be administered, especially in cases of deficiency of immune-supporting elements such as zinc, selenium, and vitamin C [8.pdf]. In addition, these patients should undergo long-term immune monitoring and be closely monitored for recurrent infections.

7. Conclusion and future perspectives

7.1 Sepsis and suppression of immune response

Septic shock is a highly complex clinical condition that requires a multifaceted approach to anesthesia management. Hemodynamic instability, organ dysfunction, and infection control are the major challenges that anesthesiologists must continually address. Fluid management, use of vasopressors and inotropes, careful selection of anesthetic agents, and perioperative hemodynamic stability are the cornerstones of anesthesia management in patients with septic shock [5].

Maintaining hemodynamic stability in these patients is one of the major challenges in anesthesia management. Stabilization of blood pressure and organ perfusion with vasopressor and inotropic agents is critical for successful surgical intervention and recovery [7]. At the same time, complications such as acute renal failure require continuous monitoring of patients' fluid balance and renal function [9].

Immune modulation and infection control are other challenges in septic shock patients both pre- and postoperatively. The use of aseptic techniques to minimize the risk of infection, broad-spectrum antibiotic therapy, and stabilization of the immune response are important components of anesthesia and intensive care management [8].

7.2 The future of pharmacological approaches

The future of anesthetic management of septic shock is aimed at optimizing existing pharmacological approaches and developing new therapeutic strategies. The effects of agents such as volatile anesthetics, both in providing hemodynamic stability and suppressing the inflammatory response, may lead to larger studies in the management of septic shock. Research into the anti-inflammatory effects of these agents may lead to better control of the immune response in sepsis.

In terms of intravenous anesthetics, drugs such as ketamine will remain an important treatment option in septic shock due to their potential to provide hemodynamic stability and reduce the inflammatory response. Similarly, the development of new dosing protocols to reduce the risk of adrenal suppression with etomidate and a better understanding of the long-term use of this agent is being sought [7].

Recent research on vasopressors and inotropic agents includes advances toward safer and more effective ways to provide hemodynamic support in patients with septic shock. In particular, combinations of norepinephrine and vasopressin have been shown to provide better outcomes in septic shock patients, and further studies are needed to determine the optimal use of these agents [10].

7.3 New treatment modalities and research

In the future, more targeted therapeutic strategies are expected to be developed for the treatment of septic shock. Immune modulation strategies are among the leading treatment modalities targeting the immune system in septic shock patients. In particular, studies on the effects of IVIG and glucocorticoids on sepsis and septic shock are investigating safer and more effective use of these agents [14].

In addition, new therapeutic modalities are being developed to accelerate the repair and recovery of organs damaged during sepsis using cellular therapies and biological agents. Research in this area may lead to more specific and personalized treatment protocols by targeting the mechanisms of sepsis that cause organ failure [15].

8. Conclusion

Septic shock is one of the most complex and challenging clinical situations encountered in anesthesia practice. Many critical factors such as hemodynamic instability, organ dysfunction, and infection control must be managed simultaneously. The selection and appropriate dosing of the pharmacologic agents used in this process plays an important role in increasing the chances of patient survival both perioperatively and postoperatively. Effective use of vasopressors, such as norepinephrine, and agents that increase cardiovascular support, such as ketamine, is key to successful septic shock management. In addition, invasive hemodynamic monitoring and strict infection control in the ICU are integral parts of the treatment process.

Future perspectives focus on the development of more effective and targeted therapeutic modalities for the management of septic shock. Immune modulation, novel biologic therapies and more advanced pharmacologic approaches may bring positive changes in the long-term management of sepsis and septic shock. These developments are seen as promising steps to improve patient recovery and reduce mortality from septic shock.

Author details

Semin Turhan
Department of Anesthesiology and Reanimation, Hitit University Erol Olçok Training and Research Hospital, Çorum, Turkey

*Address all correspondence to: smnondr@hotmail.com

References

[1] Baluch A, Janoo A, Lam K, Hoover J, Kaye A. Septic shock: Review and anesthetic considerations. Middle East Journal of Anesthesiology. 2007;**19**(1):71

[2] Yoon SH. Concerns of the anesthesiologist: Anesthetic induction in severe sepsis or septic shock patients. Korean Journal of Anesthesiology. 2012;**63**(1):3

[3] Khanna AK, Laudanski K. Septic shock and anesthesia: Much ado about nothing? Journal of Anaesthesiology Clinical Pharmacology. 2014;**30**(4):481-483

[4] Kaymak C, Basar H, Sardas S. Reactive oxygen species (Ros) generation in sepsis. FABAD Journal of Pharmaceutical Sciences. 2011;**36**(1):41-47

[5] Pinto BB, Rehberg S, Ertmer C, Morelli A. Role of ketamine and other intravenous anesthetics in septic shock: A review of pharmacological effects. Current Opinion in Anaesthesiology. 2008;**21**(2):168-177. DOI: 10.1097/ACO.0b013e3282f531a5

[6] Bughrara NF, Renew JR, Emr KS. Echocardiographic assessment in septic patients: A multicenter study of focused echocardiography in critical care. Intensive Care Medicine. 2019;**45**(5):657-667. DOI: 10.1007/s00134-018-5402-z

[7] Carsetti A, Donati A, Adrario E, Damiani E. Anesthetic management of patients with sepsis and septic shock: Clinical guidelines. Anesthesia and Analgesia. 2020;**131**(4):1322-1335. DOI: 10.1213/ANE.0000000000004598

[8] Schläpfer M, Rey C, Tafani V, Tappy L, Liaudet L. The effects of volatile anesthetics on inflammatory responses during sepsis: A review. Critical Care. 2015;**19**:45. DOI: 10.1186/s13054-015-0751-x

[9] Young CC, Harris EM, Vacchiano C. Lung-protective ventilation in septic patients under anesthesia. British Journal of Anaesthesia. 2019;**123**:898-913. DOI: 10.1016/j.bja.2019.08.017

[10] Beale RJ, Hollenberg SM, Vincent JL, Parrillo JE. Vasopressor and inotropic support in septic shock: An evidence-based review. Critical Care Medicine. 2004;**32**:455-465

[11] Bridges EJ, Dukes S. Cardiovascular aspects of septic shock: Pathophysiology, monitoring, and treatment. Critical Care Nurse. 2005;**25**(2):14-40

[12] Schwab I, Nimmerjahn F. Intravenous immunoglobulin therapy: How does IgG modulate the immune system? Nature Reviews. Immunology. 2013;**13**(3):176-189

[13] Clare S, Rowley S. Implementing the aseptic non touch technique (ANTT®) clinical practice framework for aseptic technique: A pragmatic evaluation using a mixed methods approach in two London hospitals. Journal of Infection Prevention. 2018;**19**(1):6-15

[14] Hamano N, Nishi K, Onose A, Okamoto A, Umegaki T, Yamazaki E, et al. Efficacy of single-dose intravenous immunoglobulin administration for severe sepsis and septic shock. Journal of Intensive Care. 2013;**1**:1-7

[15] Gotts JE, Matthay MA. Cell-based therapy in sepsis: A step closer. American Journal of Respiratory and Critical Care Medicine. 2018;**197**(3):280-281

Chapter 3

AI-Assisted Diagnosis and Treatment of Septic Shock

Xiaxia Yu and Yong Liu

Abstract

Sepsis is a life-threatening organ dysfunction caused by a dysregulated host response to infection. Septic shock is a severe form of sepsis characterized by persistent hypotension despite fluid resuscitation and the need for vasopressor support. Early and accurate diagnosis, along with prompt treatment, is crucial for improving outcomes in septic shock patients. Artificial intelligence (AI) has emerged as a powerful tool in the ICU, assisting in the diagnosis and treatment of septic shock through various applications, including real-time data analysis, pattern recognition, and decision support systems. This chapter discusses the integration of AI in the clinical management of septic shock, highlighting its potential to enhance diagnostic accuracy, optimize treatment strategies, and improve patient outcomes.

Keywords: sepsis, septic shock, AI-assisted diagnosis treatment, optimization ICU management, personalized medicine

1. Introduction

Sepsis is a critical global health issue, with an estimated 30 million cases annually, leading to over 6 million deaths worldwide. Despite a decline in mortality rates, the incidence of sepsis is on the rise, with an annual increase of 8–13% over the past decade, largely due to a lack of public awareness and delays in diagnosis and treatment. The condition is complex and varied, posing challenges for research and treatment. Government funding plays a crucial role in sepsis research, with the National Institute of Health (NIH) leading the way with significant investment. However, funding remains a challenge, and industry support is essential for major sepsis organizations like the surviving sepsis campaign (SSC).

In recent years, sepsis has been increasingly recognized as a disease associated with organ failure, although this may be a misinterpretation stemming from post hoc analysis. Future research should focus on detecting sepsis before organ failure occurs. As we look to the future, improving sepsis management is a priority, with a need for better drug target design and the integration of artificial intelligence (AI) in clinical trial design and personalized medicine. The PIRO framework (predisposition, infection, response, and organ dysfunction) is suggested for characterizing sepsis patients, emphasizing the use of multiple biomarkers over single values for patient selection. Advanced computational tools are necessary to support this approach.

This chapter aims to explore the fundamentals of AI in sepsis diagnosis and treatment, providing an overview of AI applications in the ICU and discussing potential strategies for implementing AI in clinical practice to enhance sepsis management.

2. Overview of AI and machine learning in sepsis diagnosis and treatment

Artificial intelligence (AI) is a dynamic field of computer science that aims to create machines capable of tasks typically requiring human intelligence, such as visual perception, speech recognition, and decision-making. AI encompasses various subfields, including machine learning (ML), deep learning, natural language processing (NLP), and robotics. In medicine, AI has the potential to transform diagnosis, treatment, and patient outcomes, particularly in areas like medical imaging and patient monitoring [1, 2].

ML, a subset of AI, empowers machines to enhance their performance on tasks by learning from data, without explicit programming. In medical applications, ML can be applied to diagnosis, prediction, and personalized treatment. ML techniques are categorized into supervised learning, which involves learning from labeled data to predict outcomes, and unsupervised learning, which identifies patterns in unlabeled data.

AI's role in sepsis management is significant, with applications in early detection and diagnosis. For instance, the Sepsis Early Risk Assessment (SERA) algorithm combines structured data with unstructured clinical notes to predict sepsis with high accuracy, providing a 12–48-hour warning before onset. This approach not only improves early detection but also reduces false positives [3].

NLP, a branch of AI, enables machines to understand and derive meaning from human language, facilitating the analysis of unstructured data such as clinical notes and radiological images. This technology has been crucial in improving the discriminatory ability of identifying infections in emergency departments [4].

However, there are challenges with large language models (LLMs), which, despite their advanced technology and algorithms, face reliability issues. Concerns about clinical information quality, evidence level, and reliability are significant, as LLMs often quote fabricated resources and are not yet suitable for regulation as medical devices [5].

Despite these concerns, LLMs have potential as assistive tools for clinicians, aiding in tasks like clinical note-taking, administrative letter writing, and summarizing patient medical records. They may also support clinical research by summarizing results and rewriting passages for different readerships, easing the burden of critical appraisal, research reporting, and peer review [2].

In summary, AI and ML are poised to play a pivotal role in sepsis diagnosis and treatment, offering innovative solutions for early detection and personalized care. As these technologies evolve, their integration into clinical practice will require careful consideration of their limitations and potential risks.

3. Early detection: Diagnosing sepsis on the ward, in the ED, and in the ICU

Artificial intelligence (AI) plays a pivotal role in the early detection and accurate diagnosis of sepsis. Roggeveen et al. [6] developed a supervised machine learning (SML) algorithm for diagnosing infections upon hospital presentation, utilizing microbiological data and blood test parameters such as C-reactive protein and white blood cell counts. They further refined this into a support vector machine (SVM) binary classifier algorithm, training and testing its diagnostic capabilities with patient profiles that included biochemistry and full blood count variables. A clinical decision support system (CDSS) was implemented, featuring ML modules to aid in antimicrobial selection and dose optimization, as well as a patient engagement module. In a 6-month study of hospitalized patients, one out of three was diagnosed with an infection within 72 hours of admission. The AUROC was 0.84 (95% CI: 0.76 to 0.91), indicating that clinicians were effective in diagnosing bacterial infections, with less than 10% not receiving appropriate treatment. However, 6% of patients without bacterial infection still received antimicrobial therapy [6].

Another validated ML algorithm, "InSight scores," used vital signs from the electronic health record (EHR) to detect and predict sepsis, severe sepsis, and septic shock in a mixed-ward population, including patients from the ED, floor units, and ICU [7]. This ML algorithm utilized data from six clinical vital signs and employed gradient tree boosting to construct the model. It outperformed common scoring systems like SIRS, Sequential Organ Failure Assessment (SOFA), and MEWS in screening for sepsis and provided predictive capabilities before sepsis onset by analyzing trends and correlations between vital sign measurements [7].

A 2017 study analyzed sepsis diagnosis in the ED through a retrospective observational cohort study, training ML algorithms to predict infections using incrementally larger subsets of features, including patient demographics, vital signs, and free-text chief complaints [3, 4]. The best-performing model incorporated free text along with vital signs and demographics [3]. Early detection and intervention are crucial for optimizing sepsis patient outcomes, with effective management in EDs and ward settings being time-dependent [5]. Transferring patients from the ED or ward to an ICU is often ineffective [5]. A meta-analysis of 28 papers found diagnostic test accuracy for predicting sepsis using AUROC ranged from 0.68 to 0.99 in the ICU, 0.96 to 0.98 in the hospital, and 0.87 to 0.97 in the ED [8]. Predictive models for sepsis can be categorized as right-aligned or left-aligned, with left-aligned models identifying patients likely to develop sepsis before a fixed time point, such as surgery, allowing for risk optimization [6].

AI has the potential to provide timely and accurate sepsis detection, outperforming current clinical warning scores that are not based on sophisticated mathematical models [5]. This technology can facilitate prompt treatment to prevent complications from delayed treatment, such as multi-organ failure and shock. ML-based early warning systems have shown high accuracy in predicting circulatory failure. Hyland et al. [7] constructed two early warning systems, circEWS and circEWS-lite, that alerted clinicians to patients at risk of circulatory failure within an 8-hour timeframe, using data from over 54,000 ICU admissions to train their systems [7]. These ML-based early warning systems could assist ICU staff in identifying sepsis patients earlier at risk for developing circulatory failure, with a lower false alarm rate than conventional alert systems, reducing alarm fatigue for staff [7, 8].

The "Haemodynamic stability index (HSI)" is a multiparameter ML model that provides early warning of hemodynamic compromise and the need for initiation of hemodynamic supports, trained by learning from thousands of clinicians' actions [9]. HSI has shown better accuracy in predicting instability than single parameters like systolic blood pressure and shock index and is a useful decision-support tool for managing circulatory shock in critical care [9, 10].

The "Recurrent Attentive And Intensive Model (RAIM)" is proposed for analyzing continuous physiological data and irregular clinical data, generating a guidance matrix to predict dynamic outputs such as the risk of physiological decompensation and/or hospital length of stay [11]. RAIM obtained over 90% AUC-ROC scores for predicting physiological decompensation with high accuracy (86.82%) for forecasting length of stay [11].

A physiology-based model using waveforms independent of other data in the EHR was able to predict sepsis within the first hour of admission with a high degree of success (AUROC = 0.92, Area under precision-recall curve = 0.90) [12]. Other tools utilizing reinforced learning have been shown to optimize the management of fluids and vasopressors in sepsis to minimize mortality, learning the optimal dosing regimen from a large training set of data on patients with sepsis in the ICU [13]. Deviation from the "AI clinician" strategy was associated with an increase in mortality in a dose-dependent fashion [14].

While AI may not be a panacea for sepsis, clinicians could use it as an aide memoire in their decision-making processes, keeping in mind that exceptions to AI-derived strategy will always exist [14]. This will enable clinicians to optimize the management of sepsis to reduce associated morbidity and mortality.

4. Pattern recognition

The heterogeneity of sepsis complicates its simplification into a singular clinical presentation, prompting a focus on AI algorithms for sepsis subtyping in recent research. According to the latest definition of sepsis (Sepsis-3), organ dysfunction is assessed using the Sequential Organ Failure Assessment (SOFA) score, which evaluates the functioning of six organ systems: respiratory, coagulation, liver, cardiovascular, central nervous system, and renal functions. These parameters are also utilized to classify sepsis subtypes, aiming to identify clinically significant variations.

Recent studies have shown that retrospective analyses of clinical variables using machine learning can classify sepsis into four phenotypes: α, β, γ, and δ [15]. Each subtype represents distinct clinical profiles with unique characteristics and patient outcomes. For instance, patients with the β phenotype tend to have a higher prevalence of chronic illnesses and renal impairments, while those with the γ phenotype often experience increased inflammation and pulmonary dysfunction. Additionally, sepsis-related acute kidney injury has been categorized into three distinct subtypes based on biochemical markers, immune patterns, and clinical outcomes [16]. While these subtyping approaches enhance our understanding of sepsis heterogeneity, they often lack mechanistic insights that could guide therapeutic interventions.

Moreover, researchers have identified two sepsis subtypes based on gene expression differences among septic patients. These subtypes demonstrate significant variations in mortality rates and responses to hormone therapy, with one category showing pronounced immune suppression and a higher mortality rate associated with hormone treatment [17].

In a similar vein, machine learning algorithms applied to secondary analyses of five randomized controlled trials have categorized acute respiratory distress syndrome (ARDS) into two subtypes: hyperinflammatory and hypoinflammatory. These subtypes exhibit distinct clinical outcomes and treatment responses [18]. Subsequent validation in a multicenter retrospective study further supported these findings [19]. Additionally, molecular phenotypes previously identified in ARDS have also been recognized in multiple sepsis cohorts, revealing varying responses to activated protein C. These molecular phenotypes may represent treatable characteristics of severe diseases that extend beyond traditional patient syndrome diagnoses [20].

The conclusions drawn from these studies, particularly regarding inflammatory responses, shed light on the heterogeneity of sepsis. Machine learning-driven sepsis subtyping broadens our understanding of disease assessment and treatment, offering novel insights for future mechanistic research and clinical diagnostics.

5. Predictive algorithms on the pathogen and antimicrobial prescribing

Machine learning (ML) algorithms are poised to revolutionize the early prediction and diagnosis of sepsis by identifying causative pathogens more swiftly than traditional methods. A study focusing on acute respiratory failure (ARF) in children [21] highlighted the challenge of distinguishing between bacterial and viral etiologies due to overlapping signs and symptoms, often leading to inappropriate antibiotic use. ML models, trained with clinical features within 24 hours of admission, showed potential in diagnosing common respiratory pathogens like adenovirus, influenza, and *Mycoplasma pneumoniae*. The model utilized nine features, including age, fever, C-reactive protein, and heart rate, to automatically predict pathogens and improve diagnostic accuracy [21].

However, not all studies have shown positive results. Lhommet et al. [22] examined the prediction of microbial causes of community-acquired pneumonia (CAP) in adults. Despite collecting comprehensive data within the first 3 hours of admission, neither experienced physicians nor an ML algorithm could accurately predict the microbial etiology of severe CAP [22]. This underscores the need for strategies like rapid molecular respiratory panel assays to provide optimal treatment options for acute respiratory infections.

The development of systems biology tools, such as metabolomics, has provided insights into the chemical environment changes in sepsis [23]. Metabolomic biosignatures have shown diagnostic value in identifying infected patients and differentiating between Gram-positive and Gram-negative bacteria [23]. This approach aligns with the need for accurate pathogen identification in sepsis.

AI also plays a role in prescribing appropriate therapies once a clinical infection is diagnosed. Case-based reasoning (CBR), a type of AI, solves new problems by adapting previous successful solutions to similar problems. A CDSS developed using CBR was integrated into the electronic health record, with ML CDSS making antibiotic selections at a similar level of appropriateness to individual clinicians but with a narrower spectrum of activity [23]. This study demonstrated the potential of ML techniques and CDSS in providing personalized prescribing and enhancing patient care [23].

Other examples include the TREAT system, a CDSS using causal probabilistic networks, which showed a 9% improvement in the appropriateness of prescribing and a trend toward improved patient survival [24]. While these systems are complex to develop and require large datasets, CBR is considered simpler and easier to implement in clinical practice [25]. Regardless of the system used, AI aids in avoiding issues of accurate recall for busy clinicians and provides access to learnings equivalent to years of clinical experience through this technology.

In summary, ML algorithms have shown potential in predicting and diagnosing causative pathogens in sepsis earlier than traditional methods, with implications for improving treatment and patient outcomes. However, challenges remain, and further research is needed to fully integrate these technologies into clinical practice.

6. AI-assisted treatment of septic shock

6.1 AI-driven clinical decision

AI-driven mechanical ventilation strategies represent a promising frontier in the management of sepsis. A systematic review [25] identified four common predictive algorithms in AI-assisted mechanical ventilation: weaning success, initiation of ventilation, complications in ventilated patients, and detection of patient-ventilator asynchrony. The "VentAI" algorithm, developed using MIMIC-III data, predicts optimal positive end-expiratory pressure (PEEP), fraction of inspired oxygen (FiO_2), and tidal volume settings, outperforming standard physician care in reducing in-hospital and 90-day mortality rates [26]. VentAI's success is attributed to its selection of lower tidal volumes (5–7.5 mL/kg), avoidance of high FiO_2 (>55%), and more frequent recommendations of PEEP levels between 5 and 7 cm H_2O and 7 and 9 cm H_2O compared to physician practices [26]. However, the algorithm's predictions must be reconciled with the practical constraints of real-world ventilation, which may limit the direct application of its strategies [26].

Jingming Liu's work introduces a two-layer LSTM network model to predict norepinephrine dosage for managing blood pressure in sepsis patients, demonstrating improved prediction accuracy over traditional methods through the MIMIC-III dataset. The results show that the LSTM model outperforms linear regression and XGBoost regression, suggesting its potential to assist in personalized treatment plans and reduce the burden on healthcare providers. Additionally, the study investigates the impact of clustering analysis on prediction accuracy, offering insights into more effective sepsis treatment strategies [9].

The study by Xuefeng Peng introduces a mixture-of-experts framework that leverages deep and kernel-based reinforcement learning to personalize sepsis treatment strategies, demonstrating improved outcomes over standard physician practices. The model dynamically switches between conservative and aggressive treatment policies based on patient history, offering a novel approach to optimize fluid and vasopressor administration in ICU sepsis patients. Further research is needed to validate these policies and explore broader clinical applications [10].

6.2 Personalized medicine

ML clustering techniques are crucial for uncovering new clinical phenotypes in sepsis, a condition marked by significant heterogeneity in host response [15]. The challenge lies in identifying distinct clinical and biological feature clusters within different patient cohorts, as patient phenotypes respond variably to treatments and carry different mortality risks [15]. Unsupervised learning protocols, such as ML algorithms, have been used to analyze datasets without labeled responses, primarily vital signs and laboratory tests collected within the first 6 hours of hospital presentation. This approach has led to the identification of four distinct sepsis phenotypes, which correlate with biomarkers and mortality [27]. These phenotypes could inform more targeted immunotherapeutic interventions when combined with additional clinical data, such as systems biology measures and novel gene expression patterns [27]. However, realizing this potential requires expanded access to patient electronic records to enable ML algorithms to analyze a broader range of data, including past medical histories and comorbidities [15]. The security and privacy concerns surrounding data access present a significant barrier to the implementation of AI in healthcare [27].

In summary, AI-driven mechanical ventilation and ML clustering techniques offer significant potential in sepsis management, from optimizing ventilation strategies to identifying new clinical phenotypes. As these technologies advance, addressing the challenges of algorithm validation, data access, and privacy will be crucial for their successful integration into clinical practice.

7. Prognosis prediction

AI's ability to predict the prognosis of patients with septic shock can provide valuable information to guide treatment decisions and family communications. A prospective study found that an AI model could predict mortality in septic shock with an accuracy of 90% when applied within the first 24 hours of ICU admission [28].

8. Barriers to AI implementation in sepsis management

As we consider the prospective deployment of AI models in sepsis management, it's clear that while retrospective trials suggest AI could revolutionize sepsis care, a cautious and gradual approach is warranted due to potential challenges in implementation [29–31]. We advocate for a strategy of "start small and move slowly," emphasizing the need for well-designed RCTs comparing AI models in conjunction with physician care to physician-only care. Broad implementation of AI models should only follow demonstrated improvements in prospective outcomes and subsequent revalidation of these findings [29, 30].

The implementation of AI in medicine must navigate political, financial, ethical, and medicine-specific barriers [29, 30]. Collaboration between healthcare providers, policymakers, and technology developers is essential to ensure responsible and effective use of AI to enhance patient outcomes [29, 30].

8.1 Political and regulatory barriers

Political and regulatory hurdles include laws and regulations restricting AI use in healthcare, lack of government funding, and patient data privacy concerns [29, 30]. The security and confidentiality of patient data when AI algorithms analyze medical records are paramount, with informed consent being fundamental yet challenging due to the complexity of some algorithms [30, 32]. The risk of data breaches, as exemplified by the 2021 cyberattack on Ireland's Health Service Executive, underscores the need for robust regulatory frameworks to address cybersecurity and protect against data misuse [30, 32].

8.2 Financial investment

Implementing AI in medicine requires significant financial investment for purchasing and maintaining AI systems, hiring trained personnel, and developing algorithms [33]. Cost-benefit analyses must be conducted, weighing initial and ongoing costs against alternative technologies to provide a solid basis for AI implementation decisions [34].

8.3 Ethical concerns

Ethical concerns revolve around bias and fairness in AI algorithms, which, if trained on biased data, could perpetuate healthcare inequalities [30]. There are also concerns about AI's role in life-or-death decision-making [35].

8.4 Medicine-specific barriers

Technical challenges in integrating AI with existing medical systems and resistance to change among healthcare providers present further obstacles [36]. Clinicians involved early in AI development are more likely to adopt the technology, emphasizing the need for healthcare staff to navigate the digitized environment, with updates to medical curricula and training to facilitate this transition [37, 38].

8.5 Communication and empathy

Clinicians must maintain emotional intelligence and compassion when conveying AI results and recommendations to patients, ensuring informed healthcare decisions [39]. Concerns about job automation due to AI are significant, but new employment opportunities in AI development and improvement may mitigate job losses [34].

9. Future directions

The future of AI in the management of septic shock holds promise for improved diagnostic accuracy, personalized treatment, and enhanced patient outcomes. Ongoing research is focused on developing more sophisticated AI models, integrating AI with other healthcare technologies, and addressing the ethical and practical challenges associated with AI implementation in the ICU [40].

10. Conclusion

While AI has made significant strides in assisting with the diagnosis and treatment of septic shock, it is essential to approach its integration into clinical practice with caution and consideration. The potential benefits of AI are substantial, but they must be balanced against the ethical and practical challenges to ensure the best possible care for patients with septic shock.

Author details

Xiaxia Yu[1] and Yong Liu[2*]

1 School of Biomedical Engineering, Shenzhen University Medical School, Shenzhen University, Shenzhen, China

2 Department of Critical Care Medicine, Shenzhen Hospital, Southern Medical University, Shenzhen, Guangdong, China

*Address all correspondence to: liuyongjoy@outlook.com

References

[1] Rawson TM, Hernandez B, Moore LSP, Blandy O, Herrero P, Gilchrist M, et al. Supervised machine learning for the prediction of infection on admission to hospital: A prospective observational cohort study. The Journal of Antimicrobial Chemotherapy. 2019;**74**(4):110815. DOI: 10.1093/jac/dky514

[2] Mao Q, Jay M, Hoffman JL, Calvert J, Barton C, Shimabukuro D, et al. Multicentre validation of a sepsis prediction algorithm using only vital sign data in the emergency department, general ward and ICU. BMJ Open. 2018;**8**(1):e017833. DOI: 10.1136/bmjopen-2017-017833

[3] Horng S, Sontag DA, Halpern Y, Jernite Y, Shapiro NI, Nathanson LA. Creating an automated trigger for sepsis clinical decision support at emergency department triage using machine learning. PLoS ONE. 2017;**12**(4):e0174708. DOI: 10.1371/journal.pone.0174708

[4] Mehrabi S, Krishnan A, Sohn S, Roch AM, Schmidt H, Kesterson J, et al. DEEPEN: A negation detection system for clinical text incorporating dependency relation into NegEx. Journal of Biomedical Informatics. 2015;**54**:213-219. DOI: 10.1016/j.jbi.2015.02.010

[5] Pepic I, Feldt R, Ljungström L, Torkar R, Dalevi D, Maurin Söderholm H, et al. Early detection of sepsis using artificial intelligence: A scoping review protocol. Systematic Reviews. 2021;**10**(1):1-7. DOI: 10.1186/s13643-020-01561-w

[6] Fleuren LM, Klausch TLT, Zwager CL, Schoonmade LJ, Guo T, Roggeveen LF, et al. Machine learning for the prediction of sepsis: A systematic review and meta-analysis of diagnostic test accuracy. Intensive Care Medicine. 2020;**46**:383-400. DOI: 10.1007/s00134-019-05872-y

[7] Hyland SL, Faltys M, Hüser M, Lyu X, Gumbsch T, Esteban C, et al. Early prediction of circulatory failure in the intensive care unit using machine learning. Nature Medicine. 2020;**26**(3):364-373. DOI: 10.1038/s41591-020-0789-4

[8] Rush B, Celi LA, Stone DJ. Applying machine learning to continuously monitored physiological data. Journal of Clinical Monitoring and Computing. 2019;**33**(5):887-893. DOI: 10.1007/s10877-018-0219-z

[9] Rahman A, Chang Y, Dong J, Conroy B, Natarajan A, Kinoshita T, et al. Early prediction of hemodynamic interventions in the intensive care unit using machine learning. Critical Care. 2021;**25**(1):388. DOI: 10.1186/s13054-021-03808-x

[10] Dung-Hung C, Cong T, Zeyu J, Yu-Shan OY, Yung-Yan L. External validation of a machine learning model to predict hemodynamic instability in intensive care unit. Critical Care. 2022;**26**(1):1-10. DOI: 10.1186/s13054-022-04088-9

[11] Xu Y, Biswal S, Deshpande SR, Maher KO, Sun J. RAIM: Recurrent attentive and intensive model of multimodal patient monitoring data. In: Proceedings of the 24th ACM SIGKDD International Conference on Knowledge Discovery & Data Mining. ACM; 2018. pp. 2565-2573

[12] Mollura M, Lehman LWH, Mark RG, Barbieri R. A novel artificial intelligence based intensive care unit monitoring

system: Using physiological waveforms to identify sepsis. Philosophical Transactions of the Royal Society A. 2021;**379**(2212):20200252. DOI: 10.1098/rsta.2020.0252

[13] Komorowski M, Celi LA, Badawi O, Gordon AC, Faisal AA. The artificial intelligence clinician learns optimal treatment strategies for sepsis in intensive care. Nature Medicine. 2018;**24**(11):1716-1720. DOI: 10.1038/s41591-018-0213-5

[14] Hassan N, Slight R, Weiand D, Vellinga A, Morgan G, Aboushareb F, et al. Preventing sepsis; how can artificial intelligence inform the clinical decisionmaking process? A systematic review. International Journal of Medical Informatics. 2021;**150**:104457. DOI: 10.1016/j.ijmedinf.2021.104457

[15] Seymour CW, Kennedy JN, Wang S, Chang CH, Elliott CF, Xu Z, et al. Derivation, validation, and potential treatment implications of novel clinical phenotypes for sepsis. JAMA. 2019;**321**:2003

[16] Chaudhary K, Vaid A, Duffy Á, Paranjpe I, Jaladanki S, Paranjpe M, et al. Utilization of deep learning for subphenotype identification in sepsisassociated acute kidney injury. Clinical Journal of the American Society of Nephrology. 2020;**15**:1557-1565

[17] Zhang Z, Pan Q, Ge H, Xing L, Hong Y, Chen P. Deep learning-based clustering robustly identified two classes of sepsis with both prognostic and predictive values. eBioMedicine. 2020;**62**:103081

[18] Sinha P, Delucchi KL, McAuley DF, O'Kane CM, Matthay MA, Calfee CS. Development and validation of parsimonious algorithms to classify acute respiratory distress syndrome phenotypes: A secondary analysis of randomised controlled trials. The Lancet Respiratory Medicine. 2020;**8**:247-257

[19] Maddali MV, Churpek M, Pham T, Rezoagli E, Zhuo H, Zhao W, et al. Validation and utility of ARDS subphenotypes identified by machinelearning models using clinical data: An observational, multicohort, retrospective analysis. The Lancet Respiratory Medicine. 2022;**10**:367-377

[20] Sinha P, Kerchberger VE, Willmore A, Chambers J, Zhuo H, Abbott J, et al. Identifying molecular phenotypes in sepsis: An analysis of two prospective observational cohorts and secondary analysis of two randomised controlled trials. The Lancet Respiratory Medicine. 2023;**11**:965-974

[21] Chang TH, Liu YC, Lin SR, Chiu PH, Chou CC, Chang LY, et al. Clinical characteristics of hospitalized children with community-acquired pneumonia and respiratory infections: Using machine learning approaches to support pathogen prediction at admission. Journal of Microbiology, Immunology, and Infection. 2023;**56**(4):772-781. DOI: 10.1016/j.jmii.2023.04.011

[22] Lhommet C, Garot D, Grammatico-Guillon L, Jourdannaud C, Asfar P, Faisy C, et al. Predicting the microbial cause of community-acquired pneumonia: Can physicians or a data-driven method differentiate viral from bacterial pneumonia at patient presentation? BMC Pulmonary Medicine. 2020;**20**:62. DOI: 10.1186/s12890-020-1089-y

[23] Zheng Y, Lan C, Wang N, Xu X, Hu T, Wu Q, et al. Machine learning algorithms identify pathogen-specific biomarkers of clinical and metabolomic characteristics in septic patients with bacterial infections. BioMed

Research International. 2020;**2020**. DOI: 10.1155/2020/5956412

[24] Paul M, Andreassen S, Tacconelli E, Nielsen AD, Almanasreh N, Frank U, et al. Improving empirical antibiotic treatment using TREAT, a computerized decision support system: Cluster randomized trial. The Journal of Antimicrobial Chemotherapy. 2006;**58**(6):123845. DOI: 10.1093/jac/dkl372

[25] Hsu JC, Chen YF, Chung WS, Tan TH, Chen T, Chiang JY. Clinical verification of a clinical decision support system for ventilator weaning. Biomedical Engineering Online. 2013;**12**(Suppl. 1):S4. DOI: 10.1186/1475-925X-12-S1-S4

[26] Peine A, Hallawa A, Bickenbach J, Dartmann G, Fazlic LB, Schmeink A, et al. Development and validation of a reinforcement learning algorithm to dynamically optimize mechanical ventilation in critical care. npj Digital Medicine. 2021;**4**(1):32. DOI: 10.1038/s41746-021-00388-6

[27] Knaus WA, Marks RD. New phenotypes for sepsis: The promise and problem of applying machine learning and artificial intelligence in clinical research. JAMA. 2019;**321**(20):1981-1982. DOI: 10.1001/jama.2019.5794

[28] Evans L, Rhodes A, Alhazzani W, Antonelli M, Coopersmith CM, French C, et al. Executive summary: Surviving sepsis campaign: International guidelines for the management of sepsis and septic shock 2021. Critical Care Medicine. 2021;**49**(11):1974-1982. DOI: 10.1097/CCM.0000000000005357

[29] Morley J, Murphy L, Mishra A, Joshi I, Karpathakis K. Governing data and artificial intelligence for health care: Developing an international understanding. JMIR Formative Research. 2022;**6**(1):e31623. DOI: 10.2196/31623

[30] Directorate General for Parliamentary Research Services Artificial Intelligence in Healthcare: Applications, Risks, and Ethical and Societal Impacts [Internet]. LU: Publications Office. 2022. Available from: https://www.europarl.europa.eu/RegData/etudes/STUD/2022/729512/EPRS_STU(2022)729512_EN.pdf [Accessed: April 12, 2023]

[31] Tachkov K, Zemplenyi A, Kamusheva M, Dimitrova M, Siirtola P, Pontén J, et al. Barriers to use artificial intelligence methodologies in health technology assessment in Central and East European countries. Frontiers in Public Health. 2022;**10**:921226. DOI: 10.3389/fpubh.2022.921226

[32] Murdoch B. Privacy and artificial intelligence: Challenges for protecting health information in a new era. BMC Medical Ethics. 2021;**22**(1):122. DOI: 10.1186/s12910-021-00687-3

[33] Wolff J, Pauling J, Keck A, Baumbach J. Systematic review of economic impact studies of artificial intelligence in health care. Journal of Medical Internet Research. 2020;**22**(2):e16866. DOI: 10.2196/16866

[34] Khanna NN, Maindarkar MA, Viswanathan V, Fernandes JFE, Paul S, Bhagawati M, et al. Economics of artificial intelligence in healthcare: Diagnosis vs. treatment. Healthcare (Basel). 2022;**10**(12):2493. DOI: 10.3390/healthcare10122493

[35] Manz CR, Zhang Y, Chen K, Long Q, Small DS, Evans CN, et al. Long-term effect of machine learning-triggered behavioral nudges on serious illness conversations and end-of-life

outcomes among patients with cancer: A randomized clinical trial. JAMA Oncology. 2023;**9**(3):414-418. DOI: 10.1001/jamaoncol.2022.6303

[36] Petersson L, Larsson I, Nygren JM, Nilsen P, Neher M, Reed JE, et al. Challenges to implementing artificial intelligence in healthcare: A qualitative interview study with healthcare leaders in Sweden. BMC Health Services Research. 2022;**22**(1):850. DOI: 10.1186/s12913-022-08215-8

[37] Blease C, Kharko A, Bernstein M, Bradley C, Houston M, Walsh I, et al. Machine learning in medical education: A survey of the experiences and opinions of medical students in Ireland. BMJ Health & Care Informatics. 2022;**29**(1):e100480. DOI: 10.1136/bmjhci-2021-100480

[38] The Topol Review [Internet]. Topol Rev.—NHS Health Educ. Engl. Available from: https://topol.hee.nhs.uk/the-topol-review/ [Accessed: April 12, 2023]

[39] Giordano C, Brennan M, Mohamed B, Rashidi P, Modave F, Tighe P. Accessing artificial intelligence for clinical decision-making. Frontiers in Digital Health. 2021;**3**:645232. DOI: 10.3389/fdgth.2021.645232

[40] Islam MM, Nasrin T, Walther BA, Wu CC, Yang HC, Li YC. Prediction of sepsis patients using machine learning approach: A meta-analysis. Computer Methods and Programs in Biomedicine. 2019;**170**:1-9

Chapter 4

Extracorporeal Blood Purification in Sepsis and Septic Shock

Girish Kumthekar, Manan Doshi and Rajasekara Chakravarthi

Abstract

We acknowledge the fact that sepsis and septic shock are induced, sustained and perpetuated with the help of circulating molecules released from various activated inflammatory cells. This has shifted focus of management of sepsis from virulence of microbes to the dysregulated host immune response. The drivers of dysregulated immune responses constitute circulating substances like cytokines, chemokines and endotoxins. Extracorporeal blood purification (EBP) is a blood purification technique where blood or its components circulate in the extracorporeal (EC) circuit with the help of a specialised or standard dialysis machine. The blood is purified with clearance of inflammatory mediators and/or toxins aimed at suppressing inflammatory mediators in the various phases of sepsis. The purified blood/component gets recirculated back to the patient. But, presently we do not have any established guidelines for the use of EBP therapies. Hence, the use of EBP therapies is largely based on the judgement of the treating physician influenced by local practice and expertise levels. The literature is hopeful about the theoretical advantages of using multiple novel extracorporeal blood purification techniques with equivocal outcomes in clinical trials.

Keywords: extracorporeal blood purification, acute kidney injury, sepsis, septic shock, sepsis biomarkers

1. Introduction

The landscape of critical care is continually evolving, with innovative concepts and algorithms emerging continuously to improve patient outcomes. Among these advancements, extracorporeal blood purification (EBP) has emerged as a promising modality.

The term EBP implies supporting the failing or failed organ artificially from outside the body wherein the device either partially or completely assumes the function of the compromised organ. Notably, the past few decades have witnessed a significant dearth of novel medications, antibiotics and pharmaceuticals. As a result, researchers have shifted their attention towards extracorporeal therapies, exploring innovative strategies to bridge the gap in conventional treatment options and improve patient outcomes. These therapies are designed to selectively remove target disease-causing or propagating substances from the body through the use of different filters, which the blood column is exposed to for a predetermined time period. While EBP is often associated with renal replacement therapy, the scope of EBP extends even beyond renal support. These modalities can be used even when renal functions are normal. EBP can be used to support one organ at a time or multiple organs at a time based on the metabolic needs of the critically ill patient. The organs that commonly require support are kidneys, heart, liver, lungs and vascular system either individually or in various combinations. One of the most prevalent and devastating conditions encountered in ICU, which can simultaneously or sequentially affect multiple vital organs, is sepsis. Sepsis often progresses to severe sepsis and ultimately septic shock, a critical condition characterised by compromised oxygen delivery to vital organs, leading to widespread tissue hypoxia and organ dysfunction. Septic shock is a continuum of sepsis syndrome where a vasopressor is required to maintain a patient's mean arterial pressure (MAP) $\geq$ 65 mmHg to avoid organ hypoperfusion indicated by a serum lactate level $\geq$ 2 mmol/L. Despite being a significant and frequently encountered clinical condition, guidelines for the use of EBP therapies in sepsis and septic shock are sparse leading to clinical decisions being based on case to case basis (**Table 1**).

1.1 The drivers of sepsis are many and poorly understood

Haemodynamic stability in sepsis leads to a complication known as septic shock. EBP techniques such as high-volume haemofiltration, coupled plasma adsorption/filtration, resin or polymer adsorbers and CytoSorb® are used to improve the shock state and reduce vasopressor requirement. EBP is an evolution in dialysis techniques where blood circulates in the extracorporeal (EC) circuit and is exposed to various specialised membranes. These membranes enable EBP to clear inflammatory mediators and/or toxins and damp their systemic expressions at various phases of sepsis [1]. As per the 'cytokine peak concentration' hypothesis, the peak of cytokine concentration during the early stage of sepsis requires optimal reduction to halt the inflammatory cascade. Once the inflammatory cascade is slowed down by removal of drivers of sepsis, the organ damage and consequent multiorgan dysfunction syndrome (MODS) can be prevented or treated [2].

Sepsis Support Systems			
Kidney Support	**Heart Support**	**Lung Support**	**Liver Support**
Intermittent haemodialysis, SLED, CRRT including CVVHDF, CVVHF, CVVHD	ECMO including VA-ECMO, VV-ECMO, IABP, intraventricular assist devices	ECCO2R, ECMO predominantly VV-ECMO, assisted ventilation (invasive and non-invasive)	Adsorbent columns like HA330, BS330, SPAD, MARS-CRRT, Prometheus, therapeutic plasma exchange
Targeted Removal of Drivers of Sepsis			
HVHF, CPFA, adsorption columns (CytoSorb™, HA 380, HA 330, polymyxin), specialised dialysis membranes (oXiris, Haemofeel PMMA).			

Table 1.
Extracorporeal organ support systems: The table illustrates available organ support systems that are used for extracorporeal blood purification. These systems include, but are not limited to, various dialysis modalities.

1.2 Sepsis and septic shock

The World Health Organisation (WHO) data from 2017 indicated morbidity and mortality related to sepsis and its complications in 48.9 million cases with 11 million sepsis-related deaths. This estimate accounts for 20% of deaths worldwide [3, 4]. The definition of sepsis, as per current understanding, is that it is a life-threatening organ dysfunction caused by a dysregulated immune response of the host to infection. Its pathophysiology involves a complex interplay between the host and the infectious agent. The host immune system may respond with an over-stimulated or under-stimulated immune response. Over-stimulation of the immune response leads to a cytokine storm (septic shock, capillary leakage and microcirculatory disturbances and MODS). On the other hand, under-stimulated immune responses lead to a protracted phase of immunoparalysis, with subsequent disseminated opportunistic infections [1]. A poorly regulated systemic inflammatory response syndrome (SIRS) and compensatory anti-inflammatory response can lead to a progressive tissue damage and potentially MODS.

2. Understanding sepsis for better management

2.1 Pathophysiology of sepsis and septic shock

Step 1: Activation of the innate immune system through binding of PAMPs and DAMPs to the specific pattern recognition receptors present on the immune cell like macrophages, monocytes, neutrophils and natural killer cells.

Step 2: Intracellular signal transduction and activation of pro-inflammatory cytokines (IL1, IL6, IL12, IL18 and tumour necrosis factor alpha (TNF-α)) [5].

Step 3: Activation of leukocytes, complement system, coagulation pathways, tissue factor production, chemokine expression and overexpression of endothelial adhesion molecules (acquired/adaptive immune system).

Step 4: Negative feedback: a compensatory anti-inflammatory response syndrome is initiated down-regulating the components of the adaptive immune system.

Coagulopathy in sepsis occurs as a result of simultaneous activation of inflammatory and haemostatic pathways. It leads to thrombin production, platelet activation and formation of fibrin clots leading to perfusion defects. Sepsis leads to suppression of natural anticoagulants like protein C, anti-thrombin, and thrombomodulin along with tissue plasminogen activator and potentiating procoagulants. This unbalanced clotting mechanism due to sepsis and its complications are implicated for microvascular coagulation, tissue hypoxia and ultimately MODS [6].

2.2 Biomarker-guided management of sepsis and septic shock

We acknowledge the fact that sepsis and septic shock are induced, sustained and perpetuated with the help of circulating molecules released from various activated inflammatory cells. These circulating molecules constitute biomarkers of sepsis. The microbiological culture and sensitivity reports often take at least 2–3 days to finalise and are not particularly conclusive especially when cultures are collected while patients are receiving anti-microbial therapy. Thus, approximately 40–50% of cases of sepsis are deemed to be culture-negative. This makes microbiological cultures less useful when therapy is required in early phases of sepsis [7]. The present management of sepsis and septic shock is based on 4 important first-line considerations, namely antibiotics, intravenous fluids, vasopressors and ventilation. The second-line considerations on management of sepsis and septic shock include electrolytes and acid-base disturbances, oxygenation, anticoagulation and glucocorticoids. In the present schema, except lactate, we find no laboratory parameter guiding the management. As we know, sepsis and its complications are induced and enhanced by immunologically active substances, which, theoretically, need their removal from the circulation. These substances might be the biomarkers influencing the decision to begin and terminate EBP therapy in patients with sepsis (**Table 2**).

Driver of Sepsis and/or Septic Shock	Molecular Weight	Possible Role in Sepsis	Available Options for Extracorporeal Removal
Interleukin-1b	18–25 kDa	Potent pro-inflammatory cytokine.	CRRT (AN-69, polysulfone) high flux, Biosky MG 350 adsorber, CytoSorb, EMic, HA 230, HA 330, Theranova ™
Interleukin –2	16 kDa	Proliferation of activated T cells, differentiation of B cells, natural killer cells, monocytes and macrophages. IL-2 also helps distinguish between foreign and 'self' antigens.	CRRT (AN-69, polysulfone) high flux, Biosky MG 350 adsorber, CytoSorb, EMic, HA 230, HA 330, Theranova ™, Biosky MG 350 adsorber
Interleukin-4	20 kDa	Development of allergic inflammation and asthma.	CRRT (AN-69, polysulfone) high flux, CytoSorb, EMic, HA 230, HA 330, Theranova ™
Interleukin-6	25 kDa	It can act in either a pro-inflammatory or an anti-inflammatory way.	CRRT (AN-69, polysulfone) high flux, CytoSorb, Haemofeel, EMic, HA 230, HA 330, Theranova ™
Interleukin-10	40 kDa	Cytokine with potent anti-inflammatory and anti-immune activity	CRRT (AN-69, polysulfone) high flux, CytoSorb, Haemofeel ™, EMic™, HA 230, HA 330, Theranova ™
Tumour Necrosis Factor-alpha	51 kDa	Apoptotic cell death, cellular proliferation, differentiation, inflammation, tumorigenesis.	CRRT (AN-69, polysulfone) high flux, CytoSorb, HVHF, Haemofeel ™, EMic™, HA 230, HA 330, Theranova ™
Interferon-gamma	33 kDa	IFN-gamma synergises with TNF-alpha and TNF-beta in inhibiting the proliferation of various cell types.	CRRT (AN-69, polysulfone) high flux, CytoSorb, HVHF, Haemofeel ™, EMic™, HA 230, HA 330, Theranova ™
Endotoxin	10 to 100 kDa	Pivotal role in initiation and perpetuation of sepsis, responsible for activation of antigen-presenting cells and direct cytotoxic damage.	oXiris™, HA 330, CytoSorb

Table 2.
Biomarkers of sepsis and septic shock and possible modalities for their extracorporeal removal.

2.3 Role of extracorporeal blood purification in sepsis

Sepsis-associated acute kidney injury (SA-AKI) is the occurrence of AKI within 7 days of sepsis onset (diagnosed according to KDIGO criteria and Sepsis 3 criteria, respectively). We suggest that sepsis-induced AKI should be considered a sub-phenotype of SA-AKI where sepsis is the predominant cause of kidney injury. Patients can present with either clinical (creatinine and urine output criteria) or subclinical AKI (injury biomarker criteria), which poses a challenge to improve outcomes. Early identification of patients at risk of new onset or worsening AKI is crucial to initiate adequate supportive measures limiting further insults to the kidney [8].

In 2018, the Surviving Sepsis Campaign (SSC) guidelines highlighted an 'Hour-1-Bundle' instead of 3- and 6-hour bundles. The 'Hour-1 Bundle' consists of 5 clinical interventions including immediate initiation of sepsis management and fluid resuscitation measures. The use of extracorporeal blood purification is not a strong recommendation in these bundles [9]. Due to rising incidence of sepsis and septic shock (11 million sepsis-related deaths worldwide in 2017), the World Health Organisation (WHO) declared sepsis a global health priority. The tools to deal with ever-increasing incidence are traditional, including management of infection, fluid and electrolytes, assisted ventilation and organ support. EBP therapies are not considered in the SSC guidelines though it acknowledged immune dysregulation as a pivotal cause of sepsis and septic shock. EBP therapies are prescribed on a case to case basis according to the prevalent practices and clinical judgement.

Organ failure in sepsis is attributed to a dysregulated host response leading to the release of pro- and anti-inflammatory cytokines and endotoxins, which have been targeted in recent decades. EBP therapies have been proposed as adjunctive options to remove excess cytokines and endotoxins, highlighting the importance of innovative approaches in managing sepsis [10]. The data on patient and EBP therapy outcomes shows promise but lacks robust recommendations on patient selection, choice of therapy and therapy end points. Nonetheless, the novel approach of modifying dysregulated immune response by removing the drivers of inflammation through EBP has attracted many investigators and clinicians.

3. Different modalities available for extracorporeal blood purification in sepsis and septic shock

EBP therapies are the strategies proposed to restore the immune balance by eliminating or deactivating the inflammatory mediators and originate as an off-shoot of renal replacement therapy (RRT).

1. High volume haemofiltration (HVHF): Tapia et al. in the article on the effectiveness of short-term 6-hour high volume haemofiltration found decrease in noradrenaline dose at 4 hours of starting the therapy in refractory severe septic shock [11]. Moreover, there was a significant improvement in metabolic and respiratory parameters as well. It was a prospective study on participants with severe septic shock treated with 6 hours of HVHF with a dose of 40 ml/kg/hr. In another study by Joannes-Boyau et al., there was no difference in haemodynamic stability, severity scores, 28-d mortality, length of stay and vasopressor-free days between two cohorts treated with either HVHF 70 mL/kg/h or standard volume haemofiltration at 35 mL/kg/h [12]. Meta-analyses also concluded that HVHF

in comparison with standard renal replacement therapy does not provide any benefit in terms of survival rate, prevention or restoration of renal function, vasopressor-free days and incidence of adverse events [13]. Two doses of HVHF with continuous haemofiltration (50–70 mL/kg/h for 24 h and 100–120 mL/kg/h intermittently for 4–8 h, also called 'pulse HVHF') were compared for efficacy in sepsis and septic shock. This was followed by conventional renal dose haemofiltration. Both groups were comparable with no remarkable superiority of one over another [14]. Several studies evaluating CPFA in sepsis and septic shock patients resulted in haemodynamic improvement compared to continuous venovenous haemofiltration (CVVH), which is CRRT modality with predominant convective clearance as HVHF. However, the evidence was weak as the patient sample size was small [15].

2. Coupled plasma filtration and adsorption (CPFA): In a prospective, randomised, multicentre parallel group trial, 192 septic shock patients underwent CPFA for cytokine and endotoxin removal with decreased mortality in patients receiving high doses of CPFA. The study revealed no difference in other parameters like length of ICU stay and new organ failures in 30 days [16]. The CPFA technique separates plasma from blood. The cytokines in the plasma component are circulated through a sorbent cartridge aimed at the removal of cytokines. Once the cytokines are adsorbed, the plasma is redirected to the dialyzer for renal replacement therapy. In CPFA, there is no direct contact between blood cells and the sorbent. This makes CPFA more biocompatible with enhanced cytokine clearance as lower plasma flow allows longer duration of contact with the resin cartridge and combined cytokine removal with renal replacement therapy by convection. CPFA therapy is a 10-hour session, for 5 consecutive days, with a plasma filtration fraction ranging between 10 and 18% [17].

3. Continuous venovenous haemofiltration (CVVH) with high cutoff membrane (HCO): It is observed that high replacement volumes enhance the lymphatic transport between the blood compartments and tissue/interstitial space. This is popularised as the 'Mediator delivery' hypothesis by Di Carlo and Alexander. CVVH with HCO is performed with high replacement volumes (around 20- to 40 -fold increase in lymphatic volumes), targeted at displacing the inflammatory mediators in the blood compartment. It has a theoretical advantage of clearing the lymphatic system and interstitial space of cytokines and endotoxins.

4. Polymyxin B hemadsorption: Polymyxin B is used as a parenteral drug to treat endotoxemia caused by Gram-negative infections. It has significant neurological and renal toxicity. In an attempt to minimise toxicity profile, a cartridge with immobilised Polymyxin B (PMX-B) for extracorporeal hemadsorption was proposed for use as an EBP therapy for Gram-negative endotoxemia and sepsis [18]. The EUPHRATES trial was performed in patients with septic shock and high levels of endotoxin in the blood. One group received standard treatment plus two endotoxin hemadsorption treatments (90–120 min) or sham within 24 h of enrolment. Endotoxin hemadsorption was not associated with a significant difference in mortality at 28 days. A post hoc analysis of this trial showed that endotoxin hemadsorption seems to be effective in improving mortality and ventilator-free days in a specific population of patients with plasma endotoxin

activity levels between 0.6 and 0.89. Further analysis showed that abnormal coagulation and hyperlactatemia in septic patients with high endotoxin activity are benefitted the most from PMX-HA [19]. Many studies have reported that polymyxin B hemadsorption could increase the expression of leukocyte surface markers such as HLA-DR making hemadsorption a 're-programming system' for the leukocytes. Another unique element proposed in this theory is that the concentration gradient from plasma to infected tissues can be restored by removing mediators from the plasma in systemic inflammation [18, 19].

5. Resin-based hemadsorption: A resin-based adsorbent cartridge known as HA330 (Jafron Biomedical, China) has also been demonstrated for its ability to eliminate cytokines. The HA330 cartridge has a pore size of 500 Da to 60 kDa and has been shown to remove molecules ranging from 10 to 60 kDa, including cytokines and complement factors, under cytokine storm conditions, such as sepsis, resulting in improved 28-day survival [20]. Huang et al. showed that EBP with HA330 resin cartridges decreased the vasopressor requirements of patients with sepsis and septic shock [21]. It is recommended that HA330 cartridges should not be used for more than 4 h for optimum benefit. Its adsorptive capacity decreases with time due to saturation, and the elimination of cytokines is negated by the shift from the interstitial to the blood compartment, which could affect the therapy outcomes.

6. Cytokine removal: Extracorporeal removal of cytokines (interleukins and leukotriene) through hemadsorption removes both pro- and anti-inflammatory cytokines from the blood. A multicentre RCT enrolling 97 patients with acute lung injury and septic shock showed that extracorporeal cytokine hemadsorption treatment was able to decrease serum IL-6 levels but without any effect on the PaO2/FiO2 ratio, organ dysfunction and mortality [22]. Modified AN69ST membrane (oXiris) is capable of removing both endotoxins and cytokines besides serving as a CRRT filter. Russell et al. used a hybrid EBP system in 15 critically ill sepsis patients utilising the oXiris filter and a CytoSorb® adsorbent cartridge. Markers of inflammation and sepsis like procalcitonin, IL6 and endotoxins were monitored at frequent intervals. Patients treated with CRRT using oXiris and CytoSorb® demonstrated better haemodynamic stability along with improved inflammatory response and renal function [23].

7. Endotoxin filters: Gram-negative bacteria release cell wall components called endotoxins with a molecular weight of 10,000 to 1,000,000 Daltons. As dialysis /ultrafiltration/convection is less efficient to remove the endotoxins from blood, ion exchange resins are the most common form of EBP for their removal from circulation [24]. In the clinical course of a specific sub-phenotype of septic shock (endotoxic shock), polymyxin B hemadsorption (PMX-HA) cartridge is recommended to bind and neutralise circulating endotoxin. The 28th Acute Disease and Quality Initiative (ADQI) suggests EBP therapies are emerging new strategies to perform immunomodulatory activities aimed at target organ recovery. This allows removing pathogen-associated molecular patterns (PAMPs) and subsequent immunomodulation by modifying the concentration of the damage-associated molecular patterns (DAMP) [8]. These filters are used with or without RRT in preferably early stages (6 to 12 hours) of diagnosis of septic shock (**Table 3**).

Technology	Indication	Modality	Target of removal	Mass separation mechanism	Comment
PAES-PVP high-flux	RRT, hyperinflammation	HD, HF, HDF	Fluids, electrolytes, middle molecules	Convection, diffusion	CRRT for kidney support
AN69-PEI-heparin	RRT, hyperinflammation, Gram-negative sepsis or endotoxemia	HD, HF, HDF	Fluids, electrolytes, middle molecules, endotoxins	Adsorption, convection, diffusion	CRRT for kidney and immunomodulatory support
AN69-ST, PMMA	RRT, hyperinflammation	HD, HF, HDF	Fluids, electrolytes, middle molecules	Adsorption, convection, diffusion	CRRT for kidney and immunomodulatory support
PAES-PVP MCO and HCO	RRT, hyperinflammation	HD	Fluids, electrolytes, middle molecules	Diffusion	CRRT for kidney and immunomodulatory support
Plasma sulfone, polypropylene (for membrane plasmapheresis)	Hyperinflammation	Centrifugation or HF	Fluids, electrolytes, middle molecules, endotoxin	Convection (membrane); gravity sedimentation (centrifuge)	Immunomodulatory support
Heparin covalently bound to polyethylene	Viraemia, bacteraemia, fungaemia	Hemadsorption	Bacteria, fungi, viruses	Adsorption	Selective immunomodulatory support
Porous polymer beads polystyrene divinylbenzene	Hyperinflammation	Hemadsorption	Protein-bound compounds, middle molecules	Adsorption	Non-selective immunomodulatory support
PMX covalently bound to polypropylene-polystyrene fibre	Gram-negative sepsis or endotoxemia	Hemadsorption	Endotoxin	Adsorption	Selective immunomodulatory support

AN, acrylonitrile; CRRT, continuous renal replacement therapy; HCO, high cutoff; HD, haemodialysis; HDF, haemodiafiltration; HF, haemofiltration, HFl, high-flux; RRT, renal replacement therapy; MCO, medium cutoff; PAES, poly(aryl ether sulfone); PEI, polyethylenimine; PMMA, poly(methyl methacrylate); PVP, polyvinylpyrrolidone.

Table 3.
Characteristics of extracorporeal blood purification therapies available for sepsis and SA-AKI [8].

3.1 Outcomes of extracorporeal blood purification in sepsis and septic shock

In critical illnesses resulting from toxic systemic inflammation, e.g., sepsis and COVID-19, EBP treatments have been deployed to reduce concentrations of inflammatory mediators (IM) in circulating blood. The goal of these treatments is to abate inflammatory organ injury and improve patient outcome. While evidence for efficacy of EBP treatment in acute inflammatory disease is lacking, it is generally considered safe [25]. But, mechanisms involving adsorbent matrix or carrier protein amplification in EBP adsorbent media could convert the adsorbent into an inadvertent bioreactor, promoting inflammatory injury and negative outcomes. The fast clearance of free cytokines principally results from renal and hepatic excretion and metabolism and receptor clearance by endocytosis. Cytokine adsorption to a matrix could 'rescue' the cytokine from renal or hepatic excretion and metabolism and prevent receptor binding and endocytosis. Cytokines adsorbed to matrices could form a 'depot of cytokines'. Removal of protective proteins, given the devices' non-specific adsorption, is also a possibility. Possible removal of certain anti-microbial drugs in critically ill infected patients by any form of EBP treatment requires close attention. The suggestion that adsorbent treatment may rapidly remove some drugs means therapeutic drug monitoring should be used and additional antibiotic doses should be considered, particularly early in treatment.

The European Society of Intensive Care Medicine (ESICM) 'EXPLORATION' survey in 2024 found, though the clinical evidence is limited, that the majority of clinicians use EBP techniques in their clinical practice and acknowledge good theoretical rationale behind it. While both cytokine adsorption and therapeutic plasma exchange (TPE) are

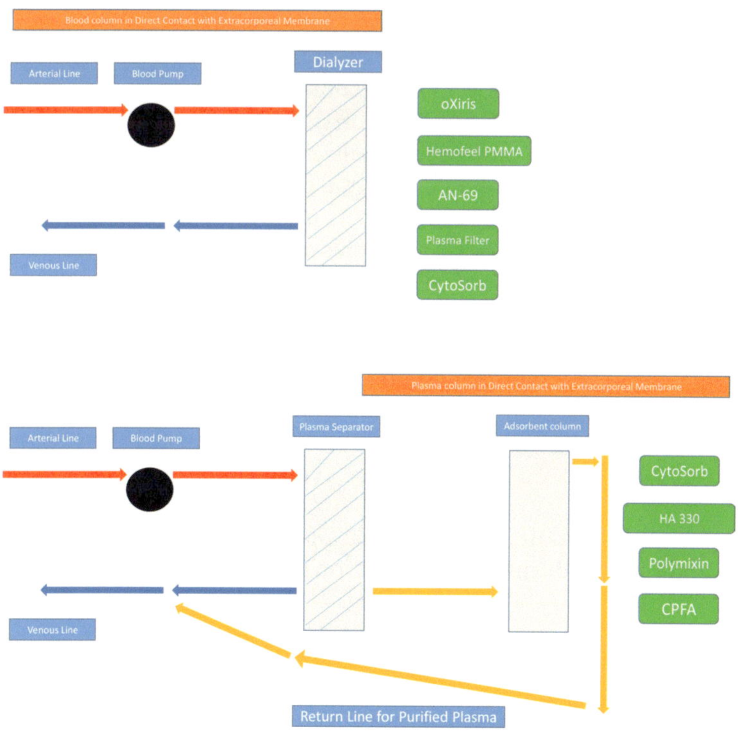

Figure 1.
Connectology for extracorporeal blood purification.

by far the most commonly used technique, both clinical evidence and future potential for further exploration in clinical trials were assessed to be the highest for TPE [26].

The literature is hopeful about the theoretical advantages of using multiple novel extracorporeal blood purification techniques with equivocal outcomes in clinical trials. The treating clinician needs to decide the therapy options on a case to case basis. The mode of therapy, its onset and conclusion are yet to be standardised. One achieved, it would affect the EBP outcomes favourable to the patients with sepsis and septic shock.

3.2 Methodology/connectology for extracorporeal blood purification

We have broadly divided EBP into two methods. First, the blood column gets directly in contact with the extracorporeal membrane and in second, the plasma removed by a plasma separator circulates through an adsorbent column. Hence, the blood corpuscles are less likely to get in contact with the adsorbent column. The CytoSorb adsorbent could be an exception where we might use either of the methods as per operator convenience and expertise (**Figure 1**). The benefits and risks involved in choosing one method over another are not clearly defined. The membranes that serve as dialyzers have the added benefit of serving as a renal support in addition to EBP for sepsis and septic shock. As illustrated in **Figure 1**, the plasma separator plays a vital role in adsorptive techniques wherein the plasma component gets cleared of the toxins leaving the cellular components unaltered.

4. Conclusions

There is an urgent need for adjuvant therapies is the management of sepsis and septic shock. With fewer new anti-microbials coming up and bacterial resistance to existing drugs increasing, we expect EBP becomes a beacon of hope in the management of sepsis. These therapies could be an offshoot of dialysis therapies, coupled with dialysis therapies or dialysis with specialised membranes. Consequently, EBP should be studied in patients with normal renal function or mild acute kidney injury with no need for renal replacement therapy. As of now, we lack complete understanding of their optimal time of initiation and goals of EBP procedures. We need robust clinical trials helping EBP therapies to be a part of standard of care in the management of sepsis and its complications. Despite promising data, let us acknowledge the presence of significant knowledge gaps in the understanding of the role of EBP in sepsis and septic shock.

Acknowledgements

I express my sincere gratitude to Dr. Suhas Mondhe and Dr. Aditi Pandey for their suggestions and support during the preparation of this manuscript.

Conflict of interest

The authors declare no conflict of interest.

Author details

Girish Kumthekar[1,2*], Manan Doshi[3] and Rajasekara Chakravarthi[2,4]

1 Nephrology and Kidney Transplantation, Symbiosis University Hospital and Research Centre (SUHRC), Symbiosis International University (SIU) Lavale, Pune, India

2 Renown Clinical Services, Hyderabad, India

3 Nephrology and Kidney Transplantation, Sahyadri Hospital, Deccan, Pune, India

4 Department of Nephrology and Kidney Transplantation, Yashoda Hospital, Hi-Tech City, Hyderabad, India

*Address all correspondence to: drgirishkumthekar@gmail.com

References

[1] Shum HP, Yan WW, Chan TM. Extracorporeal blood purification for sepsis. Hong Kong Medical Journal. 2016;**22**:478-485. DOI: 10.12809/hkmj164876

[2] Ronco C, Bonello M, Bordoni V, Ricci Z, D'Intini V, Bellomo R, et al. Extracorporeal therapies in non-renal disease: Treatment of sepsis and the peak concentration hypothesis. Blood Purification. 2004;**22**:164-174. DOI: 10.1159/000074937

[3] Organisation WH. Global Report on the Epidemiology and Burden of Sepsis: Current Evidence, Identifying Gaps and Future Directions [Internet]. Geneva, Switzerland: World Health Organization; 2020. Available from: https://apps.who.int/iris/handle/10665/334216

[4] Rudd KE, Johnson SC, Agesa KM, Shackelford KA, et al. Global, regional, and national sepsis incidence and mortality, 1990-2017: Analysis for the global burden of disease study. Lancet. 2020;**395**:200-211. DOI: 10.1016/S0140-6736(19)32989-7

[5] Hotchkiss RS, Moldawer LL, Opal SM, Reinhart K, Turnbull IR, Vincent JL. Sepsis and septic shock. Nature Reviews. Disease Primers. 2016;**2**:16045. DOI: 10.1038/nrdp.2016.45

[6] Gotur DB. Sepsis diagnosis and management. Journal of Medical Sciences and Health. 2017;**3**:1-12. DOI: 10.46347/jmsh.2017.v03i03.001

[7] Vincent JL, Sakr Y, Singer M. Et al; EPIC III investigators. Prevalence and outcomes of infection among patients in intensive care units in 2017. Journal of the American Medical Association. 2020;**323**(15):1478-1487. DOI: 10.1001/jama.2020.2717

[8] Zarbock A, Nadim MK, Pickkers P, et al. Sepsis-associated acute kidney injury: Consensus report of the 28th acute disease quality initiative workgroup. Nature Reviews. Nephrology. 2023;**19**:401-417. DOI: 10.1038/s41581-023-00683-3

[9] Levy MM, Evans LE, Rhodes A. The surviving sepsis campaign bundle: 2018 update. Intensive Care Medicine. 2018;**44**:925-928. DOI: 10.1007/s00134-018-5085-0

[10] Monard C, Rimmele T, Ronco C. Extracorporeal blood purification therapies for sepsis. Blood Purification. 2019;**47**(3):1-14. DOI: 10.1159/000499520

[11] Tapia P, Chinchón E, Morales D, Stehberg J, Simon F. Effectiveness of short-term 6-hour high-volume hemofiltration during refractory severe septic shock. Journal of Trauma and Acute Care Surgery. 2012;**72**:1228-1237; discussion 1237. DOI: 10.1097/TA.0b013e318248bc6c

[12] Joannes-Boyau O, Honoré PM, Perez P, et al. High-volume versus standard-volume hemofiltration for septic shock patients with acute kidney injury (IVOIRE study): A multicentre randomised controlled trial. Intensive Care Medicine. 2013;**39**:1535-1546. DOI: 10.1007/s00134-013-2967-z

[13] Borthwick EM, Hill CJ, Rabindranath KS, Maxwell AP, McAuley DF, Blackwood B. High-volume haemofiltration for sepsis in adults. Cochrane Database of Systematic Reviews. 2017;**1**(1):CD008075. DOI: 10.1002/14651858.CD008075.pub3

[14] Honoré PM, Jacobs R, Boer W, Joannes-Boyau O, De Regt J, De

Waele E, et al. New insights regarding rationale, therapeutic target and dose of hemofiltration and hybrid therapies in septic acute kidney injury. Blood Purification. 2012;**33**:44-51. DOI: 10.1159/000333837

[15] Ronco C, Brendolan A, Lonnemann G, Bellomo R, Piccinni P, Digito A, et al. A pilot study of coupled plasma filtration with adsorption in septic shock. Critical Care Medicine. 2002;**30**:1250-1255. DOI: 10.1097/00003246-200206000-00015

[16] Atan R, Peck L, Prowle J, Licari E, Eastwood GM, Storr M, et al. A double-blind randomised controlled trial of high Cutoff versus standard hemofiltration in critically ill patients with acute kidney injury. Critical Care Medicine. 2018;**46**:e988-e994. DOI: 10.1097/CCM.0000000000003350

[17] Govil D, Kumar GP. Extracorporeal therapy in sepsis. Indian Journal of Critical Care Medicine. 2020;**24**(Suppl. 3):S117-S121

[18] Girardis M, Coloretti I, Antonelli M, et al. Adjunctive immunotherapeutic agents in patients with sepsis and septic shock: A multidisciplinary consensus of 23. Journal of Anesthesia, Analgesia and Critical Care. 2024;**4**:28. DOI: 10.1186/s44158-024-00165-3

[19] Klein DJ, Foster D, Walker PM, Bagshaw SM, Mekonnen H, Antonelli M. Polymyxin B hemoperfusion in endotoxemic septic shock patients without extreme endotoxemia: A post hoc analysis of the EUPHRATES trial. Intensive Care Medicine. 2018;**44**(12):2205-2212. DOI: 10.1007/s00134-018-5463-7. Epub 2018 Nov 23

[20] Ankawi G, Fan W, Pomare Montin D, Lorenzin A, Neri M, et al. A new series of sorbent devices for multiple clinical purposes: Current evidence and future directions. Blood Purification. 2019;**47**(1-3):94-100. DOI: 10.1159/000493523

[21] Huang Z, Wang SR, Su W, Liu JY. Removal of humoral mediators and the effect on the survival of septic patients by hemoperfusion with neutral microporous resin column. Therapeutic Apheresis and Dialysis. 2010;**14**(6):596-602. DOI: 10.1111/j.1744-9987.2010.00825.x

[22] Schädler D, Pausch C, Heise D, et al. The effect of a novel extracorporeal cytokine hemoadsorption device on IL-6 elimination in septic patients: A randomised controlled trial. PLoS One. 2017;**12**(10):e0187015. DOI: 10.1371/journal.pone.0187015

[23] Russell JA. Vasopressor therapy in critically ill patients with shock. Intensive Care Medicine. 2019;**45**:1503-1517. DOI: 10.1007/s00134-019-05801-z

[24] Forin E, Lorenzoni G, Ferrer R, et al. Endotoxin removal therapy with Polymyxin B immobilized fiber column: A single center experience from EUPHAS2 registry. Scientific Reports. 2023;**13**:17600. DOI: 10.1038/s41598-023-44850-9

[25] Matson J, Lange P, Honore PM, et al. Adverse outcomes with extracorporeal adsorbent blood treatments in toxic systemic inflammation: A perspective on possible mechanisms. Annals of Intensive Care. 2022;**12**:105. DOI: 10.1186/s13613-022-01078-6

[26] Stahl K, Bode C, Seeliger B, et al. Current clinical practice in using adjunctive extracorporeal blood purification in sepsis and septic shock: Results from the ESICM "EXPLORATION" survey. ICMx. 2024;**12**:5. DOI: 10.1186/s40635-023-00592-6

Chapter 5

Maternal Sepsis: Updates on Diagnosis and Management

Seema Nahid, Fateen Shareef, Roshan Afsha, Azha Fatima, Umm E. Amara, Nissar Sheikh and Eynas Abdalla

Abstract

Maternal sepsis is one of the leading causes of maternal mortality all over the world. It is the occurrence of infection during pregnancy or postpartum period. If sepsis is not detected early and managed appropriately, it can progress into multi-organ dysfunction and septic shock with increased morbidity and mortality not only in the mother but in the neonate as well. The physiological changes of pregnancy often confuse and delay the diagnosis of sepsis during pregnancy. It is essential to have a high suspicion index to diagnose sepsis early. Hence, it is essential to diagnose and treat the infection and sepsis during pregnancy for better maternal and fetal outcomes. This chapter will describe the diagnosis and management of maternal sepsis with updated information in various subheadings.

Keywords: antibiotic, blood cultures, chorioamnionitis, endometritis, hypotension, maternal, pregnancy, postpartum, serum lactate, sepsis, septic shock

1. Introduction

Maternal sepsis is the 3rd leading cause of maternal death in the world [1]. Hence, it is essential to increase awareness about sepsis; its diagnosis and management are essential. Maternal sepsis is a clinical syndrome manifested by dysregulated host response to infection, causing tissue and organ injury and dysfunction during pregnancy, abortion, childbirth, and postpartum; sepsis, if not detected early and treated appropriately, can progress into more severe septic shock and MODS (Multiple organ dysfunction) [2].

The profound release of proinflammatory mediators causes infection spread and dysregulated immune response in sepsis due to virulence of the organism's local toxin release, causing complement activation [3].

Sepsis is defined as a clinical condition with physiological, biochemical, and biological abnormalities because of a dysregulated host response to the infection, leading to organ dysfunction [4]. Septic shock is a further continuation of sepsis, with the patient becoming hypotensive and not responding to fluid therapy, causing cellular hypoperfusion and oxygen deficiency [4–6].

Maternal sepsis is the sepsis occurring in women during pregnancy or puerperium and results from septic abortion, placental infection, or breast engorgement causing mastitis [7].

1.1 Epidemiology

Maternal sepsis and its mortality have been on the decline over the last 3 decades because of awareness, education, improved socioeconomic status, and early diagnosis with the availability of prophylactic antibiotics and targeted team management. Maternal sepsis is still a significant cause of maternal morbidity and accounts for 10.7% of all maternal deaths. Maternal sepsis burden is significant in low- and middle-income countries [7].

As per the WHO (World Health Organization), peripartum sepsis accounts for approximately 5.7 million cases per year, with an incidence of 4.4%. A concerning fact is that maternal mortality due to streptococcus-induced sepsis remains as high as 60% [8].

Risk factors: Various risk factors contribute to maternal sepsis for both patients as well as obstetrics factors are described in **Table 1** [2, 9, 10].

1.2 Etiology

Identifying the causes of maternal sepsis is helpful in controlling the source of infection and managing sepsis. **Table 2** describes the most frequent causes of maternal sepsis.

Chorioamnionitis is characterized by chorion, amnion, and placenta infection, causing sepsis. Endometriosis is the infection of the endometrium, myometrium, and parametrium, causing sepsis. The causative bacteria for endometriosis are commonly polymicrobial and a mixture of aerobes and anaerobic bacteria [11].

The mode of delivery of the fetus is a significant risk for maternal sepsis, as labor and ruptured membranes and the spread of infection from microbes in the lower genital tract spread during labor [11]. There is a significant increase in urinary tract infections during pregnancy due to the physiological changes and pressure on the uterus on the urinary tract system with slowing of protective peristalsis.

Risk factors for maternal sepsis	
Patient factors	**Obstetric factors**
Obesity	Emergency cesarean section
Diabetes/Impaired glucose tolerance	Prolonged rupture of membranes
Immune compromised	Prolonged labor with multiple >5 vaginal examinations
Anemia	
Chronic comorbidities (hepatic/renal/ cardiac)	Vaginal trauma/instrumental delivery
	Retained products of conception
Sickle cell disease	Cervical stitch
	Amniocentesis
History of pelvic infections	
	Invasive procedures: Amniocentesis/post chorionic villus sampling

Table 1.
Risk factors for maternal sepsis.

Causes of maternal		
Obstetric causes		
Genital tract causes	Non-genital tract causes	Non-obstetric causes
1. Chorioamnionitis	1. Lower urinary tract infections	1. Human immunodeficiency virus
2. Endometritis	2. Pyelonephritis	2. Immunocompromised (Pneumonia, Tuberculosis, Malaria)
3. Septic abortion	3. Pelvic thrombophlebitis	
4. Wound infections	4. Breast infection	

Table 2.
Common causes of maternal sepsis.

The surgical site infections, despite prophylactic antibiotics and a decrease in postoperative infection, remain a major cause of concern with a rate of 2–6% due to lower section cesarean section.

1.3 Pathophysiology

The typical host response to infection is a multifaceted mechanism that localizes and mitigates bacterial invasion while commencing the repair of damaged tissue. It entails the activation of circulating and resident phagocytic cells and the production of proinflammatory and anti-inflammatory mediators. Sepsis occurs when the response to infection becomes systemic, affecting normal tissues distant from the site of injury or infection.

A bacterial pathogen usually infiltrates a sterile location where local cells can identify the intruder and start the host reaction. The host response is activated when innate immune cells, especially macrophages, identify and attach to microbial components. Engagement of immune cell surface receptors with microbial components triggers a cascade of events leading to the phagocytosis of invading bacteria, their subsequent destruction, and debris clearance from damaged tissue. When a restricted quantity of bacteria infiltrates, the local host responses are typically adequate to eliminate the pathogens. The outcome often involves tissue repair and regeneration.

The balance of proinflammatory and anti-inflammatory mediators controls inflammatory processes, such as adhesion, chemotaxis, phagocytosis, killing bacteria, and removing tissue debris. Should the mediators equilibrate, and the initial viral challenge be surmounted, homeostasis will be reestablished [11]. The outcome will be tissue regeneration and recovery [12].

Sepsis arises when the discharge of proinflammatory mediators in reaction to an infection transcends the confines of the local environment, resulting in a more widespread response.

The etiology is probably complex, potentially encompassing the direct impact of invading microbes or their toxic byproducts, the release of substantial quantities of proinflammatory mediators, and the activation of the complement system [13, 14].

Cellular damage precedes organ dysfunction. Extensive cellular damage can arise when the immune response extends beyond the infection site, resulting in sepsis.

The precise mechanism of cellular injury has yet to be understood. Proposed mechanisms include tissue ischemia, characterized by insufficient oxygen relative to demand; cytopathic injury, which involves direct cell damage by proinflammatory

Pathogenesis of sepsis syndrome			
Septic abortion, septic peritonitis, pyelonephritis, chorioamnionitis/endometritis/Necrotizing fascitis			
Gram positive exotoxin		Gram negative endotoxin	
Neutrophils	Macrophages	Monocytes	Endothelial cells
Blood vessel			
Systemic inflammatory response (SIR)			
Myocardial effects	Vascular effects	Coagulation cascade activation	
Hypotension, metabolic acidosis, irreversible phase			
Multiorgan organ dysfunction			

Table 3.
Pathophysiology of sepsis.

mediators or other inflammatory products; and an altered rate of apoptosis, referring to programmed cell death.

Organ failure in sepsis may be attributed to diminished oxygen utilization linked to mitochondrial dysfunction and inadequate oxygen transport to tissues. Sepsis is linked to disseminated intravascular coagulation (DIC) and the activation of endothelial cells, both of which are pivotal in the onset of organ dysfunction [15].

The intravascular stimulation of coagulation with loss of localization resulting from sepsis is a characteristic of DIC, an acquired illness. Sepsis-associated disseminated intravascular coagulation (DIC) is characterized by systemic coagulation activation, inhibited fibrinolysis, and systemic inflammation, resulting in organ dysfunction.

The endothelium is crucial in exacerbating inflammation by releasing proinflammatory substances, recruiting inflammatory cells, promoting procoagulant activity, and induction of hyperpermeability.

In sepsis, platelets contribute to sepsis-induced coagulation dysfunction by releasing proinflammatory mediators, such as platelet-activating factor, and enhancing fibrin formation by producing procoagulant molecules. The mechanisms responsible for chronic thrombocytopenia in sepsis include diminished platelet synthesis, increased turnover, spontaneous platelet aggregation, and heightened platelet consumption due to microthrombi development. The mechanism of sepsis is shown in **Table 3**.

2. Sepsis-related organ-specific impacts

Organ dysfunction frequently follows cellular damage and the release of proinflammatory and anti-inflammatory mediators. All organ systems are susceptible to the effects of sepsis. The primary systems involved are the circulatory, respiratory, gastrointestinal, renal, and nervous systems.

When the immune response becomes generalized, widespread endothelial and parenchymal cellular injury may occur; cellular injury is the precursor to organ dysfunction. Hypotension due to diffuse vasodilation is the most severe expression of circulatory dysfunction in sepsis [16].

The diffuse effects of sepsis on circulatory dysfunction are the hypotensive response to diffuse vasodilatation produced by the release of vasodilators prostacyclin and nitric oxide (NO) by the endothelial cells. Hypotension may also be due to the redistribution of intravascular fluid. This results from increased endothelial permeability and reduced arterial vascular tone, increasing capillary pressure.

The capillaries, or microcirculation, may be the most important target in sepsis. Sepsis is linked to reduced functioning capillaries, resulting in an impaired capacity for maximal oxygen extraction. Widespread tissue edema, characterized by a high protein content, results from diffuse endothelial activity.

Lung: Endothelial damage in the pulmonary vasculature during sepsis disrupts capillary blood flow and increases microvascular permeability, leading to interstitial and alveolar pulmonary edema [14, 17].

Pulmonary edema follows, causing hypoxemia and a ventilation-perfusion mismatch. Lung damage is pronounced during sepsis, perhaps due to the extensive microvascular surface area of the lungs. Acute respiratory distress syndrome exemplifies these impacts.

Gastrointestinal tract: Sepsis-related circulatory abnormalities can impair the gut's barrier function, facilitating the translocation of bacteria and endotoxins into the systemic circulation, potentially through lymphatics instead of the portal vein, thereby exacerbating the septic response [18].

The first line of defense for removing germs and compounds produced by bacteria that have entered the portal system from the gut is usually the reticuloendothelial system of the liver. Liver dysfunction hinders the removal of enteric-derived endotoxin and bacterial products, thereby obstructing the necessary local cytokine response and allowing the direct entry of these potentially harmful substances into the systemic circulation [18].

Kidney: There is frequently acute renal failure in conjunction with sepsis. One mechanism involved in sepsis and endotoxemia leading to acute tubular injury is attributed to hypoperfusion and/or hypoxemia. Systemic hypotension, direct renal vasoconstriction, cytokine release (e.g., tumor necrosis factor [TNF]), and neutrophil activation by endotoxin and FMLP (a three amino acid chemotactic peptide in bacterial cell walls) may contribute to renal injury [19].

Nervous system: The most common CNS complication is an altered sensorium (encephalopathy), frequently occurring in septic patients. Due to inflammatory mediators, CNS dysfunction has been attributed to metabolism changes and cell signaling alterations. Impairment of the blood-brain barrier likely facilitates heightened leukocyte infiltration, exposure to harmful mediators, and the active translocation of cytokines across the barrier. Mitochondrial dysfunction and microvascular failure occur before functional central nervous system alterations are assessed *via* somatosensory evoked potentials [18, 19].

2.1 Management

2.1.1 Diagnostic dilemma

Reducing maternal morbidity and mortality requires early detection of maternal sepsis and timely treatment. The symptoms of peripartum sepsis are often nonspecific and can resemble other obstetric conditions, complicating the diagnostic process. Physicians and OBGYN specialists must maintain a heightened level of suspicion and evaluate all pertinent clinical and laboratory data when assessing a patient for maternal sepsis [20].

The physiological adaptations during pregnancy may lead to a less pronounced manifestation of sepsis. Pregnancy is characterized by hyperdynamic circulation, which involves increased blood volume, potentially leading to decreased blood pressure and an elevated heart rate. Tachypnea, frequently observed in sepsis, may be misinterpreted as physiological tachypnea in pregnant individuals. The similarities may confuse applying the qSOFA criteria for sepsis diagnosis. Altered mentation is uncommon in pregnant women, even in cases of severe disease, and may indicate a more specific sign of end-organ injury and sepsis when infection is present. Acute infections in pregnant patients can lead to the development of uterine contractions, a consequence of endotoxin release, which may complicate preterm delivery. Furthermore, intrauterine infection correlates with neonatal hypoxia, sepsis, or mortality.

3. Diagnosis

Early diagnosis and detection are essential to reducing mortality associated with sepsis and enhancing outcomes. Two high-profile campaigns, the Surviving Sepsis Campaign (SSC) and Sepsis Six, have suggested "bundles" of care for optimal outcomes [9]. Neither of these care packages has been specifically studied in pregnancy.

4. The SSC recommended three early screening and management tools

1. Screening and management of infection: Infection identification is conducted by assessing signs and symptoms and collecting cultures and blood samples as necessary. Subsequently, appropriate antibiotics are administered [9].

2. Assessment of organ dysfunction and sepsis management: The organ dysfunction criteria should identify patients with sepsis and septic shock, and a quick Sepsis-Related Organ Failure Assessment (q SOFA) is recommended. Although merely a quarter of infected patients exhibit 2 or more q SOFA points, they represent a significant proportion of the fatalities, accounting for three-quarters of the deaths.

3. Recognition and addressing of early hypotension: Patients presenting with infection, hypotension, or a lactate level exceeding 4 mmol/L receive 30 mL/kg of crystalloid fluid, followed by a reassessment of volume responsiveness and tissue perfusion. Our institute adheres to the protocol outlined below (**Figure 1**).

4.1 Early recognition

Timely recognition of seriously ill maternity patients who are at high risk of peripartum sepsis is essential in preventing further deterioration and reducing sepsis-associated mortality and possible death. The quick Sequential (sepsis-related) Organ Failure Assessment score (qSOFA) score and Maternal Early Warning Score (MEWS) are the two most used scores [21].

Several early warning systems are employed globally to expedite the diagnosis of sepsis for peripartum women. The modified early obstetric warning score (MEOWS), maternity SIRS (m SIRS), maternal early recognition criteria (MERC), maternal early

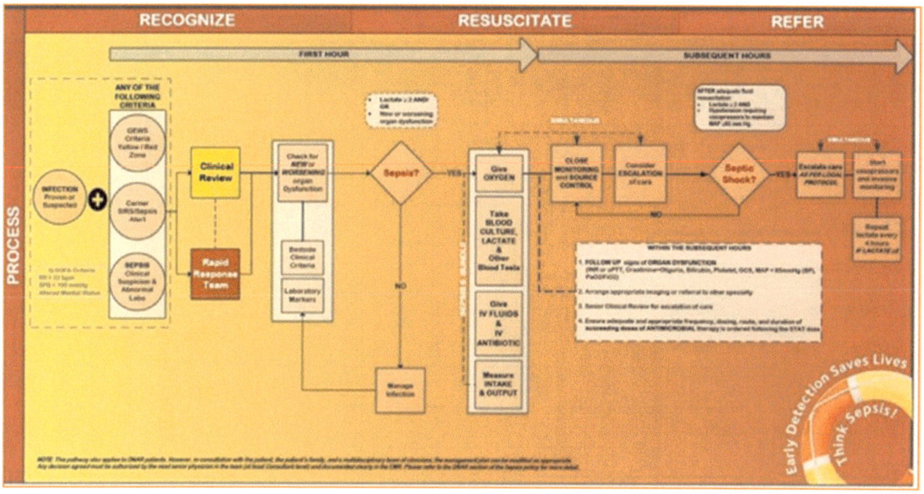

Figure 1.
Our institutional management protocol.

warning system (MEWS), SOS (Sepsis in Obstetrics Score), omq SOFA (obstetric modified quick SOFA/**Table 4**), and maternal early warning trigger (MEWT) represent a selection of these systems [21]. The common clinical presentations of sepsis are described in **Table 5**. **Table 6** shows the criteria for maternal sepsis.

qSOFA criteria	Points
Respiratory rate > 22/minutes	1
Mental status changes	1
Systolic blood pressure < 100 mmHg	1

Table 4.
Quick SOFA.

Clinical and laboratory parameters in diagnosis of sepsis	
Sign and symptoms	**Laboratory parameters**
Temperature instability (>38© or 36©)	Leukopenia or leukocytosis
Tachycardia (>110 beats/minutes)	Positive cultures
Tachypnoea (>24 breaths/Minutes)	Hypoxemia
Hypotension	Metabolic acidosis and lactatemia
Skin Mottling and/or diaphoresis	Thrombocytopenia/thrombocytosis/Coagulopathy
Nausea and vomiting	Elevated liver functions
Cerebral dysfunctions	Hyperglycemia
Oliguria and dysuria	Abnormal kidney functions

Table 5.
Clinical presentation.

General criteria
Fever or hypothermia
Tachycardia and tachypnea
Cerebral nervous system dysfunction
Hyperglycemia
Generalized edema
Inflammatory variables
Leukocytosis or leucopenia
CRP (C-Reactive protein)>7 mg/L
Raised procalcitonin
Hemodynamic variables
Hypotension
Tissue perfusion abnormalities
Lactatemia (>2 mmol/L)
Mottling or decrease capillary refilling
MODS (Multiple organ dysfunction syndrome)
Hypoxemia
Oliguria
Hyperbilirubinemia
DIC (Disseminated intravascular coagulopathy)
Ileus
Decrease in GCS (Glasgow coma scale)

Table 6.
Diagnostic criteria for sepsis in pregnant patients.

5. Investigations

Identify the source of infection and evidence of tissue dysfunction as soon as possible and, if indicated, control it surgically.

All pertinent laboratory investigations are obtained, analyzed, and reported for abnormal laboratory values. Culture findings are quickly communicated (**Table** 7).

Microscopy, culture, histopathology, and sensitivity of the following specimens guided by the clinical suspicion of the focus of infection: breast milk, wound swab, stool microscopy, culture, epidural site, or CSF culture. Request for radiologic and other diagnostic procedures if clinically appropriate (e.g., chest x-ray, pelvis-abdominal ultrasound, CT/MRI scan, lumbar puncture).

5.1 Initial management

Management objectives involve reviving the patient and addressing the root cause of the infection through the administration of suitable antibiotics and, frequently, surgical intervention. Vital Elements to Surviving Sepsis Campaign (SSC) guidelines for the management of sepsis and septic shock were divided into two phases with a

Sepsis kite compositions
Two blood culture bottles
Two specimen culture containers
Two Yellow cap tubes for Complete blood count
Purple top tube for Serum electrolytes Including kidney and liver functions test
Green top tube for serum lactate levels
Blood top tube for coagulation parameters
ABD kit
Broad spectrum antibiotics
Appropriate orders requesting forms

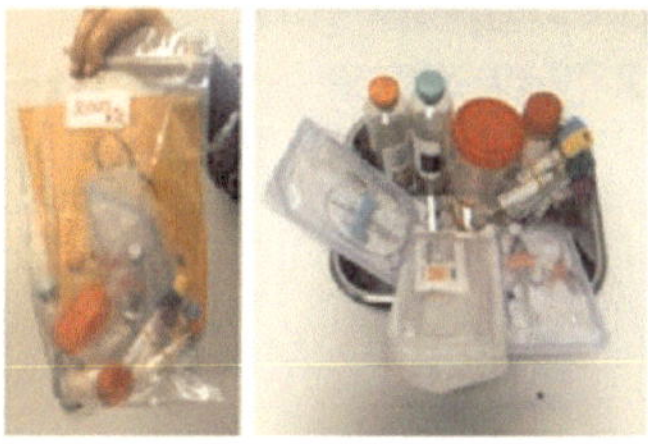

Table 7.
Investigations sampling.

multidisciplinary approach to improve patient care: the resuscitation phase and the management phase [22].

5.2 Resuscitation (sepsis six bundle)

The global directives for the management of sepsis and septic shock from 2016 to 2023 underscore the necessity of treating sepsis and septic shock as critical medical emergencies. Therefore, treatment and resuscitation must commence without delay [22].

The interventions are executed within 6 and 24 hours, respectively. The most significant recent alteration in the updated SSC bundles is the amalgamation of the 3 and 6-hour bundles into a unified "hour-1 bundle" [20]. As the literature shows, bundled compliance for sepsis management has better survival rates (**Table 8**).

3 Things to take	3 Things to give
Take blood cultures	Oxygen
blood for lactate	Broad spectrum antibiotics
Take intake and output (Monitor urine output)	Intravenous fluids
This should be done within 1 hour of suspected or diagnosis of sepsis.	

Table 8.
Sepsis six bundle.

Quick tasks to score throughout 24 hours:

1. Administer low-dose corticosteroids following established hospital protocols.

2. Ensure that glucose levels are sustained above the lower threshold of normalcy while remaining below 180 mg/dl (8.3 mmol/l).

3. Patients on mechanical ventilation need to keep inspiratory plateau pressures below 30 cm H_2O.

5.3 Antimicrobial therapy

The latest guidance from the World Health Organization regarding the treatment of maternal infections advocates for a particular class of antibiotics in the management of chorioamnionitis, specifically ampicillin and gentamicin, as well as for postpartum endometritis, which is addressed with clindamycin and gentamicin. Despite antimicrobial therapy, the origin of sepsis must be identified and addressed. They recognized that other straightforward, effective, and locally accessible antibiotics could be alternatives.

5.4 Antimicrobial choices and their considerations

Antimicrobial therapy must be tailored to the organism(s), sensitivity results once identified, and drug levels are monitored as necessary. Patients' antibiotic requirements, including type, dose, route, frequency, and duration of administration, are reviewed after initiation and de-escalated according to patients' improvement and local governing policy.

Co-amoxiclav lacks efficacy against MRSA and Pseudomonas, and its administration may increase the likelihood of neonatal necrotizing enterocolitis. It is often overlooked during pregnancy [9, 21, 22].

5.5 Fluid therapy

Following the initial fluid resuscitation with a 30 ml/kg bolus of crystalloids or albumin, subsequent fluid therapy should be directed by dynamic preload assessments, either pulse-pressure variation or passive leg-raising techniques.

Vasopressors are better in treating hypotensive septic patients who do not respond to fluid challenge. Expansion of intravascular volume, hydroxyethyl starches (HESs), and gelatin are not recommended for replacing intravascular volume.

Unfettered fluid administration to all patients, devoid of a thorough assessment of their physiological responses, may precipitate pulmonary and cerebral edema, elevate intra-abdominal pressure, and ultimately heighten mortality rates in cases of sepsis.

5.6 Role of corticosteroids

The Surviving Sepsis Campaign 2012 and 2016 recommended the intravenous infusion of 200 mg of hydrocortisone daily, which should be reserved for pressor-resistant septic shock or in patients experiencing refractory shock (those who continue to exhibit hypotension despite initial fluid resuscitation and vasopressor administration). Corticoids are given until the vasopressors are ongoing. Once vasopressors stop, the steroid is also discontinued. The administration of corticosteroid infusion in pregnant women with sepsis enhances fetal lung maturation and mitigates the risk of premature birth [22].

5.7 Prevention of deep venous thrombosis

The prevention of DVT is crucial in septic pregnant patients, given that both pregnancy and sepsis contribute to a state of hypercoagulability. Mechanical prophylaxis for venous thromboembolism is accomplished through compression stockings, intermittent lower limb compression, and pharmacological prophylaxis using low molecular weight or unfractionated heparin unless contraindicated [9, 21].

5.8 Pharmacological agents influencing vascular tone

SSC 2016 strongly recommends norepinephrine as the primary vasopressor, with vasopressin or epinephrine as alternatives to achieve the target mean arterial pressure (MAP). Dobutamine is applicable for patients experiencing persistent hypoperfusion despite sufficient fluid loading and vasopressor administration [22].

5.9 The role function of intravenous immunoglobulin (IVIG)

IVIG's immunomodulatory impact makes it a recommended treatment for severe invasive streptococcal or staphylococcal infections when other treatments have failed. High-dose intravenous immunoglobulin (IVIG) has been administered to pregnant women and demonstrates efficacy in exotoxin shock induced by streptococci and staphylococci [23].

5.10 Determination of decision

The choice to either deliver the fetus or persist with the pregnancy is determined by the patient's status, gestational age, fetal condition, presence of chorioamnionitis, and labor state. In a very unwell pregnant woman, the delivery of the infant may be deemed appropriate if it would confer advantages to the mother, the infant, or both. Mortality risk increases while attempting to deliver an unstable mother unless the source of infection is intrauterine.

During the intrapartum phase, continuous electronic fetal monitoring is recommended [23, 24].

Maternal and fetal factors are common potential indicators of delivery. Maternal causes include intrauterine infection, disseminated intravascular coagulation (DIC), hepatic and renal issues, heart failure, compartment syndrome, multifetal gestation, and acute respiratory distress syndrome (ARDS). Fetal factors encompass fetal demise and gestational age concerning a viable fetus. The decision-making process should include a collaborative discussion among obstetricians, neonatologists, microbiologists, intensivists, and anesthetists. The Early Fetus Delivery Criteria in Sepsis are described in **Table 9**.

No obstetric surgical interventions may be needed, such as surgical drainage of abscess, wound debridement, and evacuation of infected retained products to remove the source of infection.

Rapid maternal deterioration
Failure to maintain adequate blood oxygenation
Difficulty with mechanical ventilation due to gravid uterus
Multiorgan failure
Fetal compromise
Other obstetric indications

Table 9.
Criteria for early delivery in sepsis.

5.11 Complications in newborns arising from maternal sepsis

Maternal sepsis significantly affects newborn mortality, leading to a considerable number of infection-related neonatal fatalities annually. Neonatal sepsis is a significant critical complication that can lead to mortality or considerable disability despite prompt antibiotic intervention [24, 25].

5.12 Anesthesia considerations for parturient with sepsis

Surgical intervention requires an individualized decision regarding the choice between regional or general anesthesia, considering the associated risk-benefit ratio.

5.13 Regional anesthesia

Neuroaxial block is generally contraindicated in septic patients due to their potential inability to tolerate the sympathetic block and vasodilation associated with spinal anesthesia. Coagulopathy or thrombocytopenia may be present. The likelihood of developing an epidural abscess or meningitis is low in patients receiving antibiotic treatment; however, these risks should still be acknowledged in such cases.

5.14 General anesthesia

General anesthesia will probably be necessary for a septic parturient, may increase hemodynamic instability, and should be chosen with care. Advanced hemodynamic monitoring should be applied. The severity of sepsis and the altered physiology of pregnancy are considered when deciding whether to extubate or transfer to critical care. The induction of anesthesia should be slow with titrated doses of induction agents. It is recommended to avoid etomidate in septic patients. Analgesia should be maintained with paracetamol and opioids. Given altered coagulation profile and deranged renal functions in septic patients, nonsteroidal anti-inflammatory drugs are contraindicated. Postoperative oxygen therapy is desired for the increased oxygen demand. Transfer to critical care is needed in rapidly deteriorating cases, hemodynamically unstable and needing vasopressor support; mechanical ventilation is necessary for pulmonary edema, altered consciousness level, hemodialysis, multiple organ failure, or hypothermia [24, 25].

5.15 Prevention

The patient shall be placed under the appropriate isolation category, and the required infection control measures shall be implemented and adhered to. Aseptic surgical practices must also be strictly adhered to minimize the risk of infection [22, 23].

Clinical monitoring of women during labor and the postpartum period is crucial for detecting early signs of infection. Routine antibiotic prophylaxis is advised prior to skin incision for women having an emergency or elective cesarean section, as well as for those who experienced preterm rupture of the membranes, third- or fourth-degree perineal tears, or an operative vaginal birth [24].

6. Conclusion

Maternal sepsis is a leading cause of maternal mortality all over the world. The early diagnosis and appropriate management of maternal sepsis are essential for a better outcome. There are various risk factors for the occurrence of maternal sepsis, and the common etiologies for maternal sepsis are Chorioamnionitis, endometritis, septic abortion, and surgical site infections. The primary pathophysiology of sepsis is the dysregulated response to the infection. Sepsis can progress further into septic shock and multiple organ dysfunction syndrome with increased morbidity and mortality. Diagnosis of sepsis during pregnancy can be difficult due to the physiological changes of pregnancy. Various clinical criteria and scores can be useful in diagnosing maternal sepsis. The treatment of maternal sepsis is in two phases: the initial resuscitation phase and secondly the management phase. Sepsis 6 bundle and surviving sepsis protocols are useful in the early diagnosis and management of maternal sepsis. In maternal sepsis, early delivery of the fetus can be done if there is rapid maternal or fetal deterioration or difficulty in ventilation due to a gravid uterus. Maternal sepsis can be prevented by proper antibiotic prophylaxis in patients with surgical delivery, ruptured membranes, or severe degree of perineal injury patients and strictly following the infection prevention protocols.

Author details

Seema Nahid[1]*, Fateen Shareef[2], Roshan Afsha[3], Azha Fatima[4], Umm E. Amara[5], Nissar Sheikh[1] and Eynas Abdalla[1]

1 Hamad Medical Corporation, Doha, Qatar

2 Deccan College of Medical Sciences, Hyderabad, Telangana, India

3 Detroit Medical Center, Wayne State University, USA

4 Kamineni Academy of Medical Sciences and Research Centre, Hyderabad, Telangana, India

5 Apollo Institute of Medical Sciences and Research, Hyderabad, Telangana, India

*Address all correspondence to: snahid@hamad.qa

References

[1] Surviving Sepsis Campaign: International Guidelines for Management of Sepsis and Septic Shock. Iris; WHO; 2016. Available from: https://www.hsph.harvard.edu/wp-content/uploads/sites/2413/2017/08/WHO-Maternal-Sepsis-2017

[2] Singer M, Deutschmann C, Seymour C, et al. The third international consensus definitions for sepsis and septic shock (sepsis-3). JAMA. 2016;**315**(8):801-810. DOI: 10.1001/jama.2016.0287

[3] Pathophysiology of Sepsis. Available from: https://www.medilib.ir/uptodate/show/1597

[4] Sepsis–Who Cares? Available from: https://symbiosisonlinepublishing.com/pulmonology-infectious-diseases/pulmonology-infectious-diseases03.php

[5] Adams J, Lopez J, Sackner M. Whole body periodic acceleration improves survival and microvascular leak in a murine endotoxin model. PLoS One. 2019;**14**(1):e0208681

[6] Sepsis Syndromes in Adults: Epidemiology, Definitions, Clinical Presentation, Diagnosis, and Prognosis. Available from: https://medilib.ir/uptodate/show/1657

[7] Sepsis Syndromes in Adults: Epidemiology, Definitions, Clinical Presentation, Diagnosis, and Prognosis. Available from: https://medilib.ir/uptodate/show/1657/ [Accessed: September 15, 2024]

[8] Royal College of Obstetricians and Gynecologists. Bacterial Sepsis in Pregnancy. Green-Top. Guideline No. 64a. London: RCOG Press; 2012

[9] Rhodes A, Evans LE, Alhazzani W, et al. Surviving sepsis campaign: International guidelines for management of sepsis and septic shock. Intensive Care Medicine. 2017;**43**(3):304-377. DOI: 10.1007/s00134-017-4683-6. Epub 2017 Jan 18

[10] Centre for Maternal and Child Enquiries (CMACE). Saving mother's lives: Reviewing maternal deaths to make motherhood safer: 2006-2008. The eighth report on confidential enquiries into maternal deaths in the United Kingdom. BJOG. 2011;**118**(suppl. 1):1-203

[11] Parfitt SE, Bogat ML, Hering SL, Roth C. Sepsis in obstetrics: Pathophysiology and diagnostic definitions. MCN: American Journal of Maternal Child Nursing. 2017;**42**:194-198. DOI: 10.1097/NMC.00000000 00000339

[12] Hotchkiss RS, Karl IE. Pathophysiology and treatment of sepsis. The New England Journal of Medicine. 2003;**348**:138

[13] Adib-Conquy M, Cavaillon JM. Compensatory anti-inflammatory response syndrome. Thrombosis and Haemostasis. 2009;**101**:36

[14] Luce JM. Pathogenesis and management of septic shock. Chest. 1987;**91**:883

[15] Schefold JC, Hasper D, Reinke P, et al. Consider delayed immunosuppression into the concept of sepsis. Critical Care Medicine. 2008;**36**:3118

[16] McGown CC, Brown NJ, Hellewell PG, Brookes ZL. ROCK induced

inflammation of the microcirculation during endotoxemia mediated by nitric oxide synthase. Microvascular Research. 2011;**81**:281

[17] Ghosh S, Latimer RD, Gray BM, et al. Endotoxin-induced organ injury. Critical Care Medicine. 1993;**21**:S19

[18] Hassoun HT, Kone BC, Mercer DW, et al. Post-injury multiple organ failure: The role of the gut. Shock. 2001;**15**:1

[19] Takasu O, Gaut JP, Watanabe E, et al. Mechanisms of cardiac and renal dysfunction in patients dying of sepsis. American Journal of Respiratory and Critical Care Medicine. 2013;**187**:509

[20] National Institute of Clinical Excellence. Sepsis: Recognition, Diagnosis and Early Management NICE Guideline No NG51. National Institute of Clinical Excellence; 2016

[21] Bauer ME, Albright C, Prabhu M, et al. Alliance for innovation on maternal health: Consensus bundle on sepsis in obstetric care. Obstetrics and Gynecology. 2023;**142**:481

[22] International guidelines for management of sepsis and septic shock 2021. Intensive Care Medicine. 2021;**47**(11):1181-1247. DOI: 10.1007/s00134-021-06506-y. Epub 2021 Oct 2

[23] Seymour CW, Liu VX, Iwashyna TJ, et al. Assessment of clinical criteria for sepsis: For the third international consensus definitions for sepsis and septic shock (sepsis-3). JAMA. 2016; **315**:762

[24] Lewis G, editor. Saving mothers' lives: Reviewing maternal deaths to make motherhood safer – 2003-2005. In: The Seventh Report on Confidential Enquiries into Maternal Deaths in the United Kingdom. London: RCOG Press; 2007. Available from: http://www.oaa-anaes.ac.uk/assets/managed/editor/File/Reports/2003-2005_saving_mothers_full_report.pdf

[25] Blauvelt CA, Nguyen KC, Cassidy AG, Gaw SL. Perinatal outcomes among patients with sepsis during pregnancy. JAMA Network Open. 2021;**4**:e2124109-e2124109. DOI: 10.1001/jamanetworkopen.2021.24109

Chapter 6

Pathophysiology of Septic Shock

Abdullah Raheem

Abstract

Sepsis represents a critical condition marked by systemic inflammation, widespread tissue damage, and organ failure, which can lead to significant morbidity and mortality. The pathophysiology of sepsis involves a complex interplay between the immune system and pathogenic microorganisms. Upon infection, the body's immune cells recognize pathogen-associated molecular patterns (PAMPs) through pattern recognition receptors (PRRs), initiating an inflammatory response. This recognition triggers the release of a cascade of pro-inflammatory cytokines, often resulting in a "cytokine storm" that exacerbates inflammation and tissue damage. Key pathophysiological changes during sepsis include widespread vasodilation, increased capillary permeability, and microvascular thrombosis, all of which contribute to hypotension and impaired tissue perfusion. Mitochondrial dysfunction and cellular energy deficits, lead to organ failure. The condition affects multiple organ systems, including the cardiovascular, respiratory, renal, hepatic, and central nervous systems. Effective management of sepsis requires early recognition and intervention, including antimicrobial therapy, fluid resuscitation, and the use of vasopressors to stabilize hemodynamics. Despite advances in understanding and treatment, septic shock remains a significant clinical challenge, necessitating ongoing research and improved therapeutic strategies. This chapter provides a comprehensive review of the mechanisms underlying septic shock, highlighting key elements of its pathophysiology and current management approaches.

Keywords: proinflammatory cytokine, multi organ dysfunction, inflammation, coagulation, hypoperfusion, endothelial dysfunction, polymicrobial sepsis, cecal ligation and puncture

1. Introduction

Septic shock is a critical medical condition resulting from a severe and dysregulated immune response to infection, leading to systemic inflammation, tissue damage, and multiple organ failure. It is a subset of sepsis and is associated with a high mortality rate despite advances in medical care. This chapter aims to provide an in-depth understanding of the pathophysiology of septic shock, covering its initiation, immune response, vascular changes, cellular metabolism, and organ dysfunction.

2. Definition and epidemiology

Septic shock is defined as a subset of sepsis where profound circulatory, cellular, and metabolic abnormalities significantly increase mortality [1]. According to the Sepsis-3 definitions, it is characterized by persistent hypotension requiring vasopressors to maintain a mean arterial pressure (MAP) of 65 mm Hg or greater and a serum lactate level greater than 2 mmol/L despite adequate volume resuscitation [2].

Sepsis and septic shock are major healthcare challenges worldwide. The incidence of sepsis is rising, partly due to increased awareness and better diagnostic capabilities. In the United States alone, sepsis affects over 1.7 million people annually, with approximately 270,000 deaths. Globally, it is a leading cause of death in intensive care units (ICUs), with mortality rates for septic shock ranging from 25 to 50% [3].

3. Pathophysiology

3.1 Initiation of sepsis

Sepsis begins with an infection, typically bacterial, but can also be fungal or viral. Common sites of infection include the lungs (pneumonia), abdomen (peritonitis), and urinary tract (pyelonephritis). Pathogens release toxins that initiate the host immune response [4].

The innate immune system recognizes these pathogens through pattern recognition receptors (PRRs) such as Toll-like receptors (TLRs), nucleotide-binding oligomerization domain (NOD)-like receptors, and C-type lectin receptors as cleared in **Figure 1**.

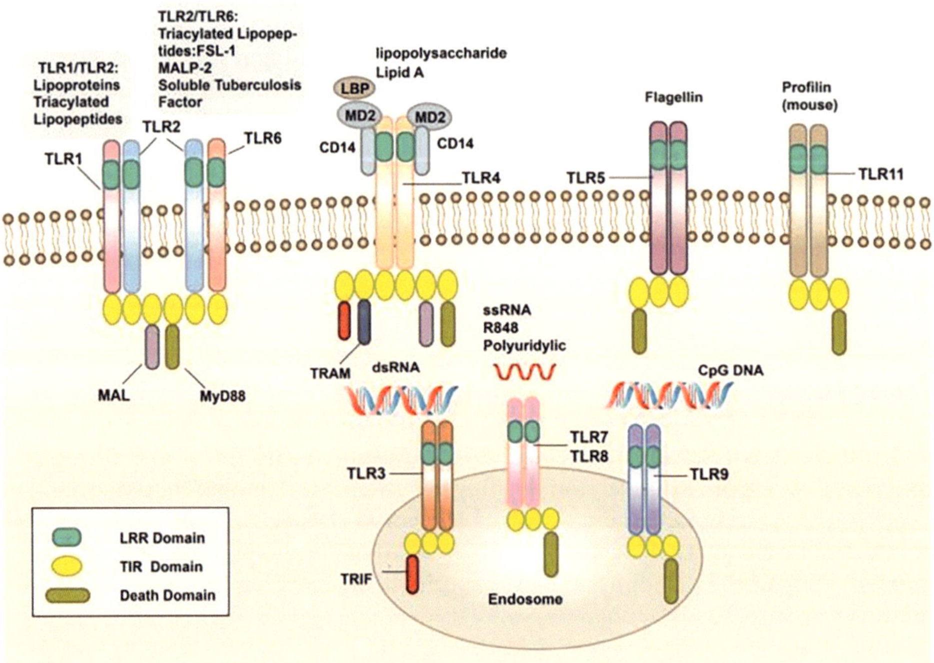

Figure 1.
The role of PRRs in recognizing pathogens [5].

These PRRs identify pathogen-associated molecular patterns (PAMPs) and damage-associated molecular patterns (DAMPs), triggering the initial immune response [6].

3.2 Immune response

The immune response in sepsis is characterized by the activation of immune cells, including macrophages, neutrophils, and dendritic cells, which release a cascade of pro-inflammatory cytokines such as TNF-α, IL-1, IL-6, and IL-8. This cytokine storm leads to widespread inflammation, which can become systemic, affecting distant organs and tissues (**Figure 2**) [8].

The immune response in sepsis involves a complex interplay between pro-inflammatory and anti-inflammatory mediators. An excessive pro-inflammatory response can cause widespread tissue damage and organ dysfunction, while an overactive anti-inflammatory response can lead to immunosuppression and increased susceptibility to secondary infections [6, 8].

3.3 Vascular changes

Septic shock involves significant alterations in vascular function, including:

- Vasodilation: Mediated by increased production of nitric oxide (NO) and other vasodilators in response to inflammatory cytokines. This leads to a drop in systemic vascular resistance and hypotension.

- Increased Capillary Permeability: Inflammatory mediators cause the endothelial cells lining blood vessels to become leaky, allowing fluids, proteins, and cells to escape into the interstitial space. This results in tissue edema and contributes to hypoperfusion.

- Microvascular Thrombosis: Activation of the coagulation cascade leads to the formation of microthrombi, which can obstruct capillaries and further impair tissue perfusion.

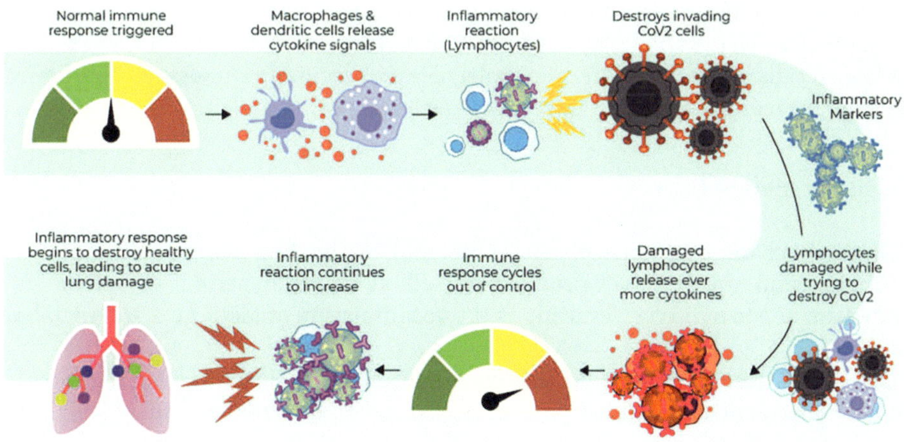

Figure 2.
Cytokine storm in septic shock [7].

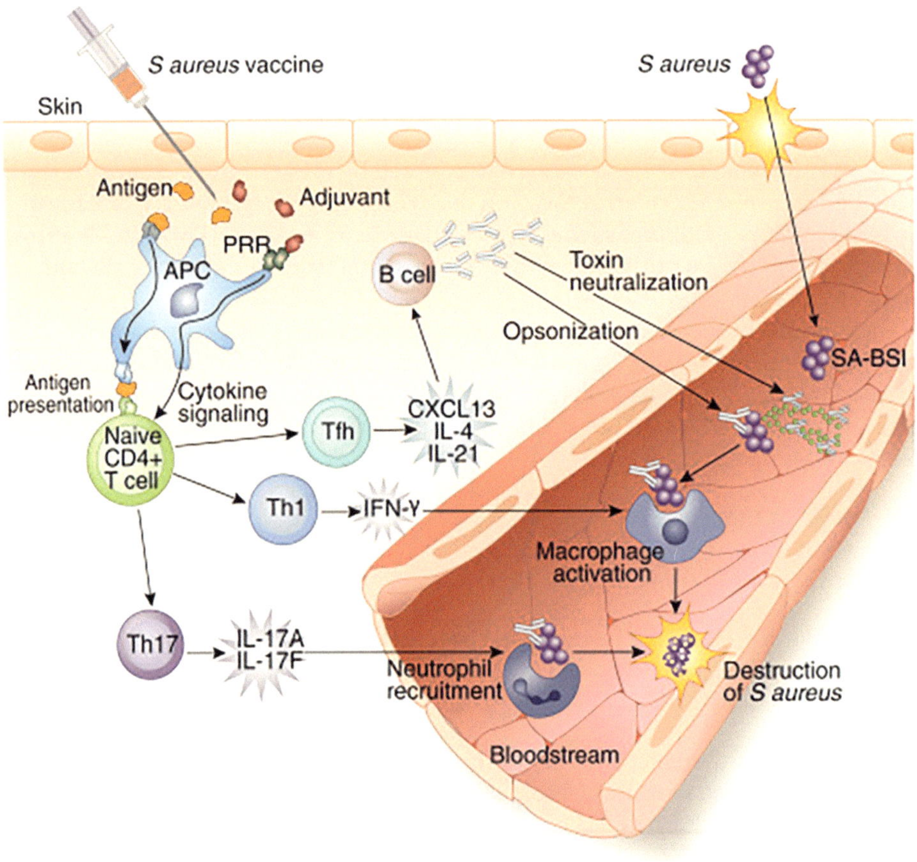

Figure 3.
Pathophysiological changes in the vasculature during septic shock [9].

This can result in disseminated intravascular coagulation (DIC), characterized by both clotting and bleeding tendencies (**Figure 3**).

Endothelial dysfunction plays a central role in these vascular changes, with endothelial cells expressing adhesion molecules that facilitate leukocyte adhesion and migration, exacerbating the inflammatory response [10].

3.4 Cellular metabolism

Septic shock disrupts normal cellular metabolism, leading to mitochondrial dysfunction and impaired ATP production. Cells switch from aerobic to anaerobic metabolism due to hypoxia, resulting in the accumulation of lactic acid and metabolic acidosis.

Oxidative stress, generated by reactive oxygen species (ROS), further damages cellular components, including lipids, proteins, and DNA. This can lead to cell death through apoptosis or necrosis (**Figure 4**). Mitochondrial damage also impairs energy production and exacerbates cellular dysfunction [12].

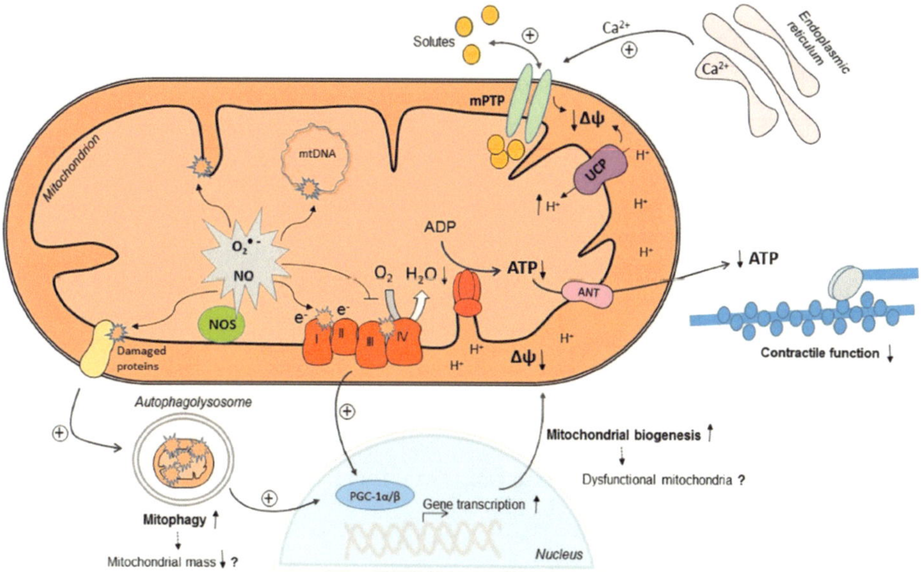

Figure 4.
Mitochondrial dysfunction in septic shock [11].

3.5 Organ dysfunction

Multiple organ dysfunction syndrome (MODS) is a hallmark of septic shock, affecting various organs, including:

Heart: Septic cardiomyopathy, characterized by reduced myocardial contractility and cardiac output. Inflammatory mediators and NO can directly depress myocardial function [13, 14].

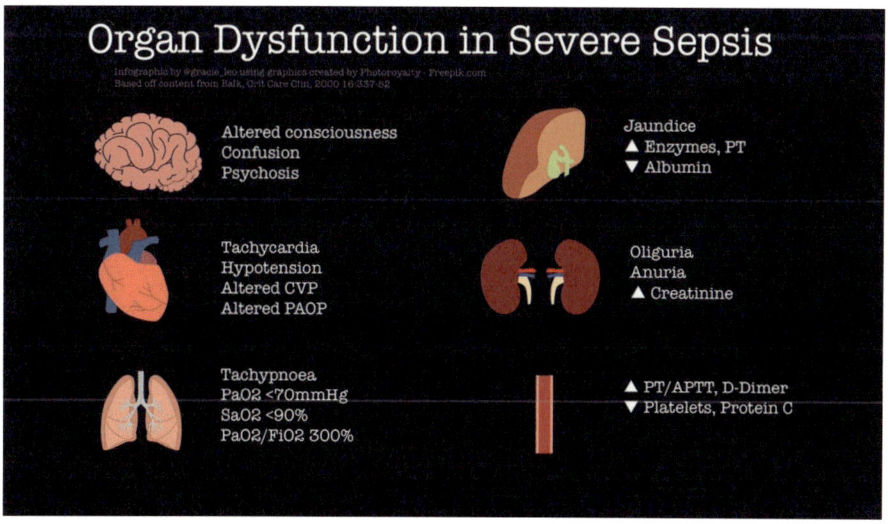

Figure 5.
Organ systems affected by septic shock [21].

Lungs: Acute respiratory distress syndrome (ARDS), with diffuse alveolar damage, increased vascular permeability, and impaired gas exchange. Patients often require mechanical ventilation [15, 16].

Kidneys: Acute kidney injury (AKI) due to hypoperfusion, inflammation, and microthrombi. This can lead to oliguria or anuria and the need for renal replacement therapy [17, 18].

Liver: Hepatic dysfunction, characterized by impaired detoxification, protein synthesis, and bile production. This can lead to jaundice and coagulopathy [19, 20].

Central Nervous System: Septic encephalopathy, presenting with altered mental status ranging from confusion to coma. Mechanisms include inflammation, impaired cerebral perfusion, and metabolic abnormalities as in **Figure 5** [22].

4. Clinical manifestations

Patients with septic shock exhibit a range of clinical symptoms and signs, including:

- Hypotension: Persistent despite fluid resuscitation, often requiring vasopressors.
- Altered Mental Status: Varying from confusion and agitation to unresponsiveness or coma.
- Oliguria: Marked decrease in urine output, indicating renal hypoperfusion and dysfunction.
- Tachypnea: Rapid breathing, often indicative of respiratory distress or compensatory response to metabolic acidosis.
- Fever or Hypothermia: Elevated or decreased body temperature due to dysregulated thermoregulation.
- Skin Changes: Mottled or cyanotic skin, warm and flushed skin due to vasodilation in early sepsis, or cool and clammy skin in later stages due to shock.

Laboratory findings may include elevated lactate levels, indicating tissue hypoxia, leukocytosis or leukopenia, thrombocytopenia, and abnormal liver and kidney function tests [23].

5. Diagnostic criteria

The diagnosis of septic shock is based on clinical criteria outlined by the Sepsis-3 definitions:

- Sepsis: Identified by infection and organ dysfunction, assessed by an increase in the Sequential Organ Failure Assessment (SOFA) score by 2 points or more.
- Persistent Hypotension: Requiring vasopressors to maintain a MAP of 65 mm Hg or greater.

- Serum Lactate Level > 2 mmol/L: Despite adequate fluid resuscitation, indicating impaired cellular metabolism and hypoperfusion.

Early recognition and diagnosis are critical for initiating timely and appropriate treatment, improving patient outcomes [24].

6. Complications

Septic shock can lead to severe and life-threatening complications, including:

- Disseminated Intravascular Coagulation (DIC): Characterized by widespread clotting and bleeding due to the consumption of coagulation factors and platelets.
- Acute Respiratory Distress Syndrome (ARDS): Severe lung injury with hypoxemia, decreased lung compliance, and bilateral infiltrates on chest imaging.
- Acute Kidney Injury (AKI): Sudden loss of kidney function, often necessitating dialysis.
- Liver Failure: Impaired hepatic function, leading to jaundice, coagulopathy, and hepatic encephalopathy.
- Secondary Infections: Increased susceptibility to infections due to immunosuppression, prolonged hospitalization, and invasive procedures.

These complications contribute to the high morbidity and mortality associated with septic shock and underscore the need for comprehensive management strategies [25].

7. Management and treatment

The management of septic shock involves a multifaceted approach to control the infection, support organ function, and modulate the immune response. Key components include:

- Antimicrobial Therapy: Early and appropriate administration of broad-spectrum antibiotics is crucial for controlling the underlying infection. Empirical therapy is often initiated based on the suspected source of infection, followed by de-escalation based on culture results and sensitivity testing.
- Fluid Resuscitation: Intravenous fluids, primarily crystalloids, are administered to restore intravascular volume and improve tissue perfusion. The goal is to achieve a MAP of at least 65 mm Hg and adequate urine output.
- Vasopressors: Norepinephrine is the first-line agent for maintaining blood pressure and perfusion. Additional agents, such as vasopressin or epinephrine, may be added if necessary.
- Source Control: Timely identification and elimination of the source of infection, such as drainage of abscesses, removal of infected devices, or surgical intervention, is essential for effective management.

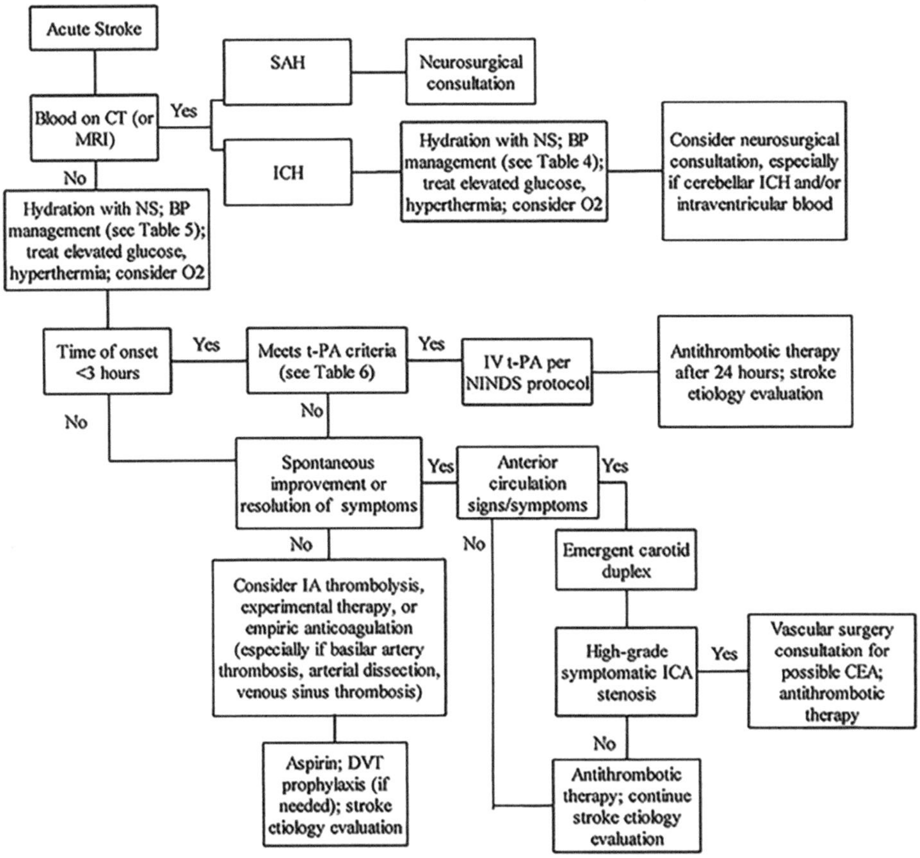

Figure 6.
Algorithm for the management of septic shock [26].

- Supportive Care: It includes mechanical ventilation for respiratory failure, renal replacement therapy for AKI, and hemodynamic monitoring to guide therapy. In addition to these measures, adjunctive therapies such as corticosteroids, immunomodulatory agents, and blood purification techniques are sometimes considered, although their roles are still being studied as in **Figure 6** [27].

7.1 Antimicrobial therapy

Early initiation of broad-spectrum antibiotics is critical in septic shock. Empirical therapy should be guided by the suspected source of infection, local antimicrobial resistance patterns, and patient-specific factors. Once culture results are available, antibiotics should be de-escalated to target the identified pathogens, reducing the risk of resistance and toxicity [28, 29].

7.2 Fluid resuscitation

Initial fluid resuscitation typically involves the rapid infusion of 30 mL/kg of crystalloids within the first 3 hours. The aim is to restore effective circulating volume, improve tissue perfusion, and reduce lactate levels. Dynamic parameters such as pulse pressure variation, stroke volume variation, and passive leg raising can help guide fluid management [28, 29].

7.3 Vasopressors

When hypotension persists despite adequate fluid resuscitation, vasopressors are initiated to maintain a MAP of at least 65 mm Hg. Norepinephrine is the first-line vasopressor due to its potent alpha-adrenergic effects, which increase vascular tone and blood pressure. Vasopressin or epinephrine may be added if additional support is needed [28, 29].

7.4 Adjunctive therapies

- Corticosteroids: Low-dose corticosteroids (e.g., hydrocortisone) may be considered in patients with refractory septic shock who do not respond to fluids and vasopressors. They are thought to reduce the inflammatory response and improve hemodynamics.

- Immunomodulatory Agents: Therapies targeting specific components of the immune response, such as anti-TNF antibodies or IL-1 receptor antagonists, are under investigation. Their efficacy and safety remain to be fully established.

- Blood Purification Techniques: Hemoadsorption and hemofiltration techniques aim to remove inflammatory mediators from the blood. These are experimental and require further validation in clinical trials [30].

8. Recent advances in research

Recent research in septic shock has focused on several key areas:

- Biomarkers: Identifying reliable biomarkers for early diagnosis, risk stratification, and monitoring treatment response. Examples include procalcitonin, presepsin, and various cytokines.

- Genomics and Proteomics: Understanding genetic and proteomic profiles to identify individuals at risk, predict outcomes, and develop personalized therapies.

- Immunomodulation: Investigating agents that modulate the immune response, such as anti-inflammatory cytokines, immune checkpoint inhibitors, and mesenchymal stem cells.

- Microbiome: Exploring the role of the gut microbiome in sepsis and its potential as a therapeutic target. Dysbiosis (microbial imbalance) may contribute to the pathogenesis of sepsis and septic shock.

- Precision Medicine: Developing personalized treatment strategies based on individual patient characteristics, including genetic, epigenetic, and metabolic profiles.

These advances hold promise for improving the diagnosis, management, and outcomes of patients with septic shock.

9. Conclusions

Septic shock is a complex and life-threatening condition resulting from a dysregulated immune response to infection. It involves profound changes in vascular function, cellular metabolism, and organ function. Early recognition, prompt treatment, and comprehensive supportive care are essential for improving outcomes. Despite advances in medical care, septic shock remains a major challenge with high mortality and long-term morbidity. Ongoing research into its pathophysiology, biomarkers, and therapeutic strategies offers hope for better management and improved survival rates.

Acknowledgements

The author acknowledges the use of ChatGPT for language polishing of the manuscript.

Author details

Abdullah Raheem
AL-Mustaqbal University, Babil, Iraq

*Address all correspondence to: abdullakraheem76@gmail.com

References

[1] Angus DC, van der Poll T. Severe sepsis and septic shock. New England Journal of Medicine. 2013;**369**(9):840-851

[2] Rhodes A, Evans LE, Alhazzani W, et al. Surviving sepsis campaign: International guidelines for management of sepsis and septic shock: 2016. Intensive Care Medicine. 2017;**43**(3):304-377

[3] Martin GS. Sepsis, severe sepsis and septic shock: Changes in incidence, pathogens and outcomes. Expert Review of Anti-Infective Therapy. 2012;**10**(6):701-706. DOI: 10.1586/eri.12.50

[4] Jarczak D, Kluge S, Nierhaus A. Sepsis-pathophysiology and therapeutic concepts. Frontiers in Medicine. 2021;**8**:628302. DOI: 10.3389/fmed.2021.628302

[5] Li D, Wu M. Pattern recognition receptors in health and diseases. Signal Transduction and Targeted Therapy. 2021;**6**:291. DOI: 10.1038/s41392-021-00687-0

[6] Brubaker SW, Bonham KS, Zanoni I, Kagan JC. Innate immune pattern recognition: A cell biological perspective. Annual Review of Immunology. 2015;**33**:257-290. DOI: 10.1146/annurev-immunol-032414-112240. Epub 2015 Jan 2

[7] Jarczak D, Nierhaus A. Cytokine storm-definition, causes, and implications. International Journal of Molecular Sciences. 2022;**23**(19):11740. DOI: 10.3390/ijms231911740

[8] Delano MJ, Ward PA. The immune system's role in sepsis progression, resolution, and long-term outcome. Immunological Reviews. 2016;**274**(1):330-353. DOI: 10.1111/imr.12499

[9] De Kock I, Van Daele C, Poelaert J. Sepsis and septic shock: Pathophysiological and cardiovascular background as basis for therapy. Acta Clinica Belgica. 2010;**65**(5):323-329. DOI: 10.1179/acb.2010.070

[10] Dolmatova EV, Wang K, Mandavilli R, Griendling KK. The effects of sepsis on endothelium and clinical implications. Cardiovascular Research. 2021;**117**(1):60-73. DOI: 10.1093/cvr/cvaa070

[11] Cimolai MC, Alvarez S, Bode C, Bugger H. Mitochondrial mechanisms in septic cardiomyopathy. International Journal of Molecular Sciences. 2015;**16**(8):17763-17778. DOI: 10.3390/ijms160817763

[12] Nedel W, Deutschendorf C, Portela LVC. Sepsis-induced mitochondrial dysfunction: A narrative review. World Journal of Critical Care Medicine. 2023;**12**(3):139-152. DOI: 10.5492/wjccm.v12.i3.139

[13] Parker MM, Shelhamer JH, Bacharach SL, et al. Profound but reversible myocardial depression in patients with septic shock. Annals of Internal Medicine. 1984;**100**(4):483-490

[14] Levy MM, Fink MP, Marshall JC, et al. 2001 SCCM/ESICM/ACCP/ATS/SIS international sepsis definitions conference. Intensive Care Medicine. 2003;**29**(4):530-538

[15] Ware LB, Matthay MA. The acute respiratory distress syndrome. The New England Journal of Medicine. 2000;**342**(18):1334-1349

[16] Bernard GR, Artigas A, Brigham KL, et al. The American-European consensus conference on ARDS. Definitions, mechanisms, relevant outcomes, and clinical trial coordination. American Journal of Respiratory and Critical Care Medicine. 1994;**149**(3 Pt. 1):818-824

[17] Bellomo R, Kellum JA, Ronco C. Acute kidney injury. Lancet. 2012;**380**(9843):756-766

[18] Singer M. The role of mitochondrial dysfunction in sepsis-induced multi-organ failure. Virulence. 2014;**5**(1):66-72

[19] Yang S, Lin S, Kelen GD, et al. A retrospective study of aged septic patients who develop progressive liver dysfunction. Surgery. 2005;**137**(1):58-64

[20] Jalan R, Williams R. Acute liver failure and multi-organ failure. Seminars in Liver Disease. 2002;**22**(3):195-203

[21] Hahmeyer MLS, da Silva-Santos JE. Rho-proteins and downstream pathways as potential targets in sepsis and septic shock: What have we learned from basic research. Cells. 2021;**10**(8):1844. DOI: 10.3390/cells10081844

[22] Mazeraud A, Righy C, Bouchereau E, Benghanem S, Bozza FA, Sharshar T. Septic-associated encephalopathy: A comprehensive review. Neurotherapeutics. 2020;**17**(2):392-403. DOI: 10.1007/s13311-020-00862-1

[23] Basodan N, Al Mehmadi AE, Al Mehmadi AE, Aldawood SM, Hawsawi A, Fatini F, et al. Septic shock: Management and outcomes. Cureus. 2022;**14**(12):e32158. DOI: 10.7759/cureus.32158

[24] Seymour CW, Liu VX, Iwashyna TJ, et al. Assessment of clinical criteria for sepsis: For the third international consensus definitions for sepsis and septic shock (Sepsis-3). Journal of the American Medical Association. 2016;**315**(8):762-774. DOI: 10.1001/jama.2016.0288

[25] Hotchkiss RS, Moldawer LL, Opal SM, Reinhart K, Turnbull IR, Vincent JL. Sepsis and septic shock. Nature Reviews. Disease Primers. 2016;**2**:16045. DOI: 10.1038/nrdp.2016.45

[26] Hernandez G, Bruhn A, Romero C, Javier Larrondo F, De La Fuente R, Castillo L, et al. Management of septic shock with a norepinephrine-based haemodynamic algorithm. Resuscitation. 2005;**66**(1):63-69. DOI: 10.1016/j.resuscitation.2005.01.009

[27] Evans L, Rhodes A, Alhazzani W, Antonelli M, Coopersmith CM, French C, et al. Surviving sepsis campaign: International guidelines for management of sepsis and septic shock 2021. Intensive Care Medicine. 2021;**47**(11):1181-1247. DOI: 10.1007/s00134-021-06506-y. Epub 2021 Oct 2

[28] Gavelli F, Castello LM, Avanzi GC. Management of sepsis and septic shock in the emergency department. Internal and Emergency Medicine. 2021;**16**(6):1649-1661. DOI: 10.1007/s11739-021-02735-7. Epub 2021 Apr 22

[29] Lagunes L, Encina B, Ramirez-Estrada S. Current understanding in source control management in septic shock patients: A review. Annals of Translational Medicine. 2016;**4**(17):330. DOI: 10.21037/atm.2016.09.02

[30] Girardis M, Coloretti I, Antonelli M, et al. Adjunctive immunotherapeutic agents in patients with sepsis and septic shock: A multidisciplinary consensus of 23. Journal of Anesthesia, Analgesia and Critical Care. 2024;**4**:28. DOI: 10.1186/s44158-024-00165-3

Chapter 7

Pathophysiology of Sepsis: A Potential Pathway for Defining Distinct Clinical Phenotypes and Potential Targeted Therapies Including Therapeutic Plasma Exchange

Philip Keith, Taylor Conrad, Jonathan Eaton and Louie Keith Scott

Abstract

Sepsis is now understood to be a syndrome affecting numerous pathways with both damage related patterns and pathogen attributed patterns. It is also becoming clear that there is a phenotypic response to those insults. We now see that sepsis requires patient specific therapy and not just a uniform therapeutic strategy. Therapeutic plasma exchange (TPE) is one phenotypic driven intervention that is being shown to improve clinical outcomes and many different clinical markers in severe cases of sepsis. As our knowledge of these phenotypes progresses, so does our understanding of the use of TPE. This chapter will briefly outline the current understanding of sepsis and begin to define severe sepsis response phenotypes while expanding on the use of TPE as a therapeutic intervention.

Keywords: endothelium, sepsis, phenotypes of sepsis, septic shock, glycocalyx, coagulopathy, therapeutic plasma exchange

1. Introduction

In the early 2000s it was recognized that sepsis, as a syndrome, had less to do with the offending microorganism and more to do with the host's response. Anyone involved in medicine has witnessed the same organism cause a slight cough in one individual and septic shock in another. So why is this the case?

Current research is confirming what we all have witnessed clinically. Sepsis is a phenotypic dependent response syndrome [1]. Therefore, should not therapy be targeted to the individual's response to sepsis and not treated as a singular disease process?

Based on current data, we can no longer accept a "one size fits all" therapeutic strategy for severe sepsis. Rather, we should significantly revise the way that we approach the treatment of sepsis and relook at our current approaches to sepsis therapy.

Sepsis trials have traditionally compared control and treatment groups as equal if they matched the usual metrics such as age, comorbidities, sex, race, time, and type of interventions, along with numerous non-specific lab results. If they matched and met a specific statistical standard, they were assumed equal. Despite these standards, to date, most sepsis intervention trials have yet to pan out over time. Why?

The answer is now becoming clear. An individual's response to sepsis is mostly about their cellular response to the infectious process, mainly their endothelial response [2]. This endothelial response is now coming into focus. Each of us possess a phenotypic response to an infectious process based on our genetic makeup.

To date, there is not an easily obtainable biomarker that can rapidly measure the health of one's endothelium as a randomization process or even to assist in a post-hoc analysis. Therefore, control and treatment groups may have seemed equivalent based on standard metrics, but without an understanding of individual phenotypic sepsis responses, were they really equal? As we now understand it, one's individual cellular response to sepsis is pivotal so we must also appreciate that equivalent study groups with true balance is almost impossible unless individual cellular response is also in a randomization formula and subsequent analysis.

This chapter hopes to explore the role of an individual's endothelial response to sepsis, and how an individual's response affects outcome. It is also our hope to discuss why some therapies may aid, some may not help, and others may even harm.

2. Sepsis as a syndrome: where things sit and where are we are going?

Sepsis was defined in 1991 by a consensus panel convened by the American College of Chest Physicians (ACCP) and the Society of Critical Care Medicine (SCCM) as a systemic inflammatory response syndrome due to infection [3]. The definition was revised in 2001 [4] and again in 2016 [5], attempting to standardize and simplify the recognition of this potentially deadly clinical syndrome. While these definitions have undoubtedly led to earlier identification and improved survival with implementation of early goal directed therapy (EGDT), the non-specific diagnostic criteria have likely contributed to "negative" outcomes observed in numerous trials over the past several decades.

Sepsis must be recognized as a syndrome—a combination of shared characteristics- not as a diagnosis. Seeking the cure for sepsis is analogous to seeking the cure for cancer. The prognosis and treatment for stage 4 pancreatic cancer is very different from the prognosis and treatment for isolated basal cell carcinoma. However, each is called cancer. Similarly, the prognosis of pneumonia with catecholamine refractory shock and multiple organ failure is different from the prognosis of acute bronchitis with fever and tachycardia, yet both are called sepsis, and using current guidelines, there would be no difference in the approach to these two, very different clinical scenarios.

One major shortcoming of prior studies has been the inability to differentiate these clinically dissimilar patients prospectively. Numerous clinical and readily available biochemical markers have been associated with poor prognosis, and some investigators have incorporated these values into predictive scoring systems [6–12].

Unfortunately, these scoring systems have since been invalidated, and clinical trials identifying "sicker" patients based on these scoring systems have largely failed to yield positive results [13, 14].

More recently, researchers and clinicians have further explored the pathophysiology of sepsis which includes a complex interaction of the endothelial glycocalyx, the inflammatory host response, and the endothelial system [15–18]. Many researchers have described these pathways in detail, and this chapter highlights some of the latest data on the cellular pathophysiology of sepsis, not just the clinical syndrome.

For a historical perspective, Rivers established early goal directed therapy (EGDT) as the standard of care for sepsis with a landmark trial published in 2001 [19]. The study included 260 patients with severe sepsis or septic shock. These patients were randomized in the Emergency Department to receive 6 hours of EGDT (which included weight-based fluids, hemoglobin transfusion goals, central venous pressure goals, mean arterial pressure goals, and mixed venous oxygen saturation goals) or standard therapy prior to ICU admission. Those patients receiving EGDT showed an improved inpatient mortality compared to standard therapy (30.5 vs. 46.5%) and EGDT became the gold standard of sepsis management. Other studies have since validated the importance of early management on survival, while debunking the necessity of targeted CVP, Hgb, and SVO2 levels [20–22]. Unfortunately, no additional or adjunct therapies have been identified since that time to further improve survival [23–27].

The PRoCESS trial was designed to compare EGDT with protocolized management and standard of care [22]. The results showed no difference in outcomes in either of these strategies. More interestingly, the investigators prospectively measured biomarkers of endothelial cell injury and other inflammatory and vascular biomarkers—both at baseline and after treatment—and found no relationship between different resuscitation strategies and biomarker profiles in sepsis. However, they did find that elevated levels of endothelial cell biomarkers of permeability and hemostasis were associated with increased mortality. These observations are important for the following reasons: First, the association of these biomarkers with increased mortality offers potential markers to better identify "sicker" patients with sepsis. Second, the observation that early therapy does not affect these values, regardless of treatment strategy, supports the concept that adjunct therapies are necessary to further improve survival in many cases of sepsis. Finally, these markers may assist in defining distinct, clinical phenotypes in sepsis and allow for patient specific interventions as opposed to the "one size fits all" approach that is currently the standard of care.

Prior trials in sepsis have targeted various points in the pathologic cascade but have selected patients based on pre-defined scoring systems and non-specific biomarkers. Apart from DIC, these therapies have not directly targeted specific clinical phenotypes, and thus the therapies may have been deemed ineffective without truly being evaluated in the subsets of patients that may benefit most from the adjunct therapy in question. More recently, investigators have begun to define distinct phenotypes of sepsis and to design individualized treatment approaches [28]. For example, previously unproven therapies such as methylene blue (in the case of excessive nitric oxide production) [29], corticosteroids (in cases of dysregulated inflammation) [26], and activated protein C (in the case of certain coagulopathies) [23] may prove beneficial in patients with distinct phenotypic profiles despite having "negative" findings in prior well-designed, prospective trials in sepsis.

Identifying these distinct phenotypes should be a focus of future research and will ultimately allow for prospective studies of individualized treatments targeting distinct points of the pathway on an individual basis. One such therapy is the use of therapeutic plasma exchange (TPE) as an adjunct intervention in sepsis related multiple organ failure with specific phenotypic characteristics.

In order to understand the rationale for the efficacy of plasma exchange in the treatment of sepsis, we first note that plasma filtration has been demonstrated to lower circulating levels of many mediators of severe sepsis in both experimental and clinical studies [30–32]. However, numerous trials with hemofiltration alone, including cytokine binding agents, have failed to yield positive clinical outcomes [33–36]. The unique clinical advantage of TPE is the simultaneous removal of these harmful mediators and replacement of acutely diseased and harmful plasma with healthy donor plasma. As such, TPE may allow the host's overwhelmed compensatory process to reestablish its footing and regulate the immune response to the host's advantage.

As mentioned above, the endothelium plays a major role in the sepsis pathway and appears to be activated by the initial cytokine storm. Hypotension results not only from inflammatory vasodilation, but also from increased vascular permeability resulting from endothelial injury [15–17]. The circulating markers of endothelial injury associated with increased mortality have been associated with electron microscopic changes to the endothelium. Interestingly, resuscitation with fresh frozen plasma (FFP) has shown to restore endothelial integrity [37]. Why is this important?

Our current understanding is that the sepsis induced endothelial activation leads to a pathologic trigger of the clotting cascade leading to a hypercoagulable microcirculatory state. Decreased ADAMTS-13 activity and increased ADAMTS-13 inhibitors are prevalent leading to increased thrombogenic ultra-large von Willebrand factor (ULvWF) multimers, ultimately resulting in diffuse microcirculatory platelet thrombosis. Increased plasminogen activator inhibitor (PAI-1) activity leads to decreased fibrinolysis and disseminated fibrin-rich microcirculatory clotting. The net result is a non-consumptive, platelet and fibrin rich microcirculatory thrombotic state with non-specific coagulation findings, often distinct from DIC, TTP, and HUS (**Figure 1**) [16, 18]. Activated protein C and thrombomodulin are among the therapies that have been investigated to reverse this process, without success [23, 27]. TPE (using plasma as replacement fluid) is unique in that it addresses both the pathologic coagulation cascade and platelet dysfunction by removing the ULvWF multimers, ADAMTS-13 inhibitors, and PAI-1 while replenishing ADAMTS-13 activity, immunoglobulins

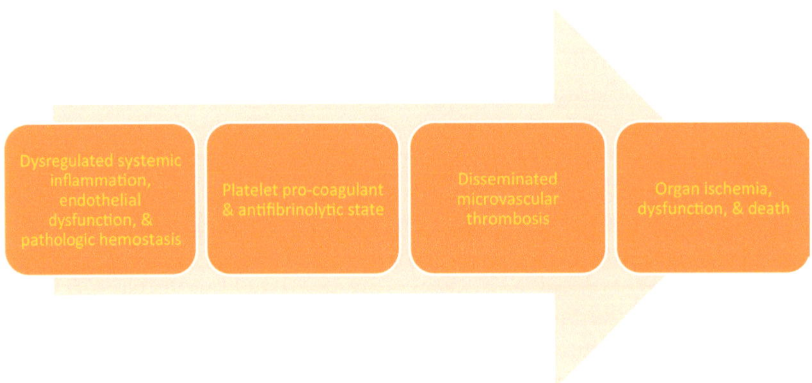

Figure 1.
Pathologic cascade of sepsis. Clinical phenotype of refractory septic shock highlighting multiple potential targets for adjunct therapies and intervention.

IgM and IgA, and coagulation factors and inhibitors such as proteins C and S and antithrombin III [18], while also restoring endothelial integrity [37].

Despite all the theoretical benefits of TPE, case reports and case series initially yielded inconsistent results on its efficacy in sepsis. The first prospective randomized controlled trial (RCT) was reported in 2002 [38]. In this trial, 106 patients with severe sepsis or septic shock were randomized to adjunct TPE or conventional therapy. The results revealed that mortality was significantly lower in those receiving TPE (33.3 vs. 53.8%). While these results were positive, the logistics of the TPE procedure could be resource intensive with many clinicians doubting the feasibility of performing the procedure broadly. These limitations have restricted the widespread use of TPE for sepsis while also contributing to the logistical difficulty of performing prospective RCTs.

2.1 Phenotypes of sepsis and TPE

Taking into consideration recent research and our expanded knowledge of the sepsis syndrome, many clinicians and researchers have attempted to identify clinical phenotypes with high predicted mortality, most in need of adjunct therapy, and most likely to respond to TPE. Noting the pathologic coagulopathy, Stegmayer reported 82% survival in 76 consecutive patients treated with adjunct TPE during a progressive course of DIC and MODS, a patient population with a historical predicted survival of <20% [39]. More recently, thrombocytopenia associated multiple organ failure (TAMOF) has been defined as a distinct phenotype of septic pediatric patients with higher organ dysfunction and mortality than other phenotypes of pediatric sepsis [18]. TAMOF is defined by (1) thrombocytopenia, (2) microangiopathic hemolysis, (3) hemodynamic failure, and (4) ischemic organ failure resulting from direct inhibition or inactivation of ADAMTS-13 (with activity <57%), leading to disseminated platelet/vWF-rich microthrombi [18, 40–42]. A small, 10-patient proof-of-concept pilot RCT demonstrated that TPE was associated with reduced organ dysfunction and mortality in children receiving TPE compared with those not receiving TPE [42].

Given the complexities and limitations of clinical trials in children, as well as a loss of clinical equipoise, additional randomized data is lacking in the treatment of TAMOF in pediatric patients. In spite of these hurdles, a network of nine quaternary PICUs in the United States collaborated and demonstrated decreased organ failure and improved survival in TAMOF patients receiving TPE compared to TAMOF patients not receiving TPE [43]. Using similar inclusion criteria as TAMOF, a single center retrospectively reported improved survival in a cohort of 40 adult patients with sepsis and MODS receiving adjunct TPE compared to propensity matched controls receiving standard therapy alone [44]. Around the same time, investigators reported improved survival in a RCT of patients with sepsis associated with DIC receiving adjunct TPE compared to groups receiving therapeutic heparin and sham therapies [45]. In addition, TPE was further found to be superior to other treatment strategies in improving markers of endothelial injury, adding more data for consideration in developing phenotypic profiles and measuring response to treatments in future trials while supporting the concept of TPE as a potential adjunct therapy.

2.2 Expanding our knowledge of sepsis phenotypes as it relates to TPE

While the endothelium and coagulation cascade have been common targets of directed therapies in sepsis, the dysregulated inflammatory response, often referred to as "cytokine storm" has also been commonly targeted. Non-specific anti-inflammatories such as corticosteroids, statins, and azithromycin have shown inconsistent results [26, 46, 47]. Cytokine removal by filtration and binding have yielded similar disappointing results [34–36] (**Table 1**). But phenotypic randomization did not occur in any of those studies. This was about to change.

In 2007 a Brazilian pediatric group was first to report a higher mortality in hyperferritinemic sepsis, with ferritin levels >500 ng/mL associated with a 3.2 relative risk of death [48]. A newly understood biomarker of pathologic inflammation was confirmed. As a follow-up, a multi-center collaborative study group reported improved survival in a cohort study of 23 children with hyperferritinemic sepsis treated with TPE compared to standard therapy [49].

The worldwide COVID-19 pandemic resulted in a massive influx of septic patients across the world, and the high observed mortality reported early during the outbreak fueled efforts to investigate additional therapies. From its onset, "cytokine storm" was felt to be a major pathologic process [50] and hyperferritinemia was identified as an independent marker of increased mortality [51–53]. TPE was proposed as a possible adjunct therapy [54], and multiple reports were published demonstrating improved survival and decreased ferritin levels with adjunct therapy [55–57]. These observations ultimately led to the first RCT of adult patients evaluating TPE for sepsis in nearly 20 years. While the study was not powered to reach statistical significance, TPE in addition to standard therapy, demonstrated a decrease in mortality in the TPE cohort compared to the standard therapy cohort (20.9 vs. 34.1%) [58]. A systematic review of 34 peer-reviewed articles, including a total of 267 COVID-19 patients treated with adjunct TPE, demonstrated decreased mortality and favorable trends in biochemical markers, including ferritin [59].

2.3 Current data on sepsis and TPE

In 2023 the American Society for Apheresis (ASFA) updated its guidelines for TPE in severe sepsis to a category III, 2A recommendation [60] based on the studies referenced above as well as evidence that continues to mount. In 2024, a systematic review and meta-analysis including 937 adult critically ill patients from 5 RCTs and 15 MCSs was published [61]. Of those enrolled in the study, 543 received adjunct TPE. The TPE

Targeted therapies	
Adrenergic system	"Decatecholaminization"
Adrenal activation/dysfunction	Corticosteroids
Endothelial dysfunction	Ascorbic acid Methylene blue
Pathologic coagulopathy	Activated protein C Heparin Thrombomodulin
Capillary leak	Fluid strategies, "massive transfusion"
"Cytokine storm"	Corticosteroids Hemofiltration Polymyxin B

Table 1.
Prior potential targeted therapies for sepsis.

group showed a significant reduction in short-term mortality, with a RR of 0.59. Of note, this study demonstrated a similar benefit in patients with sepsis due to COVID-19 infection as well as sepsis from other pathogens. Similarly, two additional meta-analyses support adjunct TPE in the setting sepsis, also regardless of the offending organism [62, 63]. Most recently, a large propensity matched analysis of 906 critically ill patients with sepsis and MODS demonstrated a reduced in-patient mortality (HR 0.38), reduced 28-day mortality (HR 0.50), and reduced 1 year mortality (HR 0.44) in patients that had undergone adjunct TPE compared to standard therapy alone [64].

Identifying patient specific pathology, and individualizing therapy based on the phenotypic profile, is the logical evolution in the management of sepsis. Biochemical information from benchside research and clinical studies alike offer valuable information that should contribute to defining these phenotypes [65]. Once these phenotypes have been defined, prospective trials using specific targeted therapies may be performed. It seems evident that phenotypic randomization is the future along with a Baysean trial design focusing on sepsis therapy, TPE or not. Currently, two separate groups are recruiting patients for separate prospective RCTs designed to investigate adjunct TPE for sepsis (EXCHANGE-2 [66], PLEXSIS [67]). The authors of this chapter are also actively designing a third trial which will include pathologic markers of endothelial activation, dysregulated inflammation, and coagulopathy in patient inclusion and analysis. The results of these three trials are certain to add valuable information to this field.

To reiterate, most trials in sepsis have treated sepsis as a specific disease rather than a complex and heterogeneous syndrome and in hindsight it should come as little surprise that these trials have, and continue to yield discouraging results. Future interventions must focus on identifying specific components of their host response. Not unlike cancer, treatment needs to be modified based on phenotype and phenotypic responses. Understanding the pathophysiology of sepsis, and identifying markers of individual abnormalities should allow for more focused research and, hopefully, ultimately to new therapies with improved outcomes.

3. Defining and understanding a host response to severe sepsis

The complexity of a host's response to sepsis is becoming increasingly difficult to put in an easily understandable format due to the enormous influx of data with focuses on endothelial dysfunction, glycocalyx degradation, metabolomic and genomic responses, coagulation disorders just to name a few. It is beyond the scope of this chapter to explore all the potential dysfunctions that occur in sepsis. Instead we will focus on the current data, what potentially lies ahead, and explore if it's possible to use readily available biomarkers to produce patient targeted therapies for severe sepsis.

3.1 Glycocalyx, exosomes and coagulation in severe sepsis

Over the past 20 years it has been debated that the endothelium should be considered an organ system and those that work in critical care are in fact Endotheliologists. Many have eloquently debated over the years, led by William Arid and others [67, 68].

The growing understanding of the immunologic, endocrine, and coagulation interactions with endothelium, and to a greater degree, the glycocalyx, is generating a better understanding of sepsis as a syndrome [5, 6]. These realizations, along with the role of exosomes, angiopoietins and many other vascular related proteins, demonstrates the need for big data and system biology to unravel the mystery of who needs what specific therapy and how to better utilize these tools for developing readily available biomarkers to guide patient targeted therapies [69, 70].

Because of the complexity of this topic, we will attempt to explore the endothelium in greater detail based on what is known thus far. However, this is not an exhaustive review as much as it is a distillation of the current data with the goal of showing the importance of phenotypic responses to sepsis and later demonstrate how differing therapies may become commonplace based on these phenotypes.

3.1.1 Glycocalyx and host defenses

The glycocalyx is a dense network of carbohydrates attached to the cell membrane of all mammalian cells that performs many functions in host defenses. Below are the known functions of the glycocalyx to date with expanding research growing daily. These essential functions relating to host defenses boiled down are:

1. Cell-cell adhesion: Carbohydrates on the glycocalyx interact with other cell surface molecules, facilitating cell-cell interactions and adhesion [71].

2. Protection from Mechanical Stressors: The thick and viscous glycocalyx forms a protective layer around cells, shielding them from shear forces, mechanical stress, and infection [72].

3. Cell signaling and receptor binding: Glycocalyx carbohydrates can bind to specific receptors on the cell surface, influencing cell signaling pathways and facilitating the interaction of growth factors, hormones, and other ligands [73].

4. Nutrient exchange: Certain carbohydrates in the glycocalyx act as binding sites for nutrient molecules, facilitating their transport into the cell [74].

5. Immune defense: The glycocalyx can interact with immune cells and molecules, regulating immune responses and preventing pathogens from adhering to the cell surface [75].

6. Cell migration: Glycocalyx carbohydrates can bind to extracellular matrix proteins, guiding cell migration during development and wound healing [76].

3.1.2 Glycocalyx, oncotic pressure and vascular integrity

The glycocalyx also plays a significant role in oncotic pressure. The degree of influence the glycocalyx has on oncotic pressure is just now coming clearer. These mechanisms involved are crucial for maintaining blood volume and preventing fluid loss from the vascular space. The Starling Forces we have all been taught are now known to be largely invalid. The glycocalyx acts as a semi-permeable barrier, allowing water and small molecules to pass through while retaining larger molecules and proteins within the blood vessels.

In pathological conditions where the glycocalyx is damaged or depleted, such as in sepsis or inflammation, oncotic pressure can decrease, leading to fluid extravasation and edema. Restoration of the glycocalyx is therefore an important therapeutic target in these conditions.

Below is just a rough synopsis what we currently understand:

1. Negative charge: The glycocalyx is negatively charged due to its abundance of sialic acid and other acidic carbohydrates [77].

2. Repulsion of anions: Negatively charged anions (such as chloride and bicarbonate ions) are repelled by the glycocalyx [78].

3. Water attraction: Water molecules are attracted to and hydrate the negatively charged glycocalyx [79].

4. Osmotic gradient: The presence of water molecules around the glycocalyx creates an osmotic gradient, drawing water into the blood vessels [80]. Putting this all together, it becomes clear the significance of the glycocalyx. Consider a blood vessel with a healthy glycocalyx. The negative charge of the glycocalyx repels chloride ions, creating an osmotic gradient that draws water into the blood vessel. This influx of water helps maintain blood pressure and prevents fluid loss into the surrounding tissues.

In contrast, if the glycocalyx is damaged or absent, chloride ions can freely enter the blood vessel, reducing the osmotic gradient. As a result, less water is drawn into the vessel, leading to a decrease in oncotic pressure and potential fluid extravasation [81].

In summary, the pro-inflammatory stimuli produced in sepsis drive the inflammatory cascade leading to glycocalyx degradation. This degradation allows the binding and extravasation of leukocytes generating von WIllebrand deposition and platelet activation. All resulting in additional inflammation and resultant thrombosis. To further exacerbate matters, this glycocalyx loss leads to capillary leaking that contributes to systemic edema and vascular hypovolemia. These cascade of events cumulatively result in hypoperfusion, microvascular blood flow and resultant organ dysfunction [82].

The complexity of these processes can not be overstated. As the field grows, so do the possibilities of identifying individual variations in sepsis responses to targeted therapies and interventions. It's the authors' belief that understanding and identifying phenotypes of sepsis response is key to not only developing targeted therapies, but also improving clinical trial design by randomizing based on these phenotypes.

3.2 Exosomes

Exosomes are extracellular vesicles formed by the fusion of multivesicular bodies and cell membranes. Exosomes effectively transport many bioactive substances such as proteins, lipids, RNA, DNA, and participate in the regulation of inflammatory and immune responses. Cytokines that are also transported by exosomes include, but not limited to, HMGB-1, IL-1β, IL-2, IL-6, IL-12, IL-15, IL-17, TNF-α and IFN-γ [83].

Within the syndrome of sepsis, it is known the Pathogen-Associated Molecular Patterns (PAMPS) and Damage-Associated Molecular Patterns (DAMPs) play a pivotal role in host defense. Exosomes are endosomal-derived vesicles, which carry proteins, lipids and nucleic acids, and facilitate intercellular communications. With sepsis, exosomes carry cytokines and DAMPs to induce inflammation. Exosomal

DAMPs include numerous pro-inflammatory cytokines such as high mobility group box 1, heat shock proteins, histones, adenosine triphosphate, and extracellular RNA [84].

Overall, the impact of exosomal participation in sepsis, particularly severe sepsis, is becoming increasingly appreciated and further research is now focusing on ways to manipulate exosomes. All that while still developing a better understanding of what intervention may help or hurt exosomal influence. Further, using exosomes as biomarkers to better identify phenotypes of a septic responses, and those that may benefit from a specific therapy and those that may not, will impact sepsis trials and therapies in the near future.

3.3 Endothelial response to sepsis

The endothelium, a thin layer of cells lining blood vessels, plays a crucial role in maintaining vascular homeostasis and regulating inflammation. Sepsis disrupts endothelial function, leading to various detrimental effects. Listed below are the major dysfunctions that occur during severe sepsis. This list is a fraction of the known dysfunctions that occur within the endothelium.

1. Increased endothelial permeability:

    - Sepsis triggers the release of inflammatory mediators such as cytokines (e.g., TNF-α, IL-1β, IL-6) and nitric oxide (NO).

    - These factors damage endothelial cell tight junctions, increasing vascular permeability.

    - Leaky endothelium allows fluid, proteins, and inflammatory cells to leak into the interstitial spaces, leading to tissue edema and organ dysfunction [85].

2. Impaired endothelial barrier function:

    - Disrupts the endothelial glycocalyx, a protective layer of glycosaminoglycans that lines the vessel lumen.

    - This impairs endothelial barrier function, allowing bacteria and toxins to penetrate the vascular space

    - Increased endothelial permeability and impaired barrier function contribute to organ failure and septic shock.

3. Hypercoagulability and thrombosis:

    - Sepsis promotes a pro-coagulant state by activating platelets, increasing the expression of tissue factor, and inhibiting fibrinolysis.

    - Endothelial damage exposes subendothelial components that trigger coagulation, leading to microthrombi formation in the microvasculature.

    - Thrombosis can further impair blood flow and tissue oxygenation.

4. Endothelial cell apoptosis:

    - Sepsis can induce apoptosis (programmed cell death) of endothelial cells.
    - Inflammatory mediators, oxidative stress, and mitochondrial dysfunction contribute to endothelial cell damage and death.
    - Endothelial cell apoptosis leads to loss of vascular integrity and further inflammation.

5. Impaired vasodilation:

    - Sepsis disrupts endothelial NO production and bioavailability.
    - NO is a potent vasodilator that promotes blood flow.
    - Reduced endothelial NO production leads to vasoconstriction, impaired tissue perfusion, and organ damage.

6. Oxidative stress:

    - Sepsis increases oxidative stress by generating reactive oxygen species (ROS), such as superoxide and hydrogen peroxide ROS damage endothelial cells, leading to impaired function and apoptosis. Consequences of Endothelial Dysfunction in Sepsis:Organ dysfunction (e.g., ARDS, kidney failure, liver failure).
    - Septic shock
    - Disseminated intravascular coagulation (DIC)
    - Increased mortality

3.4 Angiopoietin: tie-2 dysfunction on severe sepsis

The interactions between the endothelium and Angiopoietin-Tie-2 axis tends to explain much of what is seen clinically in severe sepsis. It also explains, to a certain degree, the degradation of the glycocalyx in sepsis.

As an overview, angiopoietins are a family of proteins that play a significant role in blood vessel formation and function. There are two main angiopoietins: angiopoietin-1 (Ang-1) and angiopoietin-2 (Ang-2). They have opposing effects on the health of blood vessels.

- Angiopoietin-1 (Ang-1): promotes blood vessel growth and stability, reduces leakage from blood vessels, and helps protect tissues.
- Angiopoietin-2 (Ang-2): disrupts blood vessel formation and function, increases leakage from blood vessels, and can contribute to inflammation.

3.4.1 Angiopoietins in severe sepsis

Research has shown that levels of Ang-2 are elevated in patients with severe sepsis compared to healthy individuals [85]. This increase in Ang-2 is associated with the severity of illness and increased risk of death [86]. Ang-2 may be a marker of endothelial dysfunction, a condition where the inner lining of blood vessels becomes damaged and leaky.

In a healthy state, there is a ratio of Ang-1 to Ang-2 in which Ang-1 exceeds levels of Ang-2. During inflammatory states, such as sepsis, Ang-2 levels rise through fairly complex pathways resulting in the clinical issues noted in sepsis. Angiopoietin-2 is in fact an antagonist of the endothelium-stabilizing receptor Tie-2 thus promoting vascular permeability through cellular contraction and junctional disintegration [87]. Once the signaling initiates the release of Ang-2, subsequent events cause even more issues within the syndrome of severe sepsis, along with issues of coagulopathy and thrombocytopenia [88]. The fact that Ang-2 is stored in the Weibel-Palade Bodies, along with von Willebrand factor, it becomes clear that when Ang-2 is released, so is von Willebrand factor, thus explaining, at least in some part, the related coagulopathies that develop with severe sepsis. This will be expanded on later in the chapter.

Due to the role they play in blood vessel function, angiopoietins are being investigated as potential therapeutic targets for severe sepsis. Researchers are exploring ways to:

- Increase Ang-1 levels
- Block the harmful effects of Ang-2

More research is needed to determine if targeting angiopoietins can improve outcomes in patients with severe sepsis.

3.5 Hyperferritinemia and severe sepsis

Ferritin is a protein that stores and distributes iron. In severe inflammation, cells release ferritin at various levels with varying consequences that also vary greatly from individual to individual. It has been shown that high levels contribute to tissue damage and organ failure in sepsis through numerous pathways, all affected by inflammation, macrophage activity and endothelial health to name just a few [89–91]. Further, high ferritin levels may indicate a poorer prognosis in sepsis [92, 93].

In brief, ferritin is released from various cell types depending on iron levels, as part of the oxidative stress response and by macrophages in pro-inflammatory conditions. In critically ill patients, serum ferritin levels are upregulated by cytokines independent of iron availability. However, iron is mainly transported by transferrin which is altered greatly in inflammatory states. Further, the binding affinity of transferrin to iron may be less than the binding strength of various microbes that use iron as a fuel source.

Elevated serum ferritin is an indicator of both iron storage in tissues and inflammation. All nucleated cell types express ferritin in order to store iron. Within cells, ferritin is essential to avoid iron-induced formation of reactive oxygen species, cellular toxicity and inhibit iron for microbial fuel [94]. Macrophages can either store iron in ferritin or secrete ferritin therefore considered the major source of serum ferritin.

All these factors lead to the similarities of severe sepsis with associated hyperferritinemia and of other known severe inflammatory diseases such as hemophagocytic lymphohistiocytosis (HLH) and Macrophage Activation Syndrome (MAS). Studied more in the pediatric population, MAS has typically been related to Still Diseases, LHL and other rheumatologic conditions. However, upon examining the immunologic reaction to sepsis, the similarity to MAS and secondary HLH is unavoidable [95]. Hemophagocytic disorders occur when critical pathways responsible for regulation of immune/inflammatory responses are disrupted or overwhelmed. Hemophagocytic lymphohistiocytosis is with activation of antigen-processing cells (macrophages and histiocytes) and $CD8^+$ T cells, along with proliferation and ectopic migration of T cells. Cytokine levels indicate persistently elevated levels of multiple pro-inflammatory cytokines during symptomatic disease.

All these symptoms have hyperferritinemia in common and again, its level seems to relate to the severity of disease. Thereby becoming an easily obtainable biomarker of a specific phenotypic response to sepsis that may very well lead to phenotypic driven therapies based on ferritin levels. But this is clearly only scratching the surface since more and more phenotypic biomarkers are coming into light. As mentioned, each phenotype may therefore require phenotypic-specific therapeutic interventions.

3.6 Coagulation disorders related to sepsis

Our understanding of sepsis-induced coagulopathy (SIC) has become better understood in recent years. The pathogenesis of SIC involves both protective and destructive mechanisms, with the immune response targeting pathogens while simultaneously causing endothelial injury and dysfunction. This dual response activates coagulation pathways and widespread inflammation [95–97]. The endothelial cells lining the blood vessels play a crucial role in maintaining vascular integrity, as described earlier. However, during sepsis, these cells are damaged by mechanisms such as the activation of the complement system generating membrane attack complexes and exosome release carrying DAMPs, cytokines and other inflammatory mediators, leading to significant vascular injury and the initiation of a highly dysregulated micro-thrombotic state and endotheliopathy [98–100].

The "two-path unifying theory," previously described by Chang, offers a framework for understanding SIC's pathogenesis [15]:

1. Unusually large von Willebrand factor (ULVWF) pathway activation:

    - Endothelial cells release ULVWF multimers in response to endothelial injury.

    - These multimers anchor to the endothelial surface and promote the activation, adhesion and aggregation of platelets.

    - This process, known as micro-thrombogenesis, leads to the formation of platelet-ULVWF complexes or microthrombi strings.

2. Tissue factor (TF) pathway activation:

    - The TF pathway is typically initiated by exposure to tissue factor, which is not usually present within the endothelial cells but is exposed upon vascular injury involving subendothelial tissue or extravascular tissue.

    - This pathway involves the activation of the extrinsic coagulation cascade, leading to the formation of fibrin clots/meshes.

Under normal hemostasis both pathways are activated simultaneously. This typically would result from external bodily injury/trauma but can also occur with intravascular injury/disruption. This subsequently leads to the formation of blood clots, macro-thrombogenesis, and ultimately wound hemostasis and healing with external bodily injury or venous/arterial thrombosis as seen in intravascular injury [98].

This theory suggests that pathological coagulation in SIC arises from the independent activation of the ULVWF pathway due to endothelial destruction, without the primary activation of the TF pathway. The dysregulated inflammatory response is ultimately the driving factor of this endothelial destruction. This process leads to platelet-ULVWF complexes generating microthrombi strings with excessive exocytosis of ULVWF, platelet activation, and ADAMTS13 deficiency. The ultimate result is an organ trophic or disseminated intravascular thrombosis, depending upon individual pathogen/toxin and host response dysregulation phenotype.

Clinically this is characterized as an acute and unexplained thrombocytopenia with possible associated skin findings (petechiae, purpura, and mottling). The coagulopathy may appear similar and sometimes indistinguishable from TTP or TTP-like syndromes. This may or may not include the findings of microangiopathic hemolytic anemia, but thrombocytopenia is always present and is a hallmark of SAMOF [96, 99–101]. A hemorrhagic syndrome is typically not present, as opposed to primary TF pathway activation, but may exist in later stages.

This micro-thrombogenesis is a defining feature of SIC, differentiating it from "traditional" disseminated intravascular coagulation (DIC), which is characterized by activation of the TF pathway independently. This is best understood by relating the consumptive coagulopathy of acute promyelocytic leukemia which causes DIC by release of TF into the intravascular space without activation of the endothelial pathway. Many toxins, bacteria, viruses, parasites, and other pathogens can initiate and lead to this dysregulated inflammatory/micro-thrombotic state that characterizes the sepsis syndrome. If left unchecked or worsened with therapies that lead to further endothelial destruction, the result may lead to disseminated intravascular microthrombosis (DIT), which impairs blood flow and oxygen delivery to various organs, contributing to the development of multiorgan dysfunction syndrome (MODS) [97, 99, 101].

Given that SIC is associated with a high mortality rate, emphasis should be placed on early recognition and determination of which patients may benefit from therapies such as therapeutic plasma exchange. When looking at potential coagulopathy tests, thromboelastography may potentially become useful in identifying patterns and provide a potential early signal for worsening endotheliopathy and coagulopathy that can develop in sepsis and septic shock [102, 103].

Management of SIC focuses on understanding its pathophysiology and developing effective treatments. Supportive care, including antibiotics and organ support, remains the cornerstone of therapy. Specific anticoagulant therapies, such as heparin, antithrombin, and recombinant thrombomodulin, have shown mixed results likely due to their action on the TF pathway as opposed to the ULVWF pathway. Therapeutic plasma exchange, which removes pro-coagulants and replenishes anticoagulants, offers a different approach by addressing the ULVWF pathway with removal of ULVWF and replenishment of ADAMTS13.

4. How is TPE performed

Therapeutic Plasma Exchange is a process that separates plasma from circulatory cells, discarded and replaced with donated plasma or a plasma/albumin combination.

This can be performed by two modalities. One modality is a centrifugal method where the plasma is essentially spun away from the circulatory cells. The other modality is based on a high flux membrane that sieves the plasma away from circulatory cells. Both methods are highly efficient with each having its advantages and disadvantages.

4.1 Centrifugal TPE (cTPE) vs. membrane TPE (mTPE)

Until the early 2000's, the centrifugal method of TPE was the only largely available modality. In the early 2000's, continuous renal replacement therapy (CRRT) became widely available. With this, came plasma filtration technology that could be performed on the CRRT machines. This immediately sparked debates as to which therapy was most effective. Centrifugal has shown to have less clotting issues and shorter therapy times, but otherwise there has been no real "winner" [103].

In contrast to clotting or treatment time, one advantage to the membrane method may be timing and personnel. In most healthcare systems, cTPE is a service provided by either the blood bank or the nephrology service utilizing the centrifugal method. This requires a nurse or tech at bedside throughout the procedure and is usually only available within a limited time frame. Also, the number of cTPE machines are limited within most institutions. Because of the availability of CRRT machines, mTPE may have a unique advantage on this point. The mTPE method mostly uses a standard Continuous Renal Replacement Therapy (CRRT) machine, which in most larger centers, is more readily available and can be run by the bedside nurse and initiated at any time with little delay. The timing issue may be more critical than previously thought.

All in all, the noted differences in the two modalities appear to be rather minor and there is no evidence thus far of a clinical difference except in small comparative trials [104, 105]. However, as of yet, there has not been a study looking at time points of identifying the possible need for TPE, and the patient actually receiving TPE. This may be an important comparative variable and should be investigated further.

4.2 Vascular access options to perform TPE

Vascular access for therapeutic plasma exchange can be obtained via several ways, but the two most common are central and peripheral. Each of them has benefits and drawbacks which will be discussed below. In an international apheresis survey done in 2005, peripheral venous access was shown to be more common in Europe while central venous access was more common in the United States and Asia [106]. Access for peripheral venous access is typically done with placement of dialysis-type steel needles in the peripheral veins. The veins most commonly used are those in the arms. 17-to-19-gauge needles are used in adults while 19-to-22-gauge needles are used in children. Peripheral access has a few drawbacks. One is the ability to access the peripheral veins, though this challenge has been mostly alleviated by the introduction of using ultrasound to access. The other main drawback is the blood flow rates possible with the size needles being used. A 17-gauge needle allows for a blood flow rate of 80 mL/min while a 19-gauge needle does not allow flow rates greater than 60 mL/min. Other risks of peripheral vascular access include nerve damage, hematoma formation and sclerosis of the peripheral veins [107].

Alternatively, central access can be used. As mentioned above, central access is the most common form of access used in the United States. Temporary dialysis catheters are the most commonly used form of central access used, especially for patients admitted to the hospital. These catheters are typically double or triple lumen catheters of at least 11.5 French diameter. These catheters allow for blood flow rates much higher than the peripheral access discussed above [107]. Though most of the central catheters used are temporary, tunneled catheters can also be placed for patients needing longer term TPE or for those that will be treated over time as an outpatient. The major risks associated with central catheters are well known and include (depending on location of insertion) pneumothorax, arterial puncture, central-line associated bloodstream infections, catheter occlusion and thrombus formation. Both central and peripheral access have advantages and disadvantages and the type of access selected should be based on the needs of the individual patient.

4.3 Anticoagulation strategies to perform TPE

TPE may lead to significant changes in hemostasis with a potential for bleeding and or clotting. Each individual patient's acute illness, chronic comorbidities, choice of replacement fluid, and (non-TPE procedural) anticoagulation status contribute to the net effect and make blanket recommendations impossible while leading to a fair amount of clinical variability.

Replacement with non-plasma fluid (albumin) may contribute to an increased risk of bleeding as clotting factors are removed but not replaced during the TPE procedure. As discussed previously, plasma is the preferred replacement fluid for TPE for sepsis, thus for the purpose of this discussion, patient bleeding related to TPE for sepsis is unlikely.

Regardless of replacement fluid choice, clotting of the extracorporeal circuit is possible, and anticoagulation is generally preferred. Two main options for anticoagulation are citrate and heparin.

In general, citrate is the preferred anticoagulant because of its shorter half-life, in-vitro activity, favorable safety profile, and potential for rapid reversal [108]. The in-vitro activity, confined to the extracorporeal circuit, makes clinically significant bleeding very unlikely. Citrate acts by binding ionized calcium, so clinicians should be diligent to recognize and correct signs and symptoms of hypocalcemia. Protocols often include scheduled calcium as part of the TPE order set.

Heparin offers another anticoagulant option for TPE. Similar to citrate, heparin has a short half-life and is relatively inexpensive. However, its anticoagulant effect is in-vivo and may contribute to clinically significant patient bleeding. Monitoring of therapeutic efficacy and safety, therefore, may be more challenging and monitoring of coagulation is usually required.

The third option is not to use anticoagulation at all. This is probably only possible for the filtration method because less blood is being exposed to an extracorporeal circuit and therefore less time not being exposed to the endothelium. If however, clotting is being witnessed, bolus heparin may be advisable although there are no guidelines or studies of merit that can correrbate or testify to its safety. This is where clinical discretion will be required.

All in all, given the numerous indications for TPE, the variability of replacement fluid and treatment frequency, and the infinite combination of co-morbidities and active medications, blanket guidelines do not exist for anticoagulation during TPE. A comprehensive discussion of this topic is beyond the scope of this chapter. Readers are encouraged to visit the American Society for Apheresis (ASFA) website (https://apheresis.org) for additional recommendations.

5. Conclusions

Sepsis is indeed a complex, heterogeneous syndrome and not a specific disease. Although vasomotor instability and resultant end-organ damage have related clinical features, it appears that is where it stops. With genomics, metabolomics, along with better appreciation of endothelial dysfunction within the immune response, it is clear that a sepsis response is phenotypically driven. Although clinical markers overlap, the use of currently available biomarkers allows clinical identification of many of these phenotypes and provides a path to select therapies that have been shown to improve outcomes in those phenotypes. This is in contrast to the "one size fits all" strategy that has historically driven much of the clinical management of sepsis.

Identifying sepsis response phenotypes is providing information that will clearly improve therapeutic trial design by investigating phenotype specific randomizations instead of simply using common clinical markers. As our understanding of sepsis phenotypes expands, individualized treatment strategies such as TPE can be investigated further and more accurately assign therapeutic interventions.

Biomarkers to identify those with TPE responsive phenotypes is the next step. Most likely candidates known thus far relate to endothelial dysfunction, pattern specific coagulopathies, and glycocalyx damage. However, this field is growing rapidly and should be better defined in the near future with three clinical trials on the horizon.

It is clear from the data presented, TPE has a role in the treatment of sepsis. It is also clear that its greatest benefit is to those with specific phenotypic responses. As data expands on the use of TPE in this syndrome, more questions will also need to be asked such as the timing of implementation, replacement solution composition, and identifying additional interventions that may be complementary. All in all, TPE is one intervention that is available currently with years of experience in its treatment of other conditions. Refining and defining TPE's role in sepsis is coming into focus and provides a unique, and an apparent, beneficial therapy for those with a responsive phenotype.

Author details

Philip Keith[1]*, Taylor Conrad[2], Jonathan Eaton[2] and Louie Keith Scott[2]

1 Salem Chest Specialists, Winston Salem, NC, USA

2 Louisiana State University Health Shreveport, Shreveport, LA, USA

*Address all correspondence to: pkeith97@yahoo.com

References

[1] Vincent J-L, Sakr Y. Clinical trial design for unmet clinical needs: A spotlight on sepsis. Expert Review of Clinical Pharmacology. 2019;**12**(9):893-900

[2] Fernández-Sarmiento J, Molina CF, Salazar-Pelaez LM, Flórez S, Alarcón-Forero LC, Sarta M, et al. Biomarkers of glycocalyx injury and endothelial activation are associated with clinical outcomes in patients with sepsis: A systematic review and meta-analysis. Journal of Intensive Care Medicine. 2023;**38**(1):95-105

[3] Bone RC, Balk RA, Cerra FB, Dellinger RP, Fein AM, Knaus WA, et al. Definitions for sepsis and organ failure and guidelines for the use of innovative therapies in sepsis. The ACCP/SCCM Consensus Conference Committee. American College of Chest Physicians/Society of Critical Care Medicine. Chest. Jun 1992;**101**(6):1644-1655. DOI: 10.1378/chest.101.6.1644. PMID: 1303622

[4] Levy MM, Fink MP, Marshall JC, Abraham E, Angus D, Cook D, et al. 2001 SCCM/ESICM/ACCP/ATS/SIS international sepsis definitions conference. Critical Care Medicine. 2003;**31**:1250-1256

[5] Singer M, Deutschman CS, Seymour CW, et al. The third international consensus definitions for sepsis and septic shock (sepsis-3). Journal of the American Medical Association. 2016;**315**:801-810

[6] Bakker J, Gris P, Coffernils M, et al. Serial blood lactate levels can predict the development of multiple organ failure following septic shock. American Journal of Surgery. 1996;**171**(2):221-226

[7] Haas SA, Lange T, Saugel B, et al. Severe hyperlactatemia, lactate clearance and mortality in unselected critically ill patients. Intensive Care Medicine. 2016;**42**(2):202-210

[8] Khurana D, Deoke SA. Thrombocytopenia in critically ill patient: Clinical and laboratorial behavior and its correlation with short-term outcome during hospitalization. Indian Journal of Critical Care Medicine. 2017;**21**(12):861-864

[9] Medam S, Zieleskiewicz L, Duclos G, et al. Risk factors for death in septic shock: A retrospective cohort study comparing trauma and non-trauma patients. Medicine (Baltimore). 2017;**96**(50):e9241

[10] Sanderson CM, Blyth E, et al. Predicting 30-day mortality in patients with sepsis: An exploratory analysis of process of care and patient characteristics. Journal of the Intensive Care Society. 2018;**19**(4):299-304

[11] Song JE, Kim MH, Jeong WY, et al. Mortality risk factors for patients with septic shock after implementation of the surviving sepsis campaign bundles. Infection and Chemotherapy. 2016;**48**(3):199-208

[12] Iba T, Arakawa M, Mochizuki K, et al. Usefulness of measuring changes in SOFA score for the prediction of 28-day mortality in patients with sepsis-associated disseminated intravascular coagulation. Clinical and Applied Thrombosis/Hemostasis. 2019;**25**:1076029618824044

[13] Lambden S, Laterre PF, Levy MM, Francois B. The SOFA score-development, utility and challenges of

accurate assessment in clinical trials. Critical Care. 2019;**23**(1):374. DOI: 10.1186/s13054-019-2663-7

[14] Soares M, Dongelmans DA. Why should we not use APACHE II for performance measurement and benchmarking? Revista Brasileira de Terapia Intensiva. 2017;**29**(3):268-270. DOI: 10.5935/0103-507X.20170043. Epub 2017 Sep 4

[15] Chang JC. Sepsis and septic shock: Endothelial molecular pathogenesis associated with vascular microthrombotic disease. Thrombosis Journal. 2019;**17**:10

[16] Hou PC, Filbin MR, Wang H, et al. Endothelial permeability and hemostasis in septic shock: Results from the ProCESS trial. Chest. 2017;**152**(1):22-31

[17] Johansson P, Stensballe J, Ostrowski SR. Shock induced endotheliopathy (SHINE) in acute critical illness—A unifying pathophysiologic mechanism. Critical Care. 2017;**21**:25

[18] Nguyen T, Carcillo J. Bench-to-bedside review: Thrombocytopenia-associated multiple organ failure—A newly appreciated syndrome in the critically ill. Critical Care. 2006;**10**(6):235

[19] Rivers E, Nguyen B, Havstad S, Ressler J, Muzzin A, Knoblich B, et al. Early goal-directed therapy in the treatment of severe sepsis and septic shock. The New England Journal of Medicine. 2001;**345**(19):1368-1377. DOI: 10.1056/NEJMoa010307

[20] ARISE Investigators; ANZICS Clinical Trials Group, Peake SL, Delaney A, Bailey M, Bellomo R, Cameron PA, et al. Goal-directed resuscitation for patients with early septic shock. The New England Journal of Medicine. 2014;**371**(16):1496-1506

[21] Mouncey PR, Osborn TM, Power GS, Harrison DA, Sadique MZ, Grieve RD, et al. Trial of early, goal-directed resuscitation for septic shock. The New England Journal of Medicine. 2015;**372**(14):1301-1311

[22] ProCESS Investigators, Yealy DM, Kellum JA, Huang DT, Barnato AE, Weissfeld LA, et al. A randomized trial of protocol-based care for early septic shock. The New England Journal of Medicine. 2014;**370**(18):1683-1693

[23] Abraham E, Laterre PF, Garg R, et al. Drotrecogin alfa (activated) for adults with severe sepsis and a low risk of death. The New England Journal of Medicine. 2005;**353**(13):1332-1341

[24] Dellinger P, Bagshaw SM, Antonelli M, et al. Effect of targeted polymyxin B hemoperfusion on 28-day mortality in patients with septic shock and elevated endotoxin level: The EUPHRATES randomized clinical trial. Journal of the American Medical Association. 2018;**320**(14):1455-1463

[25] Fujii T, Luethi N, Young PJ, et al. Effect of vitamin C, hydrocortisone, and thiamine vs hydrocortisone alone on time alive and free of vasopressor support among patients with septic shock: The VITAMINS randomized clinical trial. Journal of the American Medical Association. 2020;**323**(5):423-431

[26] Venkatesh B, Finfer S, Cohen J, et al. Adjunctive glucocorticoid therapy in patients with septic shock. The New England Journal of Medicine. 2018;**378**(9):797-808

[27] Vincent JL, Francois B, Zabolotskikh I. Effect of a recombinant human soluble thrombomodulin on

mortality in patients with sepsis-associated coagulopathy: The SCARLET randomized clinical trial. Journal of the American Medical Association. 2019;**321**(20):1993-2002

[28] Seymour CW, Kennedy JN, Wang S, Chang CH, Elliott CF, Xu Z, et al. Derivation, validation, and potential treatment implications of novel clinical phenotypes for sepsis. Journal of the American Medical Association. 2019;**321**(20):2003-2017

[29] Ibarra-Estrada M, Kattan E, Aguilera-González P, Sandoval-Plascencia L, Rico-Jauregui U, Gómez-Partida CA, et al. Early adjunctive methylene blue in patients with septic shock: A randomized controlled trial. Critical Care. 2023;**27**(1):110

[30] Ankawi G, Neri M, Zhang J, et al. Extracorporeal techniques for the treatment of critically ill patients with sepsis beyond conventional blood purification therapy: The promises and the pitfalls. Critical Care. 2018;**22**(1):262

[31] Busund R, Lindsetmo RO, Rasmussen LT, Røkke O, et al. Tumor necrosis factor and interleukin 1 appearance in experimental gram-negative septic shock. The effects of plasma exchange with albumin and plasma infusion. Archives of Surgery. 1991;**126**(5):591-597

[32] Janbon B, Vuillez JP, Carpentier F, et al. Removal of circulating tumor necrosis factor. Its role in septic shock treatment. Annales de medecine interne (Paris). 1992;**143**(Suppl. 1):13-16

[33] Knaup H, Stahl K, Schmidt BMW, et al. Early therapeutic plasma exchange in septic shock: A prospective open-label nonrandomized pilot study focusing on safety, hemodynamics, vascular barrier function, and biologic markers. Critical Care. 2018;**22**:285

[34] Reeves JH, Butt WW, Layton JE, et al. Continuous plasmafiltration in sepsis syndrome. Plasmafiltration in sepsis study group. Critical Care Medicine. 1999;**27**(10):2096-2104

[35] Long EJ, Taylor A, Delzoppo, et al. A randomized controlled trial of plasma filtration in severe pediatric sepsis. Critical Care and Resuscitation. 2013;**15**(3):198-204

[36] Rimmer E, Houston BL, Kumar A, et al. The efficacy and safety of plasma exchange in patients with sepsis and septic shock: A systematic review and meta-analysis. Critical Care. 2014;**18**:699

[37] Barelli S, Alberio L. The role of plasma transfusion in massive bleeding: Protecting the endothelial glycocalyx? Frontiers in Medicine (Lausanne). 2018;**5**:91

[38] Busund R, Koukline V, Utrobin U, et al. Plasmapheresis in severe sepsis and septic shock: A prospective, randomized, controlled trial. Intensive Care Medicine. 2002;**28**:1434-1439

[39] Stegmayr BG, Banga R, Berggren L, et al. Plasma exchange as rescue therapy in multiple organ failure including acute renal failure. Critical Care. 2003;**31**(6):1730-1736

[40] Bernardo A, Ball C, Nolasco L, et al. Effects of inflammatory cytokines on the release and cleavage of the endothelial cell-derived ultralarge von Willebrand factor multimers under flow. Blood. 2004;**104**:100-110

[41] Ono T, Mimuro J, Madoiwa S, et al. Severe secondary deficiency of von Willebrand factor-cleaving protease (ADAMTS13) in patients

with sepsis-induced disseminated intravascular coagulation: Its correlation with development of renal failure. Blood. 2006;**107**:528-534

[42] Nguyen TC, Han YY, Kiss JE, et al. Intensive plasma exchange increases a disintegrin and metalloprotease with thrombospondin motifs-13 activity and reverses organ dysfunction in children with thrombocytopenia-associated multiple organ failure. Critical Care Medicine. 2008;**36**:2878-2288

[43] Fortenberry JD, Nguyen T, Grunwell JR, Aneja RK, Wheeler D, Hall M, et al. Therapeutic plasma exchange in children with thrombocytopenia-associated multiple organ failure: The thrombocytopenia-associated multiple organ failure network prospective experience. Critical Care Medicine. 2019;**47**(3):e173-e181

[44] Keith PD, Wells AH, Hodges J, Fast SH, Adams A, Scott LK. The therapeutic efficacy of adjunct therapeutic plasma exchange for septic shock with multiple organ failure: A single-center experience. Critical Care. 2020;**24**(1):518

[45] Weng J, Chen M, Fang D, Liu D, Guo R, Yang S. Therapeutic plasma exchange protects patients with sepsis-associated disseminated intravascular coagulation by improving endothelial function. Clinical and Applied Thrombosis/Hemostasis. Jan-Dec 2021;**27**:1-10

[46] Afshar M, Foster CL, Layden JE, Burnham EL. Azithromycin use and outcomes in severe sepsis patients with and without pneumonia. Journal of Critical Care. 2016;**32**:120-125

[47] Chen M, Ji M, Si X. The effects of statin therapy on mortality in patients with sepsis: A meta-analysis of randomized trials. Medicine (Baltimore). 2018;**97**(31):e11578

[48] Garcia PC, Longhi F, Branco RG, Piva JP, Lacks D, Tasker RC. Ferritin levels in children with severe sepsis and septic shock. Acta Paediatrica. 2007;**96**(12):1829-1831

[49] Demirkol D, Yildizdas D, Bayrakci B, et al. Hyperferritinemia in the critically ill child with secondary hemophagocyticlymphohistiocytosis/sepsis/multiple organ dysfunction syndrome/macrophage activation syndrome: What is the treatment? Critical Care. 2012;**16**:R52

[50] Mehta P, McAuley DF, Brown M, Sanchez E, Tattersal RS, Manson JJ. COVID-19: Consider cytokine storm syndromes and immunosuppression. Lancet. 2020;**395**(10229):1033-1034

[51] Kaushal K, Kaur H, Sarma P, et al. Serum ferritin as a predictive biomarker in COVID-19. A systematic review, meta-analysis and meta-regression analysis. Journal of Critical Care. 2022;**67**:172-181

[52] Ruan Q, Yang K, Wang W, Jiang L, Song J. Clinical predictors of mortality due to COVID-19 based on an analysis of data of 150 patients from Wuhan, China. Intensive Care Medicine. 2020;**46**:846-848

[53] Zhou F, Yu T, Du R, et al. Clinical course and risk factors for mortality of adult inpatients with COVID-19 in Wuhan, China: A retrospective cohort study. Lancet. 2020;**395**(10229):1054-1062

[54] Keith P, Day M, Perkins L, Moyer L, Hewitt K, Wells A. A novel treatment approach to the novel coronavirus: An argument for the use of therapeutic plasma exchange for fulminant COVID-19. Critical Care. 2020;**24**(1):128

[55] Gucyetmez B, Atalan HK, Sertdemir I, Cakir U, Telci L. Therapeutic plasma exchange in patients with COVID-19 pneumonia in intensive care unit: A retrospective study. Critical Care. 2020;**24**(1):492

[56] Keith PD, Scott LK, Weaver KE, Day M, Choe C, Perkins L, et al. Treatment of critically ill coronavirus disease 2019 patients with adjunct therapeutic plasma exchange: A single-center retrospective case series. Critical Care Explorations. 2021;**2**(9):1-5, e0223

[57] Khamis F, Al-Zakwani I, Al Hashmi S, Al Dowaiki S, Al Bahrani M, Pandak N, et al. Therapeutic plasma exchange in adults with severe COVID-19 infection. International Journal of Infectious Diseases. 2020;**99**:214-218

[58] Faqihi F, Alharthy A, Abdulaziz S, Balhamar A, Alomari A, AlAseri Z, et al. Therapeutic plasma exchange in patients with life-threatening COVID-19: A randomised controlled clinical trial. International Journal of Antimicrobial Agents. 2021;**57**(5):106334

[59] Beraud M, Hashami SA, Lozano M, Bah A, Keith P. Role of therapeutic plasma exchange in the management of COVID-19-induced cytokine storm syndrome. Transfusion and Apheresis Science. 2022;**61**(4):103433

[60] Connelly-Smith L, Alquist CR, Aqui NA, Hofmann JC, Klingel R, Onwuemene OA, et al. Guidelines on the use of therapeutic apheresis in clinical practice—Evidence-based approach from the writing Committee of the American Society for apheresis: The ninth special issue. Journal of Clinical Apheresis. 2023;**38**(2):77-278

[61] Kuklin V, Sovershaev M, Bjerner J, Keith P, Scott LK, Thomas OMT, et al. Influence of therapeutic plasma exchange treatment on short-term mortality of critically ill adult patients with sepsis-induced organ dysfunction: A systematic review and meta-analysis. Critical Care. 2024;**28**(1):12

[62] Chen JJ, Lai PC, Lee TH, Huang YT. Blood purification for adult patients with severe infection or sepsis/septic shock: A network meta-analysis of randomized controlled trials. Critical Care Medicine. 1 Dec 2023;**51**(12):1777-1789

[63] Lee OPE, Kanesan N, Leow EH, Sultana R, Chor YK, Gan CS, et al. Survival benefits of therapeutic plasma exchange in severe sepsis and septic shock: A systematic review and meta-analysis. Journal of Intensive Care Medicine. 2023;**38**(7):598-611

[64] Yan D, Yao R, Xie X, Fu X, Pei S, Wang Y, et al. The therapeutic efficacy of plasmapheresis for sepsis with multiple organ failure: A propensity score-matched analysis based on the MIMIC-IV database. Shock. May 2024;**61**(5):685-694

[65] Stahl K, Wand P, Seeliger B, Wendel-Garcia PD, Schmidt JJ, Schmidt BMW, et al. Clinical and biochemical endpoints and predictors of response to plasma exchange in septic shock: Results from a randomized controlled trial. Critical Care. 2022;**26**(1):134

[66] David S, Bode C, Stahl K, EXCHANGE-2 Study group. EXCHANGE-2: Investigating the efficacy of add-on plasma exchange as an adjunctive strategy against septic shock-a study protocol for a randomized, prospective, multicenter, open-label, controlled, parallel-group trial. Trials. 2023;**24**(1):277

[67] Rimmer E. Therapeutic plasma exchange in septic shock: A pilot study (PLEXSIS). 2023-2026. Identifier

NCT05093075. Available from: https://clinicaltrials.gov/study/NCT05093075

[68] Hwa C, Sebastian A, Aird WC. Endothelial biomedicine: Its status as an interdisciplinary field, its progress as a basic science, and its translational bench-to-bedside gap. Endothelium. 2005;**12**(3):139-151

[69] Schouten M, Wiersinga WJ, Levi M, van der Poll T. Inflammation, endothelium, and coagulation in sepsis. Journal of Leukocyte Biology. 2008;**83**(3):536-545

[70] Joffre J, Hellman J, Ince C, Ait-Oufella H. Endothelial responses in sepsis. American Journal of Respiratory and Critical Care Medicine. 2020;**202**(3):361-370

[71] Ince C, Mayeux PR, Nguyen T, Gomez H, Kellum JA, Ospina-Tascón GA, et al. The endothelium in sepsis. Shock. 2016;**45**(3):259-270

[72] Gong T, Liu Y-T, Fan J. Exosomal mediators in sepsis and inflammatory organ injury: Unraveling the role of exosomes in intercellular crosstalk and organ dysfunction. Military Medical Research. 2024;**11**(1):24

[73] Alonso-Roman R, Mosig AS, Figge MT, Papenfort K, Eggeling C, Schacher FH, et al. Organ-on-chip models for infectious disease research. Nature Microbiology. 2024;**9**(4):891-904

[74] Kastner M, Karner A, Zhu R, Huang Q, Geissner A, Sadewasser A, et al. Relevance of host cell surface glycan structure for cell specificity of influenza a viruses. Viruses. 2023;**15**(7)

[75] Foote CA, Soares RN, Ramirez-Perez FI, Ghiarone T, Aroor A, Manrique-Acevedo C, et al. Endothelial glycocalyx. Comprehensive Physiology. 2022;**12**(4):3781-3811

[76] Offeddu GS, Hajal C, Foley CR, Wan Z, Ibrahim L, Coughlin MF, et al. The cancer glycocalyx mediates intravascular adhesion and extravasation during metastatic dissemination. Communications Biology. 2021;**4**(1):255

[77] Jacob M, Chappell D, Becker BF. Regulation of blood flow and volume exchange across the microcirculation. Critical Care. 2016;**20**(1):319

[78] Zhang H, Wang Y, Qu M, Li W, Wu D, Cata JP, et al. Neutrophil, neutrophil extracellular traps and endothelial cell dysfunction in sepsis. Clinical and Translational Medicine. 2023;**13**(1):e1170

[79] Piplani N, Roy T, Saxena N, Sen S. Bulky glycocalyx shields cancer cells from invasion-associated stresses. Translational Oncology. 2024;**39**:101822

[80] Hamrangsekachaee M, Wen K, Yazdani N, Willits RK, Bencherif SA, Ebong EE. Endothelial glycocalyx sensitivity to chemical and mechanical sub-endothelial substrate properties. Frontiers in Bioengineering and Biotechnology. 2023;**11**:1250348

[81] Yu H, Song Y-Y, Li X-H. Early diabetic kidney disease: Focus on the glycocalyx. World Journal of Diabetes. 2023;**14**(5):460-480

[82] Levick JR, Michel CC. Microvascular fluid exchange and the revised Starling principle. Cardiovascular Research. 2010;**87**(2):198-210

[83] Jacob M, Chappell D. Reappraising starling: The physiology of the microcirculation. Current Opinion in Critical Care. 2013;**19**(4):282-289

[84] Chappell D, Jacob M, Becker BF, Hofmann-Kiefer K, Conzen P, Rehm M, et al. A newly discovered "great barrier reef". Der Anaesthesist. 2008;**57**(10):959-969

[85] Iba T, Levy JH. Derangement of the endothelial glycocalyx in sepsis. Journal of Thrombosis and Haemostasis. 2019;**17**(2):283-294

[86] Wautier JL, Wautier MP. Vascular permeability in diseases. International Journal of Molecular Sciences. 2022;**23**(7):3645-3660

[87] Ong T, McClintock DE, Kallet RH, Ware LB, Matthay MA, Liu KD. Ratio of angiopoietin-2 to angiopoietin-1 as a predictor of mortality in acute lung injury patients. Critical Care Medicine. 2010;**38**(9):1845-1851

[88] Lukasz A, Hillgruber C, Oberleithner H, Kusche-Vihrog K, Pavenstädt H, Rovas A, et al. Endothelial glycocalyx breakdown is mediated by angiopoietin-2. Cardiovascular Research. 2017;**113**(6):671-680

[89] Kernan KF, Carcillo JA. Hyperferritinemia and inflammation. International Immunology. 2017;**29**(9):401-409

[90] Fang YP, Zhang HJ, Guo Z, Ren CH, Zhang YF, Liu Q, et al. Effect of serum ferritin on the prognosis of patients with sepsis: Data from the MIMIC-IV database. Emergency Medicine International. 2022;**2022**:2104755

[91] Missano Florido M, Assunção M, Mazza B, Jackiu M, Freitas F, Bafi A, et al. Evaluation of iron, transferrin and ferritin serum levels in patients with severe sepsis and septic shock. Critical Care. 2012;**16**(1):P424

[92] Karakike E, Giamarellos-Bourboulis EJ. Macrophage activation-like syndrome: A distinct entity leading to early death in sepsis. Frontiers in Immunology. 2019;**10**:55

[93] Carcillo JA, Shakoory B, Castillo L. Secondary hemophagocytic lymphohistiocytosis, macrophage activation syndrome, and hyperferritinemic sepsis-induced multiple-organ dysfunction syndrome in the pediatric ICU. In: Mastropietro CW, Valentine KM, editors. Pediatric Critical Care: Current Controversies. Cham: Springer International Publishing; 2019. pp. 245-255

[94] Imashuku S, Hibi S. Cytokines in hemophagocytic syndrome. British Journal of Haematology. 1991;**77**(3):438-440

[95] Boeddha NP, Bycroft T, Nadel S, Hazelzet JA. The inflammatory and hemostatic response in sepsis and meningococcemia. Critical Care Clinics. 2020;**36**(2):391-399

[96] Diehl JL, Borgel D. Sepsis and coagulation. Current Opinion in Critical Care. 2005;**11**(5):454-460

[97] Kaplan KL. Coagulation activation in sepsis. Critical Care Medicine. 2000;**28**(2):585-586

[98] Jacobi J. The pathophysiology of sepsis-2021 update: Part 1, immunology and coagulopathy leading to endothelial injury. American Journal of Health-System Pharmacy. 2022;**79**(5):329-337

[99] Levi M, van der Poll T. Coagulation and sepsis. Thrombosis Research. 2017;**149**:38-44

[100] Bui-Thi HD, Le Minh K. Coagulation profiles in patients with sepsis/septic shock identify mixed hypo-hypercoagulation patterns based on rotational thromboelastometry:

A prospective observational study. Thrombosis Research. 2023;**227**:51-59

[101] Cox D. Sepsis—It is all about the platelets. Frontiers in Immunology. 2023;**14**:1210219

[102] Tsao CM, Ho ST, Wu CC. Coagulation abnormalities in sepsis. Acta Anaesthesiologica Taiwanica. 2015;**53**(1):16-22

[103] Luo C, Hu H, Gong J, Zhou Y, Chen Z, Cai S. The value of thromboelastography in the diagnosis of sepsis-induced coagulopathy. Clinical and Applied Thrombosis/Hemostasis. 2020;**26**:1076029620951847

[104] Keklik M, Çelik S, Yıldızhan E. Comparison of centrifugal and membrane filtration modalities on therapeutic plasma exchange. Journal of Clinical Apheresis. 2022;**37**(3):217-222

[105] Yetimakman AF, Kesici S, Bayrakci B. Plasma filtration versus centrifugation in pediatric therapeutic plasma exchange: Should the diagnosis define the method?†. Therapeutic Apheresis and Dialysis. 2020;**24**(1):85-89

[106] Malchesky PS, Koo AP, Roberson GA, Hadsell AT, Rybicki LA. Apheresis technologies and clinical applications: The 2005 international apheresis registry. Therapeutic Apheresis and Dialysis. 2007;**11**(5):341-362

[107] Ipe TS, Marques MB. Vascular access for therapeutic plasma exchange. Transfusion. 2018;**58**(2):580-589

[108] Shunkwiler SM, Pham HP, Wool G, Ipe TS, Fang DC, Biller E, et al. The management of anticoagulation in patients undergoing therapeutic plasma exchange: A concise review. Journal of Clinical Apheresis. 2018;**33**(3):371-379

Chapter 8

Clinical and Laboratory Parameters as Biomarkers for Diagnosis and Prognosis of Sepsis in Patients Admitted to Intensive Care Units

Eduardo Almeida de Souza Minuzzo,
Pauline Brendler Goettems Fiorin, Vítor Antunes de Oliveira,
Mirna Stela Ludwig and Matias Nunes Frizzo

Abstract

The Intensive Care Unit (ICU) has the highest incidence of patients with various infectious processes. Sepsis, a systemic inflammatory response syndrome associated with infections, is characterized by inflammatory cytokine production, innate immune system activation, mitochondrial damage, and severe organ dysfunction. Early diagnosis is crucial for appropriate therapeutic interventions and reducing mortality. Various biomarkers have been studied for diagnostic and prognostic purposes, including lactate, interleukins, C-reactive protein, and procalcitonin. Immune-inflammatory biomarkers, such as leukogram, leukocyte ratios, neutrophil variation index, and leukocyte morphological parameters, provide valuable information about sepsis severity and progression. Additionally, redox state and cellular stress response biomarkers contribute to understanding sepsis pathophysiology and organ dysfunction stratification. The combined use of these biomarkers allows for more accurate diagnoses, early treatment, reduced hospital stays, minimized sequelae, and decreased sepsis mortality risk. This chapter describes the applicability of clinical and laboratory parameters as biomarkers for diagnosing and prognosing infectious processes and sepsis in ICU patients.

Keywords: sepsis, intensive care unit (ICU), biomarkers, diagnosis, prognosis

1. Introduction

The Intensive Care Unit (ICU) is a hospital unit designed to receive critically ill patients in order to monitor, diagnose, and treat them through intensive care provided by a specialized team proficient in the use of specific equipment, technologies, and treatment of severe clinical decompensations. Among the pathologies treated in the

ICU are infections, which can be associated with sepsis, resulting from the interaction of pathogenic microorganisms with susceptible individuals, leading to inflammatory organic alterations with local or systemic repercussions [1].

The Surviving Sepsis Campaign's 2021 guidelines define sepsis as a life-threatening organ dysfunction secondary to a dysregulated host response to infection. In sepsis, the infection generates reactions against its own organs and tissues, causing high rates of morbidity and mortality, especially when not correctly diagnosed and treated. Sepsis and its complication, septic shock, impact millions of people worldwide, potentially causing death in every six to every three of ten affected individuals [2, 3].

The World Health Organization estimates that sepsis affects approximately 48.9 million people annually, resulting in about 11 million deaths worldwide. There are significant regional differences in incidence, with 85% of sepsis-related deaths occurring in low- and middle-income countries. In Brazil, there were 463 thousand deaths from sepsis between 2010 and 2019, with an average standardized death coefficient of 22.8 per 100,000 inhabitants, predominantly in the elderly followed by the 50- to 59-year-old age group. Analyzing sepsis mortality rates in Brazilian regions, the southeast had the highest rate, observed in São Paulo with 34.2 deaths/100,000 inhabitants; in the south, the state of Rio Grande do Sul had the highest rate with 30.8 deaths/100,000 inhabitants; in the north, Amazonas showed the highest rate with 16.2 deaths/100,000 inhabitants; in the northeast, the state of Pernambuco presented the highest rate with 27.8 deaths/100,000 inhabitants, and in the Midwest, the highest rate was observed in Mato Grosso with 22.6 deaths/100,000 inhabitants [4].

Early identification and establishment of appropriate measures in the initial hours of sepsis development improve outcomes, while negative outcomes are observed when diagnosis and treatment are delayed. Despite the importance of early detection, there is no established gold standard for diagnosis, and sepsis screening tools are designed to promote early identification, being used in various locations, such as in-patient wards, emergency departments, or intensive care units [2]. Tools for sepsis screening are based on various clinical parameters, and the most recommended currently for early identification of infection-induced organ dysfunction are the systemic inflammatory response syndrome (SIRS) criteria, with better sensitivity compared to the quick Sequential Organ Failure Assessment (qSOFA) [5].

In addition to clinical parameters, host response biomarkers play an important role in both the diagnosis and recognition of infections and organ dysfunction, as well as in risk stratification, prognosis, and patient management. Laboratory parameters include acute-phase proteins, cytokines, chemokines, damage-associated molecular patterns (DAMPs), endothelial cell markers, leukocyte surface markers, noncoding RNAs, miRNAs, soluble receptors, as well as metabolites and gene expression changes. These laboratory parameters are used as inflammatory biomarkers, including proteins and cellular molecules related to nucleic acids, although their high cost minimizes their greater use [6].

Considering the definition of sepsis, which is based on the presence of inflammation-induced organ dysfunction resulting from the imbalance between tissue perfusion and metabolic tissue needs, global tissue hypoperfusion leads to various clinical manifestations, such as arterial hypotension, decreased capillary refill time, cold skin, and extremities, which can be used as defining clinical parameters of sepsis [7]. In this context, lactate already has a well-defined association with mortality in patients suspected of infection and sepsis, and it is suggested to be used for screening in undifferentiated adult patients with suspected sepsis. The presence of elevated or normal lactate levels significantly increases or decreases the suspicion of the final diagnosis of sepsis in suspected patients, and it can even be used as a perfusion biomarker [2].

Another important factor involved in the pathogenesis of sepsis is the production of reactive oxygen species (ROS), which include hydrogen peroxide (H_2O_2), superoxide (O_2^-), and hydroxyl radicals (HO^-). ROS are produced by the activated NADPH oxidase complex and prepare the immune cell for response to aggressive microorganisms; however, excessive activation and production of these reactive species promote endothelial injury, cell damage, and organ failure [8].

In association with oxidative stress present in sepsis, heat shock proteins (HSPs) can also be considered biomarkers associated with sepsis and modulation of the immune-inflammatory state. Heat shock proteins, including the most phylogenetically conserved, the 70 Kilodalton protein (HSP70), play important roles in the intracellular milieu as chaperone activity, correction of damaged proteins, and assist in protein folding and unfolding, exerting a cytoprotective effect. However, when located in the extracellular milieu, they have a pro-inflammatory effect. In the case of sepsis, when immune cells are exposed to bacterial toxins, there is increased export to the extracellular milieu, increasing their serum concentration, especially modulating the immune-inflammatory picture, as during fever related to bacterial infection [9].

Furthermore, the pathophysiology of sepsis also includes a hyper-inflammatory phase, in which immune cell destruction by apoptosis occurs and an increase in regulatory T cells expression, which leads to complement system stimulation, coagulation system activation, vascular endothelium, neutrophils, and platelets activation, which play an important role in the inflammatory responses that occur in sepsis, justifying the importance of using immunohematological biomarkers in evaluating this clinical condition, as well as in its follow-up. Among these alterations, an increase in neutrophil counts, appearance of immature granulocytes, immature granulocyte index (IG or Delta Neutrophil Index—DNI), and leukocyte morphology evaluation are observed. In addition, leukocyte quantitative analysis using detection of neutrophil-lymphocyte ratio (NLR), monocyte-lymphocyte ratio (MLR), platelet-lymphocyte ratio (PLR), mean platelet volume-platelet count (MPV/PC) ratio, and mean platelet volume-platelet distribution width (MPV/PDW) ratio may play an important evaluation role in both diagnosis, prognosis, and patient monitoring [10, 11]. The use of these parameters can aid in both diagnosis and monitoring of sepsis, such as the appearance of immature cells and their relationship with leukocyte consumption, platelet activation, and risk for disseminated intravascular coagulation (DIC) development, and also infer about cell apoptosis [12].

Considering the prevalence of sepsis and its high mortality rate, early identification and institution of appropriate treatment are essential to achieve success in the outcome of patients with sepsis. Adequate treatment includes the initiation of broad-spectrum antibiotic therapy directed to the possible focus of infection. Despite this recommendation, the prevalence of infection by multidrug-resistant germs in patients with sepsis is not well established, nor is the use of laboratory biomarkers that assist in early diagnosis and also have prognostic capacity. In this sense, we understand that the increase in these biomarkers in the evaluation of patients with infectious processes and sepsis may allow correct, early diagnosis, as well as the introduction of early appropriate treatment, ensuring the patient shorter hospital length of stay as well as reduction of sequelae and lower risk of sepsis-related mortality. Thus, this chapter aims to describe the applicability of clinical and laboratory parameters as diagnostic and prognostic biomarkers in infectious processes and sepsis in patients admitted to the ICU.

2. The intensive care unit (ICU)

The Intensive Care Unit (ICU) is a specialized hospital unit dedicated to the treatment of patients who require life support and those at high risk of organ failure and death, providing care for severely ill patients such as those with respiratory failure, acute kidney injury, cardiovascular disorders, and sepsis, among others [13]. Effective life support requires a personalized approach, following pre-established standards aimed at recovering the sick individual, with flexible decisions within the ICU. Fundamental elements of intensive care therapy include therapeutic procedures, frequent and continuous reassessment, and timely correction throughout the patient's evolving course [6].

This unit is classified in levels, standing level 1 for the unit capable of providing oxygen, noninvasive monitoring, and more intensive nursing care. Level 2 ICU is the unit that can provide invasive monitoring and basic life support for a short period, and level 3 ICU provides a full spectrum of monitoring and life support technologies [14].

The ICU also is classified according to the type of assistance. Medical ICU (MICU) is the unit that provides assistance to severe medical illnesses like diabetes, seizures, and chronic obstructive pulmonary disease. Cardiac ICU is dedicated to the treatment of severe heart diseases (heart attack, congestive heart disease, etc.). Neuro ICU being the unit designated to treat patients with stroke and other neurological conditions. Surgical ICU (SICU) offers care to unstable, severely, or potentially severely ill patients in the perioperative setting [15, 16].

According to Resolution CFM No. 2156/2016, which defines criteria to improve the flow of care in the ICU, admission to the sector should be given primarily to patients requiring life support interventions, with a high probability of recovery and no limitation of therapeutic support. Thus, patients diagnosed with infectious processes, who have a high probability of recovery, are given priority for admission, if they are not associated with irreversible terminal diseases or conditions without the possibility of recovery [17].

3. Infectious processes

Infectious diseases have been a constant companion of humanity since time immemorial, decimating populations through epidemics and everyday infections. Robert Koch and contemporaries demonstrated that certain microorganisms are the cause of various human diseases and that these infectious processes confer the leading cause of morbidity and mortality [18].

From the perspective of infectious diseases, any microorganism capable of causing disease is a pathogen. The classification of pathogens is not absolute because it continues to evolve and adapt, with microorganisms included in one of the following groups: commensals, obligate pathogens, opportunistic pathogens, zoonotic pathogens, and environmental pathogens. Pathogenic microorganisms do not have the same degree of virulence, meaning they do not have the same likelihood of causing disease, being influenced by factors of the host itself such as immunity and nutritional status, among others.

Representatives of pathogenic microorganisms include bacteria, protozoa, helminths, fungi, and viruses, with their disease-causing abilities related to degrees of virulence and their relationships with host factors. Among the main causative agents of infectious processes, particularly severe ones like sepsis, are bacteria. In bacteria, surface structures are phylogenetically conserved, such as lipopolysaccharides (LPS) in Gram-negatives and lipoteichoic acid and lipopeptides in Gram-positives, which are commonly considered the main triggers of the host's inflammatory response to bacterial infection. However, these differences cannot explain why some bacteria cause more severe infections and a higher frequency of sepsis than others, with bacterial virulence potentially mediated by toxins, which are responsible for the progression and outcome of sepsis [19].

4. Sepsis

4.1 Concept

Sepsis is a condition that has significant impact on the health of affected individuals, as well as on healthcare systems, and thus efforts to define it have been expended. In the consensus of 1992, ratified in 2003, sepsis was defined as a systemic inflammatory response syndrome caused by an infectious process. This concept was revised in 2021, and the Surviving Sepsis Campaign's guidelines define sepsis as a life-threatening organ dysfunction secondary to a dysregulated host response to infection, Septic shock corresponds to circulatory, cellular, and metabolic abnormalities severe enough to increase mortality [2, 20].

4.2 Etiology

According to the new definition of sepsis, an infectious process corresponds to the triggering factor for the host's dysregulated response with consequent organ dysfunction [21]. The infectious diagnosis is essential and will guide a significant part of the management of sepsis. The clinical symptoms of sepsis and infection are many and can be nonspecific, such as fever, chills, and malaise. Specific symptoms may arise according to the infectious focus, such as productive cough in pneumonia and pain and discomfort when urinating in urinary tract infection. Once the infection and sepsis progress, symptoms of organ dysfunction begin to appear, including confusion, reduced urine output, and dyspnea, among others, depending on the compromised organs [22].

In addition to the importance of recognizing and treating infections related to sepsis, it is also necessary to emphasize the association with multidrug-resistant germs, as they require broad-spectrum antibiotics to ensure effective therapy. Methicillin-resistant *Staphylococcus aureus* (MRSA) accounts for approximately 5% of positive culture infections in critically ill patients, with regional variations in incidence (approximately 2% in Eastern Europe to 10% in North America). Individual characteristics and risk factors also occur, including a history of previous MRSA infection or colonization, recent use of intravenous antibiotics, previous recurrent skin infection or chronic wounds, presence of invasive devices, hemodialysis, recent hospitalization, and disease severity [2].

Gram-negative infections also play an important role in public health, affecting both healthy individuals and those with preexisting comorbidities but are particularly dangerous in vulnerable populations such as the elderly and hospitalized patients. The association of sepsis with gram-negative germ infection should also be considered when there is evidence of previous infection or colonization by antibiotic-resistant microorganisms in the past year, local prevalence of multidrug-resistant germs, healthcare-associated infections, use of broad-spectrum antibiotics in the last 90 days, concomitant use of selective digestive tract decontaminants, and recent hospitalization. Some individuals may be at particular risk for fungal infections, such as those with febrile neutropenia, who fail to defervesce after 4–7 days of broad-spectrum antibiotic therapy, or those with immunosuppression. Sepsis and septic shock associated with fungi are most commonly observed in ICUs and are associated with worse outcomes (**Figure 1**) [23].

4.3 Pathogenesis

The inflammatory imbalance is the cornerstone of sepsis pathogenesis. The host's initial response to invasive pathogens includes macrophage phagocytosis and the production of various pro-inflammatory cytokines, which can trigger a cytokine storm and activation of the innate immune system, mediated by pattern recognition receptors (PRRs), initiating activation in immune cells by detecting damage-associated molecular patterns (DAMPs) or pathogen-associated molecular patterns (PAMPs). This activated immune response involves PRRs interactions with exogenous factors derived from pathogens and endogenous factors released by damaged cells. In addition to changes in innate immune response, dysfunctions in cellular and humoral immune responses occur, manifested by low production of cytokines such as tumor necrosis factor (TNF), and interleukins 1 (IL-1) and 6 (IL-6), as well as the apoptosis of T and B cells and dendritic cells, contributing to a shift in the immune system toward developing an immune suppressive anti-inflammatory response [21].

Mitochondrial damage is another important factor evidenced in sepsis, where cellular metabolic disturbances, insufficient energy production, and oxidative stress are observed, promoting the apoptosis of cells composing the organs as well as immune cells, resulting in immune disturbances, multiple organ failure, and death. Additionally, autophagy occurs in the cellular environment, inducing cell death through a catabolic process involving lysosomal degradation and recycling of cytoplasmic components, which promotes further tissue function loss [24].

In addition to inflammatory changes, there is an imbalance between tissue perfusion and metabolic needs, caused by inflammation-induced cardiac dysfunction and redistribution of blood volume, associated with impaired tissue oxygen utilization. These alterations manifest clinically as arterial hypotension, decreased capillary refill time, the presence of cutaneous mottling, and cold extremities [7].

Hypotension arises as a result of injury, microcirculatory dysfunction, and increased capillary permeability promoting greater fluid extravasation, also mediated by the release of inflammatory molecules. Some individuals also experience a state of systemic vasodilation that prevents perfusion despite adequate resuscitation. Arterial and venous vasodilation is caused by failure of contraction of smooth muscle in the vascular wall and results in reduced pressure gradient, hindering proper venous

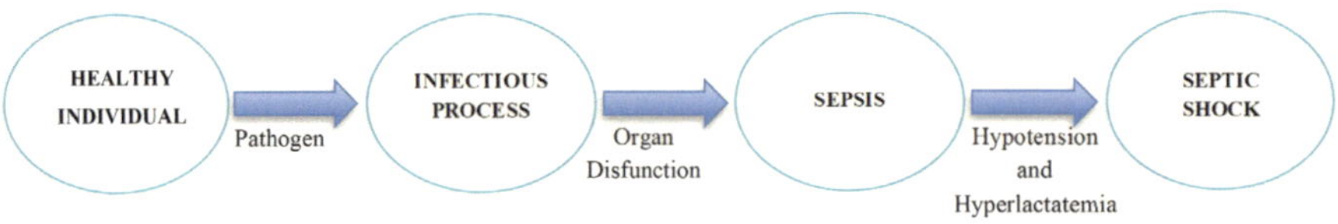

Figure 1.
Diagram for infectious process and sepsis. Flowchart of the development from infectious processes to sepsis. Source: Prepared by the authors.

return and thus compromising cardiac output. In these patients, adequate resuscitation with fluids and vasopressors allows hemodynamic stabilization, increasing venous return and promoting a hyperdynamic state characterized by increased cardiac output and low systemic vascular resistance. However, inflammatory cytokines can also cause myocardial depression with impaired contraction due to mitochondrial dysfunction in myocytes, manifested by left ventricular dysfunction, leading to hypokinesis and reduced stroke volume [7].

Cellular lesions result from reduced oxygen supply with incomplete oxidative reactions, leading to increased production of free radicals and impairment of the antioxidant system machinery. In parallel, exposure to DAMPs or PAMPs induces the release of inflammatory cytokines by activated leukocytes, causing increased production of reactive nitrogen species (RNS) such as nitric oxide, resulting in irreversible inhibition of the electron transfer chain and worsening of mitochondrial damage. Finally, mitochondrial matrix expansion and rupture occur, initiating apoptosis and autophagy [21].

As a result of changes in immune response, hypotension, and circulatory alterations, coagulation disorders occur, impacting the development of organ failures, manifested through disseminated intravascular coagulation, an acquired syndrome characterized by intravascular coagulation activation with loss of localization and potential microcirculation damage. Coagulation disorders occur as a consequence of impairment of one or more of the three physiological anticoagulation systems: the tissue factor inhibitor system, the protein C activation system, and the antithrombotic system (**Figure 2**) [21, 25].

4.4 Pathophysiology

Infection triggers a complex cascade of changes in order to recognize the infection, control pathogen spread, and initiate the repair mechanisms. Most processes resolve with localized inflammation (heat, redness, and swelling), but more severe infections or those caused by more virulent pathogens can trigger systemic responses with signs such as fever, tachycardia, tachypnea, and progress to involve tissues at other sites, causing organ dysfunction, and consequently shock. The most common sites of infection are pulmonary, abdominal, and urinary tract [26].

The host's innate immune system's initial detection after infection is to recognize pathogen-associated molecular patterns, mediated by PRRs, including Toll-like receptors (TLRs), retinoic acid-inducible gene 1-like receptors, NOD-like receptors, and C-type lectin receptors. For most infections, the host's innate immune system can eliminate the pathogen through pro-inflammatory responses, including: release of cytokines and chemokines such as tumor necrosis factor (TNF) and interleukins 1β, 12, and 18; recruitment of phagocytes; and local activation of complement and coagulation systems. Among patients with sepsis, pathogens cannot be eliminated by the host's immune system, leading to immune system homeostasis disruption, resulting in excessive inflammation and immune suppression [27].

The excessive inflammation in sepsis is mediated through the release of pro-inflammatory mediators by leukocytes, parenchymal cells, endothelium, and platelets. Injury to leukocytes and parenchymal cells results in the release of damage-associated molecular patterns, subsequently disrupting the host's response through the activation of various PRRs, which can also recognize pathogen-associated molecular patterns, triggering a vicious cycle involving injury and organ dysfunction. Moreover, the coagulation system, complement system, neutrophils, and vascular

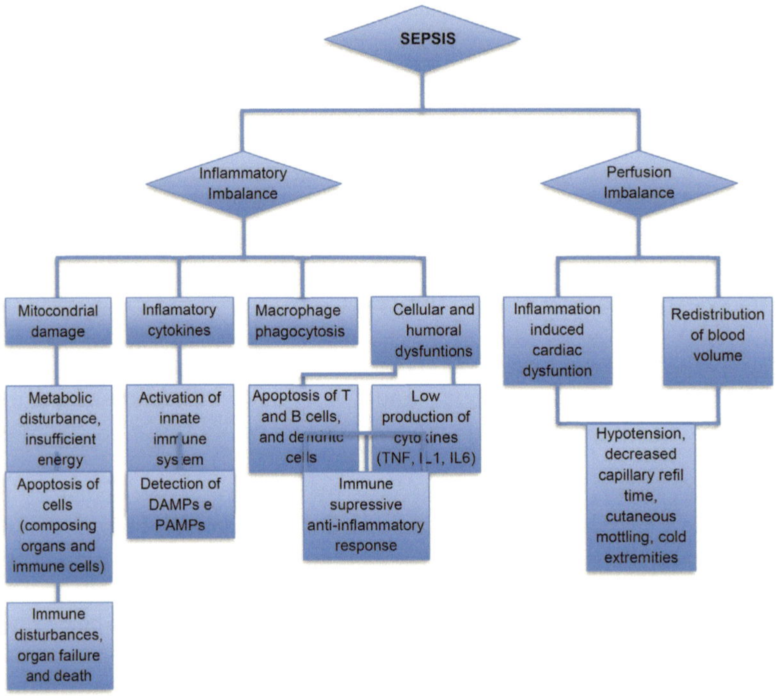

Figure 2.
Diretrizes de conscientização sobre sepse do CDC. Flowchart of the sepsis awareness guidelines from CDC considering leadership commitment, accountability, multi-professional expertise, action, tracking, reporting, and education. Source: Prepared by the authors.

endothelium are also activated in this phase. In the immune suppression stage, both innate and adaptive immune systems are involved. This phase is characterized by apoptosis of T cells, B cells, and dendritic cells, T cell exhaustion, and expansion of regulatory T cells and myeloid-derived suppressor cell populations. Patients with sepsis have an increased number of myeloid-derived suppressor cells, which are immature myeloid cells that can hinder immune responses, particularly T cell function. Reprogramming of antigen-presenting cells leads to reduced expression of HLA-DR and decreased ability to produce pro-inflammatory cytokines. In this sense, in the septic clinical picture, the most important findings are delayed neutrophil apoptosis and the appearance of immature band neutrophils in peripheral blood, which have deficient antimicrobial function [27].

4.5 Diagnosis

Sepsis presents with various clinical manifestations, and depending on the origin of the initial infection, it may not be evident until more advanced stages of the disease course, when its signs and symptoms become obvious. Also, the existence of other health conditions that can mimic sepsis should be considered, such as acute pulmonary embolism, acute myocardial infarction, acute pancreatitis, transfusion reactions, adrenal crisis, alcohol withdrawal, and thyrotoxicosis [28].

Early determination of sepsis to ensure appropriate treatment has a significant impact on morbidity and mortality. Tools for sepsis detection are established to promote its early identification and consist of methods that utilize clinical variables such as the criteria of systemic inflammatory response syndrome (SIRS), vital signs, signs of infection, quick sequential organ failure assessment (qSOFA), sequential organ failure assessment (SOFA) criteria, National Early Warning Score (NEWS), or Modified Early Warning Score (MEWS). These tools should be capable of assessing and detecting sepsis in various healthcare settings, such as hospital wards, emergency departments, or intensive care units [2, 29].

Currently, qSOFA is not recommended for sepsis identification due to its low sensitivity (despite high specificity) when compared with SIRS criteria for early sepsis diagnosis. To determine the presence of SIRS, two or more of the following criteria are necessary: (1) - body temperature above 38 or below 36 degrees Celsius; (20 - heart rate above 90 beats per minute; (3) - respiratory rate above 20 breaths per minute or partial pressure of carbon dioxide (CO_2) less than 32 mmHg; and (4) - white blood cell count above 12,000 or below 4000 per cubic millimeter (mm^3) or above 10% immature forms [2, 29].

4.6 Prognosis, monitoring, and outcome

Early diagnosis and appropriate treatment instituted have a significant impact on the prognosis and outcome of patients with sepsis, which can also be influenced by other factors such as disease severity, assessed through severity scales (e.g., APACHE II, SAPS III, SOFA, qSOFA), the presence of hypotension and elevated serum lactate, the presence of comorbidities (chronic obstructive pulmonary disease, asthma, coronary artery disease, hypertension, diabetes, liver cirrhosis, cancer, and chronic kidney disease), as well as the topography of the infection associated with the septic condition. Thus, it is observed that mortality at 28 days is higher among individuals with sepsis accompanied by hypotension, with or without hyperlactatemia, and these patients have a worse prognosis [30].

Early treatment improves mortality and outcome of patients with sepsis, and therefore, the identification of those at higher risk is essential. The Sequential Organ Failure Assessment (SOFA) score was designated to measure organ dysfunctions in patients admitted to the ICU, showing a good correlation with the prognosis of sepsis. Among adults with suspected infection admitted to the ICU, an increase of 2 or more points in the SOFA score had higher prognostic accuracy for determining in-hospital mortality [31, 32].

The identification of patients with infection and organ dysfunctions, factors that characterize sepsis, is a major challenge and of great importance, as it will lead to the recognition of individuals at higher risk of unfavorable outcomes. In this context, the qSOFA has been used as a tool for early identification of these patients to promote adequate resuscitation and treatment and reduce mortality. The qSOFA consists of three parameters: low systolic blood pressure ($\leq$100 mmHg), tachypnea ($\geq$22 breaths/minute), and altered mental status (Glasgow Coma Scale <15). The maximum score is three points, and a score of two points or more provides a 3- to 14-fold increase in mortality risk [33].

In addition to qSOFA, lactate is a biomarker used as a prognostic assessment tool in patients with sepsis, with low levels or within the normal range associated with less severity. Serum lactate concentrations above 4 mmol/L are related, with 96% specificity, as a predictor of hospital mortality in patients without hypotension. Comparing the predicted mortality rate by serum lactate with the predicted mortality rate by qSOFA showed a positive relationship but with the superiority of lactate accuracy in determining short-term prognosis and long-term mortality. Furthermore, qSOFA has lower sensitivity but similar specificity to lactate in predicting mortality, and they can be used together as tools for prognosticating patients with sepsis [32].

Despite the availability of evidence-based guidelines for sepsis, success of several large-scale quality improvement initiatives, and growing interest in clinical decision support, much work remains to ensure optimal sepsis care in hospitals. For this reason, the Core Elements contain the efforts to improve sepsis identification, management, and outcomes, intended to monitor and optimize hospital management, and helps facilitate implementation of guideline-recommended care practices that apply to a broad range of persons with sepsis.

According to CDC, the Hospital Sepsis Program Core Elements include:

- Hospital Leadership Commitment: dedicating the necessary human, financial, and information technology resources;

- Accountability: appointing a leader or co-leaders responsible for program goals and outcomes;

- Multi-Professional Expertise: engaging key partners throughout the hospital and healthcare system;

- Action: implementing structures and processes to improve the identification of, management of, and recovery from sepsis;

- Tracking: measuring sepsis epidemiology, management, and outcomes to assess the impact of sepsis initiatives and progress toward program goals;

- Reporting: providing information on sepsis management and outcomes to relevant partners;

- Education: providing sepsis education to healthcare professionals, patients, and family and caregivers.

5. Biomarkers in sepsis

5.1 Perfusion biomarkers

Lactate is the product of glucose and pyruvate metabolism, and in sepsis, the inflammatory response leads to increased glycolysis and/or reduced pyruvate dehydrogenase activity, preventing pyruvate from participating in Krebs cycle metabolic reactions. Additionally, tissue perfusion may be compromised in sepsis and associated with shock states, leading to increased serum lactate and the emergence of other signs of hypoperfusion such as prolonged capillary refill time [2, 34].

Serum lactate should be collected in every patient with suspected or confirmed sepsis, as its association with mortality is well established and it plays an important role as a guide in the initial resuscitation of the patient, and should be reassessed every 2 to 4 hours until normalization [2, 34]. Another important aspect is that lactate can also be used to assess treatment response and prognosis and, when found in elevated levels after adequate resuscitation, defines septic shock, correlating with increased morbidity and mortality, while decreasing values correlate with improved circulation and better outcomes [34, 35].

Analyzing serum lactate levels associated with qSOFA provides greater sensitivity and specificity for predicting 30-day mortality. Additionally, lactate clearance has also been shown to be useful in predicting mortality, although it is compromised in patients with hepatic insufficiency and cannot be reliable in this group of patients, as lactate metabolism depends on the liver for its clearance [36, 37].

In addition to serum lactate, perfusion can also be assessed through capillary refill time, as the skin is accessible in all patients for bedside microcirculation assessment. This assessment is based on the fact that the skin and muscles are the first tissues to have their blood flow compromised in sepsis and the last to be perfused after resuscitation. Capillary refill time (CRT) is defined as the time required for the distal capillary bed to regain its color, after pressure has been applied for 10 seconds, considered abnormal when above 3 seconds [34, 38].

In addition to lactate and capillary refill time, renal injury and failure are frequently encountered complications in critically ill patients and are associated with higher mortality, especially when associated with sepsis. In this sense, clinical and laboratory criteria are markers that define renal injury, using reduced urine output and elevated serum creatinine. Sepsis is associated with about 50% of cases of renal injury, and more than 60% of septic patients meet criteria for renal insufficiency. Furthermore, independent risk factors or clinical consequences of sepsis and renal injury, such as hypovolemia and exposure to nephrotoxic drugs, impair the relationship between the two clinical conditions, but it is known that the inflammatory cascade triggered by sepsis contributes to renal injury, significantly increasing mortality compared to patients with sepsis (without renal injury). It is believed that renal hypotension and associated ischemia lead to primary injury caused by sepsis, but there is also a relationship with tubular injury, inflammation, and apoptosis [39].

5.2 Inflammatory and defense biomarkers

Sepsis is a disorder involving a variety of alterations, from complex reactions until systemic inflammation, resulting in the elevation of various blood biomarkers, including immune cells and cytokines. Leukocytes, interleukin-6, and acute-phase proteins are among the key biomarkers, and it is crucial to assess their association with morbidity and mortality [40].

In recent years, some biomarkers of systemic inflammation, including those related to sepsis, have become available in major blood analyzers as part of a complete blood count or as parameters measured in researches. Among these new parameters are neutrophil CD64 expression, mean neutrophil and monocyte cellular volume, immature granulocyte fraction, neutrophil delta index, and monocyte volume variation width (MDW). Many of these markers could potentially be useful in identifying patients at risk of bacterial sepsis, although there are currently no studies confirming their effectiveness. Another potential application of data derived from complete blood count would be using formulas such as neutrophil-to-lymphocyte ratio (NLR), platelet-to-lymphocyte ratio (PLR), and monocyte-to-lymphocyte ratio (MLR) as adjuncts to assess the extent of inflammation [41, 42].

Interleukin-6 is a cytokine synthesized by T lymphocytes, fibroblasts, endothelial cells, and monocytes, secreted in conditions of infection, inflammation, or neoplastic diseases, and also acts as an important mediator during the acute phase of the inflammatory response in sepsis. Although its pro-inflammatory effects are well recognized, it also plays a role as an anti-inflammatory or protective molecule in many situations. It is also essential for both innate and adaptive immunities, required for efficient pathogen clearance, and plays a significant role in humans by regulating the acute-phase response, hematopoiesis, metabolic rate, lipid homeostasis, and neural development [41, 43].

C-reactive protein (CRP) and procalcitonin are widely used to facilitate diagnosis, but their prognostic values are limited. CRP is produced in the liver due to IL-6 production and release and is one of the most widely used acute-phase proteins, helping differentiate inflammatory conditions from other diseases. Procalcitonin's advantage lies in its high specificity for bacterial sepsis, with minimal or no increase in viral infection, cardiogenic shock, or noninfectious systemic inflammatory response [44]. A recent study has showed that serum interleukin-6 levels have greater diagnostic value for infection in patients with organ dysfunction compared to CRP and procalcitonin [43]. To improve specificity and sensitivity in interpreting IL-6, CRP, and procalcitonin, hematological parameters, including leukocyte counts, are also used.

Total leukocyte count and absolute neutrophil count are qualitative and quantitative parameters used for evaluating patients with infection and routinely performed in hospital settings. Inflammation alters the dynamics of neutrophil production, circulation, and migration, and during infection and sepsis, there is a significant increase in proliferation and migration into circulation, with large quantities of immature forms found in peripheral blood. Neutrophils are the first cells to migrate through the endothelium and reach the site of infection, stimulated by inflammatory cytokines; however, in sepsis, the neutrophilic response may be compromised and inadequate to eliminate the infectious agent [40, 45].

In addition to the increase in neutrophil count, infectious processes and sepsis may be related to the appearance of immature granulocytes, assessed by the neutrophil variation index or delta neutrophil index (DNI), and also by the immature granulocyte index (IG%). These biomarkers have a significant association with severity and mortality, with DNI calculated by subtracting the polymorphonuclear fraction from the neutrophil and eosinophil fraction, divided by the percentage of promyelocytes, myelocytes, and metamyelocytes in peripheral blood. In addition to IG% and DNI, band neutrophil counts and the corresponding left shift are also biomarkers of the body's response to aggressors and may be important in sepsis evaluation [46].

Characteristic morphological changes in leukocyte cell size, nucleus density, appearance of nuclear lobes, presence of toxic granulations, vacuolization, and Döhle bodies can occur in sepsis. Identifying these changes in peripheral blood depends on the examiner's experience, but they are early detected characteristics of sepsis that, when identified and quantified, can significantly contribute to the diagnosis and monitoring of infectious processes and sepsis [47].

The management of critically ill individuals depends on the intensity of insult as well as the intensity of the inflammatory response. Determining biomarkers for immune response in these patients is challenging, but some leukocyte parameters derived from complete blood count have been investigated as potential tools [10].

In this sense, the analysis of leukocyte parameters allows for the detection of the neutrophil-to-lymphocyte ratio (NLR), monocyte-to-lymphocyte ratio (MLR), platelet-to-lymphocyte ratio (PLR), and mean platelet volume-platelet count (MPV/PC), which are related to the prognosis of patients affected by infection and sepsis [10, 12].

Absolute neutrophil count has already been widely used in the laboratory evaluation of infectious and septic patients, with neutrophilia being common in patients treated in the ICU during hospitalization, probably related to associated bacterial infection. Remarkably, ICU patients tend to develop neutrophilia during hospitalization, showing higher average neutrophil levels than those observed in those who do not require intensive care, with neutrophilia associated with increased risk of death. Overall, neutrophils show hyposegmented nuclei, in some cases with pre-apoptotic chromatin and hypergranular cytoplasm, sometimes with hypogranular basophilic areas. This dysmorphism appears to be related to accelerated and disordered granulopoiesis associated with hyperinflammation. These morphological anomalies generally precede the increase in reactive lymphocytes [48].

The neutrophil-to-lymphocyte ratio (NLR) is an inflammatory biomarker that can be used as an indicator of systemic inflammation, which is defined by the absolute number of neutrophils divided by the absolute number of lymphocytes. It is a simple measure and adds no additional cost to routine complete blood count tests, which are routinely performed in hospitals. The NLR has been considered a reliable marker in cases of systemic inflammation and infection and is studied as a predictor of bacterial infection, including respiratory syndromes and pneumonia. Furthermore, the NLR has already been used as a guide for the prognosis of various diseases, such as cancer and community-acquired pneumonia. Moreover, the NLR is considered an independent predictor of hospital mortality in sepsis patients, being another recent biomarker that deserves careful evaluation in sepsis [12].

Furthermore, an increase in PLR is related to tumor size, lymph node infiltration, metastasis, and prognosis, and it can be used as a potential inflammatory indicator for pneumonia diagnosis. Platelets circulate in their inactive form and can be quickly activated at the site of vascular injury or in response to pro-inflammatory cytokines or infectious factors. Considered as a new inflammation index, PLR mainly reflects the level of systemic inflammation. Previous studies have confirmed that PLR is closely related to tumors, diabetes, coronary artery disease, and connective tissue diseases. The advantage of using PLR is that this marker relates to platelet aggregation and the inflammatory reaction and may be more valuable in predicting various inflammations than platelet or lymphocyte counts alone [42].

PLR has been proposed as a biomarker capable of reflecting the severity of inflammation during the treatment of some inflammatory and/or infectious diseases. Comparing PLR changes during treatment, it was found that the greater the variation of PLR, the longer the hospital stay. In this sense, in COVID ICU studies, changes in the platelet/lymphocyte ratio in peripheral blood during hospitalization were observed, which reflected disease progression and the prognosis of COVID-19 patients. The greater the variation of PLR, the more severe the cytokine storm, and the longer the hospital stay, the worse the prognosis [42].

Regarding platelet count in infectious processes and sepsis, platelets actively participate in the immune response in addition to playing an important role in hemostasis, coagulation, maintenance of vascular integrity, angiogenesis, innate immunity, inflammatory response, tumor biology, and so on. Changes in their number and activity are closely related to a wide variety of diseases. Platelet activation by inflammatory and/or infectious mechanisms, even without vascular damage, indicates new platelet functions, such as participation in inflammation and immune regulation. Additionally, platelets' pro-inflammatory activity is mediated by their interaction with other circulating leukocytes, followed by the release of cytokines and chemokines during the inflammatory process. In sepsis, platelets play an important role in determining sepsis-related organ dysfunction, as they catalyze the development of hyperinflammation, disseminated intravascular coagulation, and microthrombosis, leading to multiple organ dysfunctions. Platelet dysfunction is considered an independent risk factor for the prognosis of sepsis patients [48].

The key role of platelets in critical illness is a consequence of their interaction with endothelial cells leading to organ failure. Platelet markers, such as platelet distribution width (PDW) and mean platelet volume (MPV), are altered in sepsis and are easily accessible, being available in a complete blood count, but are still underutilized. Additionally, coagulation disorders are also common during sepsis, characterized by pro-coagulant states induced by inflammatory cytokines (IL-6) and determined through platelet dysfunction and other markers such as fibrinogen, prothrombin time, and activated partial thromboplastin time (PT and APTT) [25].

5.3 Biomarkers of redox state

The triggering of the host response to the presence of an infectious aggressor constitutes a basic defense mechanism in which inflammatory phenomena occur, including cytokine activation, nitric oxide production, reactive oxygen species (ROS), and adhesion molecule expression in the endothelium. It should be understood that all these actions have the physiological purpose of combating infectious aggression and restricting the agent to the site where it is present. Regarding the increase in ROS production/generation in sepsis, both extrinsic factors (endotoxins, viruses, fungi, etc.) and intrinsic factors (inflammatory mediators) that determine sepsis induce a complex cascade of cellular events resulting in the release of pro- and anti-inflammatory mediators, including oxidants and antioxidants, which under normal conditions are in balance [49].

Oxidative stress occurs when oxidant levels exceed antioxidant levels, contributing to the process of sepsis and potentially leading to organic dysfunction. The inflammatory response and persistent oxidative stress observed during sepsis-induced organ failure lead to mitochondrial dysfunction and cell death. Excessive oxidative stress is a characteristic of sepsis, compromising redox homeostasis [49].

Reactive oxygen species (ROS) regulate cellular homeostasis and act as modulators of cellular dysfunction, contributing to the pathophysiology of the disease. Reactive oxygen species are byproducts of numerous enzymatic reactions in various cellular compartments, including the cytoplasm, cell membrane, endoplasmic reticulum, mitochondria, and peroxisome, as part of basic metabolic functions. Inflammatory and metabolic diseases are associated with altered ROS production by mitochondria [50].

The mitochondrial electron transport chain present in the inner membrane of the mitochondria consists of five oxidative phosphorylation complexes, in which electrons are transferred from complex I to II-IV, leading to adenosine triphosphate (ATP) generation in complex V (ATP synthase). When there is defective reduction of O_2 to H_2O_2, the result is an excessive generation of superoxide, which is usually converted to hydrogen peroxide (H_2O_2) by manganese-containing superoxide dismutase (Mn-SOD) and then to H_2O by catalase (CAT). Several oxidative stress biomarkers involved in the sepsis process include an increase in the SOD/CAT ratio, resulting in H_2O_2 accumulation in cells, decreased glutathione levels, increased malondialdehyde levels, and an increase in protein carbonyl groups. Thus, any alteration in the SOD/CAT ratio, such as CAT inhibition or SOD overexpression, will lead to increased oxidative stress and morbidity in sepsis. Selenium-containing glutathione peroxidase also plays a role in the catalytic conversion of H_2O_2 to water [49].

In addition to causing increased ROS production, oxidative stress in sepsis also leads to attenuation of endogenous antioxidants, preventing complete neutralization of ROS, further increasing their accumulation [48].

5.4 Cellular stress response biomarkers (HSP70)

Alterations that induce cellular stress are associated with various processes such as DNA-damaging agents that activate specific repair processes for different types of genetic lesions; heat shock proteins or chemotaxins, which cause protein denaturation; hypoxia and respiratory intoxication, which cause mitochondrial stress; nutrient deprivation with activation of cellular autophagy; and infectious agents that induce stress through the activation of receptor recognition patterns. Most of these mechanisms involve paracrine and endocrine signals that communicate a potential threat to the organism and contribute to maintaining systemic homeostasis. These processes of intercellular communication include changes in cell morphology and its connections with the microenvironment, exposure to surface molecules, and the release of bioactive factors such as ions, small metabolites, intracellular proteins, cytokines, or microvesicles [44].

Heat shock proteins (HSPs) are chaperones that act in response to stress and play different roles in the body. Among them, one of the most well-known HSPs is the 70 Kilodalton heat shock protein (HSP70), whose role is to facilitate protein folding and prevent the secretion of inflammatory mediators. HSP70 also plays anti-apoptotic and anti-inflammatory roles as demonstrated in animal models and decreases the expression of pro-inflammatory genes by disrupting the phosphorylation of transcription factors and inhibiting nuclear factor κB (NF-κB), which plays an important role in the pathophysiology of sepsis.

The progression and worse prognosis of sepsis include changes in HSP70, in its both intracellular (iHSP70) and extracellular (eHSP70) expression levels. iHSP70 acts as a chaperone, correcting protein damage by assisting in protein folding and refolding, modulating the inflammatory response, playing an important role in the cellular stress response and protection against sepsis, preventing intestinal, pulmonary, and leukocyte apoptosis and inflammation. However, when this protein is observed in immune cells exposed to bacterial endotoxins (lipopolysaccharides—LPS), there is an increase in the rate of iHSP70 export to the extracellular environment (eHSP70). Serum concentration of eHSP70 and levels of oxidative stress are elevated in patients with sepsis, and these two variables may be considered biomarkers of sepsis severity and mortality [9].

Considering that eHSP70 has a pro-inflammatory role and iHSP70 does the opposite, the extracellular to intracellular ratio of HSP70 (also known as the HSP70 state index) is related to the immune-inflammatory balance and may act as a marker of subclinical tissue and systemic injury processes.

6. Treatment

Standard operating procedures used in sepsis include approach protocols with components forming the sepsis bundle, early identification, serum lactate measurement, and culture collection, early initiation of antibiotics, and fluids. The systematization of care for individuals suspected of sepsis, from identification to treatment, through the use of protocols, is associated with decreased morbidity and mortality, as observed in hospitals with higher adherence to sepsis bundles [2].

6.1 Volume replacement

Effective volume resuscitation is crucial for stabilizing sepsis-induced tissue hypoperfusion. Retrospective analysis of adults with sepsis or septic shock shows higher mortality, slower resolution of hypotension, and longer ICU stay among patients who did not receive crystalloid fluid therapy in the early hours of sepsis onset. The goal of intravenous fluid administration is to reduce tissue hypoperfusion by increasing circulating blood volume, enhancing preload, and, consequently, cardiac output, improving oxygen delivery to peripheral tissues and reducing metabolic derangements.

6.2 Vasoactive drugs

For patients with septic shock unresponsive to fluid administration, the use of vasopressor drugs is recommended to maintain a target mean arterial pressure (MAP) above 65 mmHg. MAP is the primary determinant of mean systemic filling pressure, which, in turn, is the main driver of venous return and cardiac output. Its increase results in improved tissue blood flow, ensuring greater tissue perfusion. Norepinephrine is the recommended first-line vasopressor agent for treating patients with septic shock, which is a potent agonist of α-1 and β-1 adrenergic receptors, resulting in vasoconstriction and increased MAP with minimal effects on the heart [2].

6.3 Antibiotic therapy

The early administration of appropriate antibiotics is one of the most effective interventions, along with fluid therapy and the use of vasopressors, with an impact on reducing mortality in patients with sepsis. This approach should be treated as an emergency, especially in patients with septic shock. Antibiotic administration should commence within the first hour after suspicion of sepsis, without delay for sample collection or other procedures. The choice of treatment should be based on risk factors, probable site of infection, among other factors [2].

Moreover, early recognition and appropriate empiric antimicrobial treatment are crucial in changing the current scenario of high mortality rates. Considering such suspicions is critical because therapeutic options for the treatment of multiresistant organisms, especially concerning resistant gram-negatives, are limited as antibiotics available for this class are restricted. Infections caused by *Acinetobacter baumannii*, *Pseudomonas aeruginosa*, and *Klebsiella pneumoniae* have become increasingly frequent worldwide, and in some settings, these agents have become the leading cause of sepsis in intensive care units, followed by Gram-positives and fungi [51].

7. Final considerations

Sepsis remains a major challenge in clinical practice due to its high rates of morbidity and mortality. Early diagnosis and immediate treatment are crucial for improving patient outcomes. In this context, biomarkers play an essential role by providing valuable information about the physiological and pathological processes underlying sepsis, allowing clinicians to diagnose the condition more accurately and rapidly. The assessment of clinical and laboratory parameters, especially hematological biomarkers, can aid in the identification, stratification, prognosis, and prediction of adverse outcomes in sepsis.

Furthermore, the combination of various clinical and laboratory biomarkers enhances diagnostic accuracy and provides a comprehensive understanding of the patient's condition. This integrated approach facilitates the early detection of sepsis, enabling healthcare professionals to initiate treatment protocols before the onset of severe complications. The use of these biomarkers also allows for the evaluation of therapeutic intervention effectiveness and the adjustment of treatment plans according to the patient's progression, thereby optimizing care and clinical outcomes.

Author details

Eduardo Almeida de Souza Minuzzo[1], Pauline Brendler Goettems Fiorin[2], Vítor Antunes de Oliveira[3], Mirna Stela Ludwig[4] and Matias Nunes Frizzo[5*]

1 Program in Integral Health Care - PPGAIS, Regional University of Northwestern Rio Grande do Sul State - UNIJUÍ, Brazil

2 Health Sciences (UFCSPA), Graduate Program in Comprehensive Health Care, PPGAIS - UNIJUÍ/UNICRUZ/URI, Brazil

3 Biological Sciences - Toxicological Biochemistry, UFSM, Graduate Program in Comprehensive Health Care, PPGAIS - UNIJUÍ/UNICRUZ/URI, Brazil

4 Biological Sciences - Physiology (UFRGS), Graduate Program in Comprehensive Health Care, PPGAIS - UNIJUÍ/UNICRUZ/URI, Brazil

5 Biochemist and Biomedical, Cellular and Molecular Biology (PUCRS), Graduate Program in Comprehensive Health Care, PPGAIS - UNIJUÍ/UNICRUZ/URI, Brazil

*Address all correspondence to: matias.frizzo@unijui.edu.br

References

[1] Brasil. Ministério da Saúde. Agência Nacional de Vigilância Sanitária. Resolução N° 7, de 24 de fevereiro de 2010. Dispõe sobre os requisitos mínimos para funcionamento de Unidades de Terapia Intensiva e dá outras providências. Brasília-DF: Agência Nacional de Vigilância Sanitária; 2010

[2] Evans L, Rhodes A, Alhazzani W, Antonelli M, Coopersmith CM, French C, et al. Surviving sepsis campaign: International guidelines for management of sepsis and septic shock 2021. Intensive Care Medicine. 2021;**47**:1181-1247

[3] Fleischmann C, Scherag A, Adhikari NKJ, Hartog CS, Tsaganos T, Schlattmann P, Angus DC, Reinhart K. Avaliação da incidência global e mortalidade de sepse tratada em hospital. American Journal of Respiratory and Critical Care Medicine. 2016;**193**(3):259-272

[4] Almeida NRC, Pontes GF, Jacob FL, Deprá JVS, Porto JPP, Lima FR, et al. Analysis of trends in sepsis mortality in Brazil and by regions from 2010 to 2019. Revista de Saúde Pública. 2022;**56**:1-12

[5] Serafim R, Gomes JA, Salluh J, Povoa P. A comparison of the quick-SOFA and systemic inflammatory response syndrome criteria for the diagnosis of sepsis and prediction of mortality. Chest Journal. 2018;**153**(3):646-655

[6] Pinsky MR, Teboul JL, Vincent JL. Hemodynamic Monitoring. 1st ed. Alemanha: Editora Springer; 2019

[7] Caraballo C, Jaimes F. Organ dysfunction in sepsis: na ominous trajectory from infection to death. Yale Journal of Biology and Medicine. 2019;**92**:629-640

[8] Kumar S, Gupta E, Kaushik S, Srivastava VK, Mehta S, Jyoti A. Evaluation of oxidative stress and antioxidant status: Correlation with the severity of sepsis. Scandinavian Journal of Immunology. 2018;**87**:1-11

[9] Sulzbacher MM, Ludwig MS, Heck TG. Oxidative stress and decreased tissue HSP70 are involved in the genesis of sepsis: HSP70 as a therapeutic target. Revista Brasileira de Terapia Intensiva. 2020;**32**(4):585-591

[10] Djordjevic D, Rondovic G, Surbatovic M, Stanojevic I, Udovicic I, Andjelic T, et al. Neutrophil-to-lymphocyte ratio, monocyte-to-limphocyte ratio, platelet-to-lymphocyte ratio, and mean platelet volume-to-platelet count ratio as biomarkers in critically ill and injured patients: Which ratio to choose to predict outcome and nature of bacteremia? Mediators of Inflammation. 2018;**1**:1-15

[11] Doganyigit Z, Eroglu E, Akyuz E. Inflammatory mediators of cytokines and chemokines in sepsis: From bench to bedside. Human & Experimental Toxicology. 2022;**41**:1-11

[12] Ni J, Wang H, Li Y, Shu Y, Liu Y. Neutrophil to lymphocyte ratio (NLR) as a prognostic marker for in-hospital mortality of patients with sepsis. Medicine. 2019;**98**:1-5

[13] Ervin JN, Kahn JM, Cohen TR, Weingart LR. Teamwork in the intensive care unit. The American Psychologist. 2018;**73**(4):468-477

[14] Marshall JC, Bosco L, Adhikari NK, Connolly B, Diaz JV, Dorman T, et al.

What is na intensive care unit? A report of the task force of the world Federation of Societies of intensive and critical care medicine. Journal of Critical Care. 2017;**37**:270-276

[15] Dudzinski DM, Januzzi JLJR. The evolving medical complexity of the modern cardiac intensive care unit. Journal of the American College of Cardiology. 2017;**69**(16):2008-2010

[16] Rohrig SAH, Lance MD, Faisal MM. Surgical intensive care – Current and future challenges? Qatar Medical Journal. 2020;**2**:1-4

[17] Brasil. Conselho Federal de Medicina. Resolução CFM N° 2.156, de 17 de novembro de 2016. Estabelece os critérios de admissão e alta em unidade de terapia intensiva. Brasília-DF: Conselho Federal de Medicina; 2016

[18] Standing up to infectious disease. Nature Microbiology. 2019;**4**:1-1

[19] Cheung GYC, Bae JS, Liu R, Hunt RL, Zhenh Y, Otto M. Bacterial virulence plays a crucial role in MRSA sepsis. PLoS Pathogens. 2021;**17**:1-18

[20] Salomão R, Ferreira BL, Salomão MC, Santos SS, Azevedo LCP, Bruniatti MKC. Sepsis: Evolving concepts and challenges. Brazilian Journal of Medical and Biological Research. 2019;**52**:1-14

[21] Huang M, Cai S, Su J. The pathogenesis of sepsis and potential therapeutic targets. International Journal of Molecular Sciences. 2019;**20**:1-31

[22] Huerta LE, Rice TW. Pathologic difference between sepsis adn bloodstream infections. Journal of Applied Laboratory Medicine. 2019;**3**(4):654-663

[23] Holmes CL, Anderson MT, Mobley HLT, Bachman MA. Pathogenesis of gram-negative bacteremia. Clinical Microbiology Reviews. 2021;**34**:1-20

[24] Remy S, Gossez M, Belot A, Hayman J, Portefaix A, Venet F, et al. Massive increase in monocyte HLA-DR expression can be used to discriminate between septic shock and hemophagocytic lymphohistiocytosis-induced shock. Critical Care. 2018;**22**:1-2

[25] Iba T, Levy JH, Warkentin TE, Tachil J, Van Der Poll T, Levi M. Diagnosis and management of sepsis-induced coagulpathy and disseminated intravascular coagulation. Journal of Thrombosis and Haemostasis. 2019;**17**:1989-1994

[26] Jacobi J. The pathophysiology of sepsis – 2021 update: Part 1, immunology and coagulopathy leading to endotelial injury. American Journal of Health-System Pharmacy. 2022;**79**(5):329-337

[27] Gu X, Zhou F, Wang Y, Fan G, Cao B. Respiratory viral sepsis: Epidemiology, pathophysiology, diagnosis and treatment. European Respiratory Review. 2020;**26**:1-12

[28] Gauer R, Forbes D. Sepsis: Diagnosis and management. American Academy of Family Physicians. 2020;**101**(7):409-418

[29] Chakraborty RK, Burns B. Systemic Inflammatory Response Syndrome. Treasure Island (FL): StatPearls Publishing; 2022

[30] Qu Z, Zhu Y, Wang M, Li W, Zhu B, Jiang L, et al. Prognosis and risk factors of sepsis in chinese ICUs: A retrospective analysis of a cohort database. Shock. 2021;**56**(6):921-926

[31] Li Y, Yan C, Gan Z, Xi X, Tan Z, Li J, et al. Prognostic values of SOFA score, qSOFA score, and LODS score for patients with sepsis. Annals of Palliative Medicine. 2020;**9**(3):1037-1044

[32] Liu Z, Meng Z, Li Y, Zhao J, Wu S, Gou S, et al. Prognostic accuracy of the serum lactate level, the SOFA score and the qSOFA score for mortality among adults with sepsis. Scandinavian Journal of Trauma, Resuscitation and Emergency Medicine. 2019;**27**:1-10

[33] Brink A, Alsma J, Verdonschot RJCG, Rood PPM, Zietse R, Lingsma HF, et al. Predicting mortality in patients with suspected sepsis at the emergency department; a retrospective cohort study comparing qSOFA, SIRS and National Early Warning Score. PLoS One. 2019;**14**:1-14

[34] Hernandez G, Bellomo R, Bakker J. The tem pitfalls of lactate clearance in sepsis. Intensive Care Medicine. 2019;**45**:82-85

[35] Nolt B, Tu F, Wang X, Ha T, Winter R, Williams DL, et al. Lactate and immunosuppression in sepsis. Shock. 2018;**49**(2):120-125

[36] Matos SINS. Nível de lactato como indicador prognóstico de mortalidade e morbilidade hospitalar. Dissertação (Mestrado em Medicina). Porto: Instituto de Ciências Biomédicas Abel Salazar, Universidade do Porto; 2021

[37] Silva LMF, Diogo LP, Vieira LB, Michielin FC, Santarem MD, Machado MLP. Performance of scores in the prediction of clinical outcomes in patients admitted from the emergency servisse. Revista Latino-Americana de Enfermagem. 2021;**29**:1-10

[38] Miranda AC, Menezes IAC, Junior HC, Luy AM, Nascimento MM. Monitoring peripheral perfusion in sepsis associated acute kidney injury: Analysis of mortality. PLoS One. 2020;**15**:1-14

[39] Poston JT, Koyner JL. Sepsis associated acute kidney injury. BMJ. 2019;**364**:1-14

[40] Xie Y, Huang P, Zhang J, Tian R, Jin W, Xie H, et al. Biomarkers for the diagnosis of sepsis-associated acute kidney injury: Systematic review and meta-analysis. Annals of Palliative Medicine. 2021;**10**(4):4159-4173

[41] Mcelvaney OJ, Curley GF, Rose-J ohn S, Mcelvaney NGM. Interleukin-6: Obstacles to targeting a complex cytokine in critical illness. The Lancet Respiratory Medicine. 2021;**9**:643-654

[42] Rayes J, Bourne JH, Brill A, Watson SP. The dual role of platelet-innate immune cell interactions in thrombo-inflammation. Research and Practice in Thrombosis and Haemostasis. 2019;**4**(1):23-35. Published 2019 Oct 17. DOI: 10.1002/rth2.12266

[43] Song J, Park DW, Moon S, Cho H-J, Park JH, Seok H, et al. Diagnostic and prognostic value of interleukin-6, pentraxin 3, and procalcitonin levels among sepsis and septic shock patients: A prospective controlled study according to the Sepsis-3 definitions. BMC Infectious Diseases. 2019;**19**:1-11

[44] Godínez-Vidal A, Alcántara-Gordillo R, Aguirre-Rojano VI, López-RomeroSC,González-CalatayudM, González-Perez LG, et al. Evaluación de la proteína C reactiva, la procalcitonina y el índice PCR/PCT como indicadores de mortalidad systemic homeostasis. Nature Reviews. Molecular Cell Biology. 2018;**19**(11):731-745

[45] Resende CB, Borges I, Gonçalves WA, Carneiro R, Rezende BM, Pinho V,

et al. Neutrophil activity in sepsis: A systematic review. Brazilian Journal of Medical and Biological Research. 2020;**53**:1-6

[46] Kim SB, Lee KH, Lee JU, Ann HW, Ahn JY, Jeon YD, et al. Long pentraxin 3 as a predictive marker of mortality in severe septic patients who received successful early goal-directed therapy. Yonsei Medical Journal. 2017;**58**(2):370-379

[47] Arora P, Gupta PK, Lingaiah R, Mukhopadhyay AK. Volume, conductivity, and scatter parameters of leukocytes as early markers of sepsis and treatment response. Journal of Laboratory Physicians. 2019;**11**:29-33

[48] Zhao L, Zhao L, Wang YY, Yang F, Chen Z, Yu Q, et al. Platelets as a prognostic marker for sepsis: A cohort study from de MIMIC-III database. Medicine. 2020;**99**:1-9

[49] Nagar H, Piao S, Kim C-S. Role of mitochondrial oxidative stress in sepsis. Acute and Critical Care. 2018;**33**(2):65-72

[50] Forrester SJ, Kikuchi DS, Hernandes MS, Xu Q, Griendling KK. Reactive oxygen species in metabolic and inflammatory signaling. Circulation Research. 2018;**122**(6):877-902

[51] Gomes MZR, Braga DQ, Pinheiro DOPB, Verduc RCAS, Dos Reis LV, De Lima EM, et al. Predictive score for carbapenem-resistant gram-negative bacilli sepsis: Single-center prospective cohort study. Antibiotics (Basel). 2022;**12**:1-21

Chapter 9

Sepsis-Induced Coagulopathy: From Pathophysiology to Patient Care

Abdelrahman Balal, Ahmad M. Obeidat, Khalid Y. Fadul, Wala Sati, Sara M.I. Ahmed, Mohamed Elgassim and Seema Nahid

Abstract

Sepsis is a potentially life-threatening complication of infection, leading to sequential events that can result in widespread organ dysfunction. Sepsis triggers strong activation of the coagulation system and its regulatory cells, resulting in a wide spectrum of hemostatic abnormalities, ranging from subclinical activation of coagulation and hypercoagulability to sustained systemic clotting activation leading to consumption of clotting factors and platelets and the development of overt DIC. SIC is a major complication of sepsis, and it represents a variant of non-overt DIC that involves intravascular coagulation induced by inflammatory-mediated TF expression and is associated with an increased risk of thrombosis, worsening organ dysfunction, and increased mortality. The pathogenesis of SIC is multifactorial. Contributors include hyperinflammation, dysregulated immune response, and altered coagulation. The dysregulated coagulation activation, disruption of the body's natural anticoagulant systems, and impairment of fibrinolysis represent a basic pathogenic process that drives the emergence of coagulopathy in sepsis. Treatment of DIC depends on treating the underlying condition. Early goal-directed therapy is essential to avoid morbidity and mortality. The considered use of blood component therapy, alongside prompt management of the underlying infectious source, may represent a reasonable therapeutic approach for improving outcomes in these high-risk patients.

Keywords: sepsis, sepsis-induced coagulopathy, SIC, sepsis-associated DIC, disseminated intravascular coagulation, coagulopathy, coagulation abnormalities

1. Introduction

Historically, sepsis has been defined as a systemic inflammatory response syndrome due to infection. In 2016, sepsis was redefined by the Third International Consensus Definitions for sepsis as a life-threatening organ dysfunction caused by a dysregulated host response to infection [1]. Current understanding now focuses on the potential for significant morbidity and mortality due to the dysregulated host response rather than the infection itself. Organ dysfunction is defined as an increase in the SOFA score of at least two points. Sepsis-induced coagulopathy is a complication of sepsis, and it is considered to be responsible for organ dysfunction in this setting.

Sepsis-induced coagulopathy (SIC) is a serious complication in sepsis patients. SIC is considered an early stage of DIC—it encompasses most clinically apparent cases of overt DIC [2]. Early identification of SIC is crucial, as SIC is associated with increased mortality risk by two-fold [3]. Activation of the coagulation system is an integral part of the host response to infection; however, excessive activation may be detrimental to the host [4]. Sepsis triggers immunological, inflammatory, and coagulation responses that activate the coagulation pathway [5]. The dysregulated host response leads to a series of pathological reactions, including alterations in the coagulation system, manifesting as SIC, DIC, and multiple organ dysfunction [6]. Sepsis triggers a strong activation of the coagulation system and its regulatory cells, resulting in a wide spectrum of hemostatic abnormalities. These abnormalities range from isolated thrombocytopenia or subclinical activation of coagulation (hypercoagulability) to sustained, systemic clotting activation leading to microthrombi with intravascular fibrin deposition and consumption of platelets eventually resulting in the diffuse bleeding as well as the development acute DIC [7]. Sepsis-associated DIC carries a high mortality risk [8]. Therefore, the early recognition and management of this complication are crucial to improving the prognosis for these patients.

2. Epidemiology of sepsis-induced coagulopathy

The incidence of SIC may vary according to the definition used, the patients studied, and the diagnostic criteria applied. While extensive large-scale data are limited, existing evidence showed that SIC occurs in approximately 21–29% of sepsis patients with an associated mortality rate at 28 days ranging from 23 to 44% [9]. Moreover, sepsis-associated DIC has been proven to have an incidence of 30–50% in critically ill patients with sepsis [10]. In a Japanese multicenter observational study of 1895 sepsis patients who were admitted to intensive care units (ICU), 29% had SIC [8]. In a secondary analysis of two randomized controlled trials conducted in Europe, the SIC prevalence was 22.1% (the HYPRESS trial) and 24.2% (the SISPCT trial) [3].

Thrombocytopenia is present in up to 35–50% of critically ill medical patients [11]. Platelet counts typically decline during the first four days of ICU admission. Sepsis is a well-known risk factor for thrombocytopenia in critically ill patients, and the severity of platelet reduction directly correlates with sepsis severity [12]. The main factors contributing to thrombocytopenia in sepsis patients include impaired platelet production, increased platelet consumption or destruction, and sequestration of platelets within the spleen or at the endothelial level [10]. A prolonged global coagulation time, measured by prothrombin time (PT) and the activated partial thromboplastin time (aPTT), is observed in 14–28% of sepsis patients. Several other coagulation test abnormalities are often observed in these patients, such as increased fibrin degradation products (in 99% of patients with sepsis) and decreased levels of coagulation inhibitors, such as antithrombin and protein C (90% of sepsis patients) [10].

3. Risk factors for sepsis-induced coagulopathy

Sepsis is a serious and relatively common condition and represents the leading cause of mortality among critically ill patients in noncardiac intensive care units worldwide [13]. Coagulopathy is a prevalent complication among sepsis patients, and its occurrence is associated with poorer clinical outcomes [14]. Furthermore, sepsis-induced coagulopathy is associated with an increased risk of thrombosis, worsening of organ dysfunction, and increased mortality [11]. Early recognition of risk factors predisposing to coagulopathy is crucial to implementing appropriate prevention and treatment strategies. However, the literature provides limited insight into the risk factors associated with the development of SIC.

Coagulopathy occurs with higher frequency in older patients, which might be explained by age-related changes in coagulation and fibrinolysis [15]. In 2022, a large retrospective observational study also identified several risk factors for developing DIC in patients with sepsis. These included serum albumin levels ≤2.5 g/dL, respiratory tract infection, and more than 1-hour delay in antibiotic treatment [16]. Other studies have found that the respiratory system is the most common site for infection leading to sepsis and DIC [17–19]. Pneumonia has been specifically associated with a prothrombotic state and coagulation abnormalities [19]. In 2023, a retrospective cohort study including patients with confirmed SIC showed that higher SOFA, total bilirubin levels, lactate levels, lower platelet counts, and increased international normalized ratio (INR) values were independently associated with SIC [20]. In contrast, variables such as age, Acute Physiology, and Chronic Health Evaluation II (APACHE II) scores, the presence of diabetes mellitus, bloodstream infections, procalcitonin, C-reactive protein, creatinine, fibrinogen, and D-dimer were not independently associated with an increased risk of SIC [20]. The PT/INR has also been found to be an accurate prognostic variable for 30-day all-cause mortality in sepsis and severe septic shock. Research has specifically demonstrated that a PT/INR value >1.5 is associated with an increased risk of all-cause death at 30 days in this patient population [21]. With the presence of these findings, identifying high-risk individuals, such as those with poor nutritional support (low albumin), respiratory tract infection as an inciting event, high SOFA scores, impaired organ function, and coagulation abnormalities, may enable earlier detection of SIC.

Bacterial endotoxin is a potent activator of the coagulation and fibrinolytic systems, which may play an important role in both SIC and DIC, especially in Gram-negative bacterial infections. DIC was observed in 10% of a cohort study among 612 individuals with Gram-negative bacteremia [22]. However, there have also been many reports in which DIC developed in patients with Gram-positive bacterial sepsis or systemic fungal infection or infections by other pathogenic microorganisms [23]. Viral infections also contribute to the development of coagulopathy *via* multiple mechanisms like the direct viral cellular effects, generation of autoimmune antibodies against platelets, and overproduction of procoagulant factors such as tissue factor and von Willebrand [24].

Many reports during the 2009 H1N1 influenza pandemic described thrombotic events in hospitalized patients, including deep vein thrombosis, pulmonary emboli, acute myocardial infarctions, and thrombotic microangiopathy [25, 26]. Similarly, patients with severe COVID-19 infection due to SARS-CoV-2 also have an increased risk for thromboembolic events [27]. The coagulation profile seen in these patients with SARS-CoV-2 infection and a clinically significant thromboembolic event is marked by very high levels of fibrinogen, elevated D-dimers, mild reductions platelet counts as well as antithrombin III consistent with an overall prothrombotic state without overt evidence of consumptive coagulopathy [28]. Notably, D-dimer levels above 1 μg/mL were associated with an increased mortality risk, and levels greater than 2 μg/mL prognosticated an even higher mortality risk in these patients [29].

4. Pathophysiology of sepsis-induced coagulopathy

Sepsis results in a complex derangement in many systems, including the coagulation cascade. SIC is a complex condition characterized by a severe hyperinflammatory and procoagulant state resulting from an immune response to infection, leading to widespread inflammation and coagulation abnormalities, ranging from subclinical coagulopathy to overt DIC [30]. In recent years, the underlying mechanisms contributing to the pathological disruption of the coagulation system in patients with sepsis have become increasingly well-understood [31]. Multiple mechanisms at different sites in the hemostatic balance act simultaneously to contribute to a hypercoagulable state [31].

The coagulation system has two main components: the procoagulant pathway initiates and maintains blood clotting and the anticoagulant pathway which regulates the procoagulant pathway by preventing the excessive formation of clots. During the early stages of infection, the coagulation process functions as a natural defense mechanism that aims to confine the responsible pathogen and prevent its spread into a systematic circulation [32]. In sepsis, however, this physiological response becomes dysregulated, leading to overwhelming coagulation activation on one end while inhibiting anticoagulant mechanisms on the other [33].

4.1 Pathogenesis of sepsis-induced coagulopathy

SIC pathogenesis is multifactorial, with contributors including hyperinflammation, dysregulated immune response, and altered coagulation system [34]. This is manifested by hyperactivated coagulation cascade, dysfunction of natural anticoagulant mechanisms, and suppression of fibrinolytic processes [32]. These derangements act cumulatively, leading to the development of SIC and DIC. Also, the activation of coagulation and inflammatory systems is central in mediating a progression to organ dysfunction during sepsis [33]. The increased expression of tissue factor (TF) on both the endothelial cells and monocyte surface is also an essential mechanism that results in SIC due to excessive activation of the extrinsic coagulation pathway [33]. This is accompanied by dysfunctional natural anticoagulant systems, such as the protein C pathway, which worsens the procoagulant state [33]. Finally, the upregulated production of inflammatory cytokines like tumor necrosis factor-alpha (TNF-alpha) and interleukin-6 (IL-6) can also stimulate the coagulation cascade and impair the regulatory functions of the natural anticoagulant mechanisms [35].

4.2 Role of inflammatory cytokines in SIC

Most pro-inflammatory cytokines have been shown to stimulate the activation of the coagulation cascade in *in vitro* studies [36]. TNF is one of the first mediators detected, followed by a rise in levels of several interleukins, with IL-6 and IL-1 being prominent [36]. There is an increased understanding of the bidirectional crosstalk between inflammatory and coagulation pathways, where inflammation activates a procoagulant state, and the coagulation process also significantly impacts inflammatory activity [37]. Notably, the procoagulant state of sepsis can persist even after the inflammatory response has subsided, which causes a vicious cycle of inflammation, coagulation, and organ dysfunction [36].

Tumor necrosis factor (TNF), the first cytokine detected in plasma during bacterial infection and known for its potent procoagulant activities, was initially thought to mediate hemostatic activation in sepsis [36]. However, in subsequent trials utilizing various strategies to block TNF activity, it was found that while the endotoxin-induced increase in TNF could be completely prevented, the activation of the coagulation system remained unaffected [38]. In line with this, studies investigating the use of an anti-TNF monoclonal antibody in individuals with sepsis did not reveal any significant benefits [39, 40]. Interestingly, further research has revealed that intervention with anti-IL-6 alone completely suppressed endotoxin-triggered coagulation cascade activation [41]. These observations may indicate that IL-6 is the primary mediator of cytokines-induced hemostatic changes rather than TNF.

4.3 Activation of coagulation in sepsis

Sepsis-induced acute inflammatory responses impair the antithrombotic functions of vascular endothelial cells. This is due to decreased nitric oxide and prostaglandin I2 production and disruption of the endothelial glycocalyx layer [42]. Disruption of the vascular endothelium also releases thrombogenic factors, including von Willebrand factor (VWF) and adhesion molecules, which promote platelet adhesion and aggregation [43]. Platelets further contribute to the host immune response by promoting thrombus formation by expressing adhesion molecules on their surface and releasing granular components, such as platelet factor 4 (PF4) and von Willebrand factor (VWF) [44]. These responses result in the formation of intravascular microthrombi (immunothrombosis) as a defense mechanism against the infecting pathogen [42]. The increased production of plasminogen activator inhibitor 1 (PAI 1) results in the suppression of fibrinolytic processes, which is a crucial characteristic of the coagulation disturbances observed in sepsis (Fibrinolytic shutdown) [42]. Moreover, the increased vascular permeability during sepsis leads to extravasation of natural anticoagulant factors (e.g., AT and protein C), affecting their regulatory role in the coagulation cascade [45]. The combined effect of coagulation activation, impairment of anticoagulant mechanisms, and suppression of fibrinolysis leads to the procoagulant state and the development of SIC.

The onset of sepsis is triggered when pathogenic microbial components (PAMPs), such as lipopolysaccharide or endotoxin from Gram-negative or peptidoglycan from Gram-positive bacteria, bind to pattern recognition receptors (PRR) like Toll-like receptor (TLR) 4 or nucleotide-binding oligomerization domain receptors (NOD) [46]. TLRs not only respond to PAMPs but also transduce the binding signals from host-derived stress molecules, known as damage-associated molecular patterns (DAMPs). This interaction triggers a vicious cycle of inflammation and coagulation [47]. The recognition of these pathogen-associated molecular patterns (PAMPS) by PRR triggers a signaling cascade that stimulates the transcription of genes involved in inflammatory and immune responses, often mediated through the nuclear factor-kB signaling pathway, leading to rapid and massive production of inflammatory mediators and thereby establishing a hyperactive inflammatory response [48]. The endothelial and epithelial cells and innate immune cells like neutrophils, macrophages, and lymphocytes generate potent pro-inflammatory mediators such as TNF-alpha, IL-6,

IL-1, and IL-8 [49]. The coagulopathy of sepsis is mediated by the modulating effects of inflammatory cytokines on the hemostatic system. The activated inflammatory cells, particularly monocytes and neutrophils, express tissue factors on their surface, thereby initiating the extrinsic coagulation cascade [30]. Furthermore, activated monocytes secrete extracellular vesicles containing procoagulant tissue factor and phosphatidylserine. This releases the tissue factor into the blood and activates the extrinsic coagulation cascade [30]. Moreover, Neutrophils also play a major role in activating the coagulation cascade by releasing neutrophil extracellular traps (NETs). These NETs are composed of histones, procoagulant DNA, and other DAMPs released in response to invading pathogens. Although NET formation is essential for clearing pathogens, the overproduction of NETs in sepsis can induce inflammation and lead to tissue injury. In addition, NETs are highly prothombogenic, further enhancing the hypercoagulable state with sepsis (**Figure 1**) [42].

The tissue factor-dependent extrinsic coagulation pathway is considered a crucial element in the initiation of systemic activation of coagulation during sepsis [30]. The extrinsic coagulation cascade begins when tissue factor, normally stored in the vascular endothelium, is exposed to circulating blood after injury, and the process

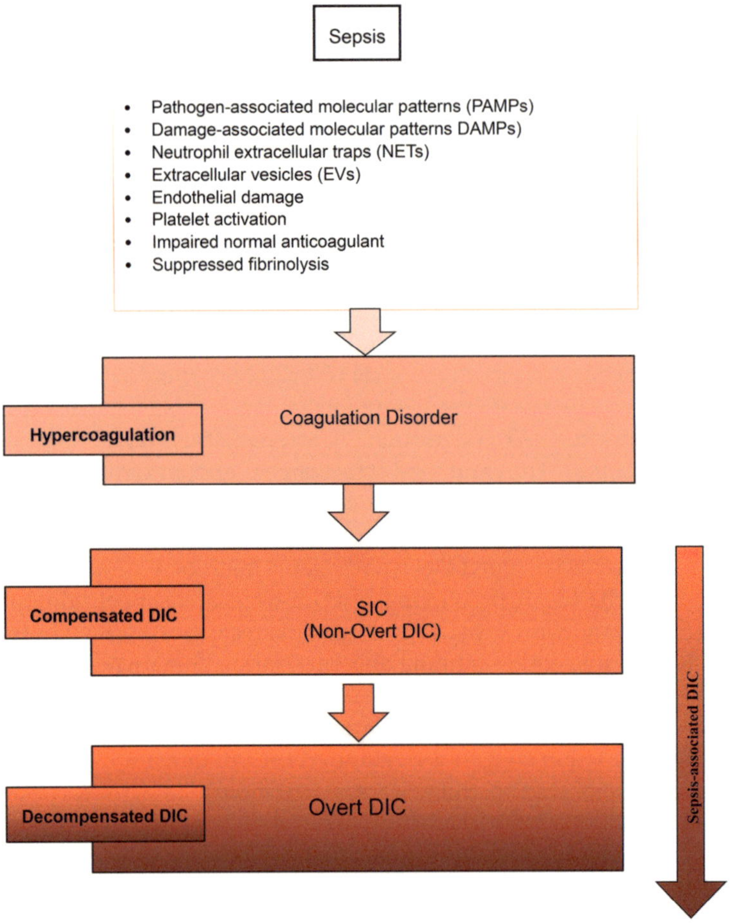

Figure 1.
The initiation and progression of thromboinflammation in sepsis. Modified from Iba et al. [42].

of initiation starts. Inflammatory cells, mainly monocytes, and other circulating macrophages, also express tissue factors. Sepsis-induced inflammation enhances the tissue factor (TF) expression on endothelial cells and circulating monocytes, which is a major mechanism promoting a procoagulant state [50, 51]. *In vivo*, thrombin generation consists of three sequential phases: initiation, amplification, and propagation [50, 52]. Thrombin (factor IIa) is a serine protease that plays a critical role in coagulation. It converts the soluble fibrinogen into insoluble fibrin strands, which are blood clots' main structural components. Thrombin is also a potent activator of platelets, and it extensively promotes systemic coagulation by positive feedback mechanisms [53].

The coagulation cascade begins on cells that express the procoagulant protein tissue factor, such as monocytes, endothelial cells, or platelets. Tissue factor binds to and activates factor VII, converting it to its active form [54]. The enzymatic action of the tissue factor/activated factor VIIa complex results in the activation of small quantities of both factor IX and factor X, thereby initiating the common coagulation pathway. Activated factor IX can activate factor V, which binds to activated factor X to form the prothrombin complex [54]. The initial stage of the coagulation cascade produces a small quantity of thrombin, which is not enough to maintain a large clot but is necessary to stimulate the amplification of the clotting process. The amplification phase increases the small amount of thrombin generated during the initiation phase. Thrombin stimulates the activation of platelets, increasing their surface area for further coagulation processes to occur. Additionally, platelet activation and degranulation enhance the coagulation cascade by providing substrates including activated clotting factors as well as phospholipid membranes. Propagation phase—this is mainly a result of the synthesis and release of large amounts of thrombin that converts fibrinogen to fibrin [54]. Fibrin monomers immediately polymerize to form a stable fibrin mesh that traps platelets, red blood cells, and other cellular components, giving rise to a robust blood clot [55].

4.4 Impairment of anticoagulant mechanisms

Generally, the activation of the coagulation cascade is regulated by three principal anticoagulant mechanisms: the Antithrombin, Protein C, and tissue factor pathway inhibitor (TFPI) [35]. However, during the sepsis-induced hypercoagulable state, the functioning of all three of these regulatory pathways can become impaired. This impairment can occur due to decreased synthesis, consumption, or proteolytic degradation of these regulatory pathways [56]. Additionally, Antithrombin is a key anticoagulant; it inhibits the enzymatic activity of thrombin and factor Xa, but its function may be impaired by decreased antithrombin levels or impaired activity [57]. Sepsis-induced inflammation downregulates the expression of thrombomodulin and endothelial protein C receptor (EPCR) on endothelial cells, thereby impairing the protein C anticoagulant pathway [57]. The protein C system is typically activated when thrombin binds to thrombomodulin on the surface of endothelial cells. Activated protein C, bound to its cofactor protein S, inactivates factors Va and VIIIa, thereby inhibiting thrombin generation. The tissue factor pathway inhibitor, which normally limits the activity of the tissue factor-factor VIIa complex, can also be functionally impaired during sepsis [56].

4.5 Suppression of fibrinolysis

Another consideration in SIC is the impairment of fibrinolysis, which is primarily driven by increased levels of PAI-1. The activation of thrombin-activatable fibrinolysis inhibitors represents an early characteristic of sepsis and may precede the onset of thrombocytopenia [58]. This impaired fibrinolytic activity, in combination with the procoagulant state, leads to excessive intravascular fibrin deposition and the development of microvascular thrombosis, which contributes significantly to the pathogenesis of SIC [59]. Inhibition of plasminogen activation in the early stages of sepsis leads to an acute shutdown of fibrinolysis, a process associated with increased mortality in septic patients [59]. The resulting thrombotic microangiopathy, described by platelet-dense clots in the microvasculature, causes poor tissue perfusion and multi-organ failure [60]. In summary, the dysregulated coagulation activation, the disruption of the body's natural anticoagulant systems, and the impairment of fibrinolysis represent a basic pathogenic process that drives the emergence of coagulopathy in sepsis.

5. Diagnosis of sepsis-induced coagulopathy

Diagnosis and monitoring of SIC is an integral part of the overall assessment of organ function in septic patients [32]. SIC presents as a subclinical form of DIC in the context of sepsis. The diagnosis of SIC can be made using a combination of routine laboratory tests, including platelet count, prothrombin time (PT), activated partial thromboplastin time (aPTT), and fibrinogen levels [32, 33]. The Japanese Ministry of Health and Welfare developed the initial diagnostic criteria for DIC in 1983, which combined clinical findings with laboratory components, including platelet count, prothrombin time, fibrin/fibrinogen degradation products, and fibrinogen. In 2017, the International Society on Thrombosis and Hemostasis further refined this concept with a screening tool termed sepsis-induced coagulopathy (SIC) score to objectively assess disease severity [61, 62]. The SIC score is a set of criteria that allows for the easier and earlier detection of sepsis-associated coagulopathy. Unlike other DIC screening methods, for example, ISTH overt DIC score and Japanese Association for Acute Medicine (JAAM) score, SIC entirely relies on sepsis-related Sequential Organ Failure Assessment (SOFA) scoring—platelet count, international normalized ratio, or prothrombin time [61].

In sepsis-associated DIC, the reduced tissue perfusion due to microvascular thrombosis often leads to organ dysfunction. In non-sepsis-related DIC, the suppression of fibrinolysis is uncommon, and systemic bleeding is more prevalent [63]. Thus, decreased fibrinogen levels are not a typical or specific finding of SIC, unlike the more common observations of thrombocytopenia and prolonged PT. The SIC does not include the evaluation of fibrinogen level (a component of the ISTH score) and D-dimer plasma concentrations (a component of the ISTH and JAAM scores) [61]. FDPs and d-dimers were excluded from the SIC score, as they lacked correlation with the severity of sepsis [64]. A fundamental distinction between SIC and overt DIC is the degree of consumption of platelets and coagulation factors. According to ISTH DIC diagnostic criteria, elevated fibrin degradation products or D-dimer levels, reduced platelet count, prolonged PT, and decreased fibrinogen concentrations indicate overt DIC (**Table 1**) [62]. The SIC score has higher sensitivity (74.3%) compared to the modified ISTH (mISTH) scoring system (49.5%); however, its specificity in identifying SIC is limited in identifying coagulopathy associated with sepsis [66].

Typical laboratory findings in SIC include elevated markers of procoagulant activity (TF) and thrombin generation (thrombin-antithrombin TAT), combined with moderate reductions in anticoagulant factors (ATIII) [59]. Platelet counts often decline in the early stage of the disease's course, while fibrinogen levels are typically

Item	Score	Overt DIC range	SIC range
Platelet count (x10^9/L)	2	<50	<100
	1	≥50, <100	≥50, <100
FDP/D-dimers	3	Strong increase	—
	2	Moderate increase	—
Prothrombin time (PT ratio)	2	≥6 s	>1.4
	1	≥3 s, <6 s	>1.2, <1.4
Fibrinogen (g/ ml)	1	< 100	
SOFA score	2	—	≥2
	1	—	1
Total score for DIC or SIC		≥5	≥4

Abbreviations: DIC—disseminated intravascular coagulation; SIC—sepsis-induced coagulopathy; FDP—fibrin degradation products; SOFA—Sequential Organ Failure Assessment.

Table 1.
International society on thrombosis and hemostasis criteria for DIC and SIC [65].

within the normal range or increased at the time of ICU admission [67]. Persistent dysregulation of the immune-thrombotic response can lead to the progression from SIC to overt DIC, with severe depletion of fibrinogen, platelets, and antithrombotic proteins, leading to a coagulopathy that can manifest as thrombotic, fibrinolytic, or a mixed clinical picture (**Figure 2**) [69].

5.1 Conventional coagulation assays and biomarkers in sepsis

Generally, the assessment of the coagulation system in septic patients involves conventional hemostatic tests, such as platelet count and PT, aPTT, and fibrinogen. Though these tests give a clue about the overall status of coagulation in patients, interpreting them in SIC can be challenging [32].

5.2 Standard coagulation tests

Prothrombin time and activated partial thromboplastin time are traditional coagulation laboratory tests that have long been used to evaluate the hemostatic status of patients with sepsis. The prothrombin time (PT) and activated partial thromboplastin time (aPTT) measures the number of seconds that plasma must clot after the addition of calcium and an extrinsic or intrinsic pathway coagulation activator, respectively [70]. However, in sepsis, these assays may not reflect the global hemostatic picture due to the simultaneous activation of both pro- and anticoagulant pathways and the presence of coagulation inhibitors [71]. Abnormal results of the standard coagulation parameters appear only at a later stage of sepsis (when more advanced hypocoagulable hemostasis develops). Second, these tests only evaluate part of the hemostatic mechanism as they focus on plasma-based coagulation components and do not directly assess the critical role of cellular elements [71]. Thus, understanding the multiple processes involved in SIC remains necessary for interpreting traditional hemostasis assays.

	Thrombosis		Bleeding
	Non-Over DIC (SIC)	Overt DIC	
Plasma Marker		Thrombotic	Fibrinolytic
Procoagulant			
Tissue Factor	↑↑	↑↑↑	↑↑↑
Fibrinogen	↔↑	↔/↓	↓↓↓
Platelets	↓	↓↓	↓↓↓
TAT	↑↑	↑↑	↑↑↑
Anticoagulant			
Antithrombin III	↓↓	↓↓↓	↓↓↓
Thrombomodulin	↓↓	↓↓	↓↓↓
Protein C	↓↓	↓↓↓	↓↓↓
TFPI	↓↓	↓↓	↓↓
Antifibrinolytic			
PAI-I	↑↑	↑↑	↑↑
Fibrinolytic			
tPA	↔/↑	↔/↑	↑↑↑
D-dimer/FDP	↔/↑	↑↑	↑↑↑

Figure 2.
Clinical laboratory features and trends in SIC. Reproduced from Williams et al. [68] SIC is a variant of non-overt DIC in septic patients that involves intravascular coagulation induced by inflammatory-mediated TF expression, leading to TAT and mild-to-moderate consumption of platelets and endogenous anticoagulants (ATIII). Moreover, PAI-1 is markedly increased, leading to the early inhibition of fibrinolysis. The coagulopathy in SIC can develop into overt DIC associated with a thrombotic phenotype, marked by excessive clotting and worsening consumption. Finally, Elevated tPA antigen and fibrinolysis markers (D-dimer) suggest overt disseminated intravascular coagulation with a predominant fibrinolytic phenotype [68]. Abbreviations; ↔ = no change, ↑ = mild changes, ↑↑ = moderate changes, and ↑↑↑ = severe changes, ATIII—Antithrombin III; DIC—disseminated intravascular coagulation; FDP—fibrin degradation products; PAI-1—plasminogen activator inhibitor-1; SIC—sepsis-induced coagulopathy; TAT—Thrombinantithrombin complex; TF—tissue factor; TFPI—tissue factor pathway inhibitor; tPA—tissue plasminogen activator.

5.3 Platelet count

Thrombocytopenia is a common finding in sepsis and is often one of the earliest indicators of sepsis-induced coagulopathy. The pathogenesis of sepsis-induced thrombocytopenia is multifactorial, involving platelet sequestration, increased platelet consumption, and decreased platelet production [72]. Commonly defined as a platelet count of less than 150,000 cells per microliter, thrombocytopenia is an independent predictor of poor outcomes in sepsis patients. It is associated with increased mortality rates and prolonged duration of ICU admissions in these patient populations [72, 73]. Therefore, a lower platelet count has been incorporated into widely used risk assessment scoring systems, including the SOFA score.

5.4 Fibrin degradation products

Fibrin degradation products (FDPs) derive mainly from the proteolytic clearance of three major subjects of the fibrinogen-fibrin cycle: fibrinogen, soluble precursor fibrin, and cross-linked fibrin, which is considered a final stable form [30]. D-dimer is a product of the breakdown of cross-linked fibrin and the subsequent degradation of the fibrin clot by the fibrinolytic enzyme plasmin [74]. Although d-dimers are FDPs and are associated with fibrinolysis, elevated concentrations reflect concurrent activation of the coagulation system. As such, the circulating levels of D-dimer may reflect the activation of both the coagulation and fibrinolytic pathways [74]. In early sepsis, D-dimer levels are commonly elevated due to the simultaneous activation of the coagulation system and increased fibrinolysis. However, in later stages of sepsis, D-dimer levels may return to normal as the fibrinolytic mechanisms become significantly suppressed [30], even though a high amount of fibrin continues to be produced. Interestingly, it has been reported that among patients admitted to an ICU for severe sepsis or septic shock, a normal level of D-dimer on presentation was associated with a higher risk of death as well as decreased fibrinolytic activity [75].

5.5 Fibrinogen

An acute-phase protein, fibrinogen, typically increases secondary to inflammation. In sepsis, initial fibrinogen levels are usually normal or high, resulting from this acute-phase reaction [76]. Nevertheless, in fulminant DIC, a consumption of fibrinogen leads to hypofibrinogenemia. Consequently, testing for fibrinogen levels alone does not accurately diagnose SIC. More recently, a study concluded that fibrinogen levels decreased in the ICU were associated with a high mortality rate among septic patients despite non-overt DIC diagnosis [67].

5.6 Nonconventional hemostatic tests and markers in sepsis

Thromboelastography (TEG) and rotational thromboelastometry (ROTEM) are viscoelastic, point-of-care tests that provide a more comprehensive evaluation of the dynamic process of clot formation, stabilization, and lysis, including the interactions between cellular and plasmatic components of coagulation [77]. Unlike the conventional coagulation parameters, TEG and ROTEM can help differentiate between hypercoagulable, hypocoagulable, and fibrinolytic states, which may be helpful as a diagnostic tool for evaluating SIC [78]. Viscoelastic testing (VET) can identify the early activation of the coagulation system that results in a hypercoagulable state, even when conventional coagulation tests remain within the normal range [78]. Both a hypocoagulable and a hypercoagulable hemostatic profile, as measured by RTOEM, have been associated with a significantly elevated risk of mortality in septic patients [79]. Although viscoelastic tests provide a similar assessment of the *in vivo* hemostatic process compared to standard coagulation tests, they do not fully account for the significant influence of other critical elements in the physiological environment, such as blood flow and the endothelium [71].

The number of septic patients with hemostatic abnormalities detected in TEG or ROTEM results varies from 43 to 100% [78]. The timing of TEG (or ROTEM) is important when considering the dynamic aspect of coagulation in sepsis; serial measurements of these tests may provide a more precise picture of the evolution over time from initial hypercoagulability to eventual hypocoagulability and DIC [80]. In addition, Using VET for the management of SIC has been focused on guiding blood product administration [81]. VET parameters can give critical information about the evolving process of clot formation, such as the initiation (R time), the rate of clot formation (α angle), and maximum strength. Sepsis has been linked to a hypercoagulable state with significantly higher clot firmness and formation rate, as reflected by a shorter EXTEM clotting time compared to healthy controls [82]. Enhanced EXTEM clotting time has been correlated with increasing severity of sepsis [82]. While in septic shock, ROTEM has revealed a normal but prolonged clot formation, with significantly diminished fibrinolytic activity [82]. In addition, patients with overt DIC exhibited decreased maximum clot firmness (MCF) compared to patients with sepsis without DIC. Moreover, MCF shows high sensitivity to diagnose DIC in sepsis [83]. These alterations in ROTEM parameters indicate a general picture of hypercoagulability early in sepsis that progresses to a hypocoagulable state and consumptive coagulopathy as the disease progresses.

MCF depends on platelets and fibrinogen levels. A reduction in MCF indicates that both components are likely decreasing because of their continuous activation and consumption during the evolution of coagulopathy [68]. A hypocoagulable state (lower MCF) was also an independent risk factor for mortality in patients with sepsis [84]. In conclusion, VETs provide a greater assessment of hemostatic abnormalities in sepsis than conventional coagulation tests and may help guide clinical management by aiding outcome prediction [85].

6. Treatment of sepsis-induced coagulopathy

The 2016 Surviving Sepsis guidelines emphasize an early, goal-directed therapeutic approach to improve mortality outcomes in patients diagnosed with sepsis. This includes the administration of antibiotics to treat the underlying infection, intravenous fluids resuscitation, and the use of vasoactive medications to maintain adequate perfusion pressure [86]. According to the British clinical practice guidelines for diagnosis and management of disseminated intravascular coagulation, 'the cornerstone of the treatment of DIC is treatment of the underlying condition' [87]. Early initiation of therapy is critical, as delays in treatment have been associated with increased morbidity and mortality [86]. The 2021 update to the Surviving Sepsis Campaign recommendations highlights the importance of promptly addressing infection source control in sepsis and septic shock patients [88]. Source control should be implemented as soon as possible following the diagnosis [88]. Based on these guidelines, the use of pharmacological thromboprophylaxis with low molecular weight heparin is strongly recommended for patients with sepsis or septic shock.

Specific recommendations for the management of SIC are limited, as most trials have focused on DIC rather than earlier stages of SIC. For SIC progressing to overt DIC and a bleeding phenotype, the recommended interventions include transfusion of red blood cells (strong recommendation) for anemia (Hb <7.0 g/dL), administration of plasma for active bleeding or before invasive procedures (weak recommendation), and platelet transfusion (weak recommendation) for platelet counts less than 50 × 10^9/L [86]. For cases of SIC progressing to overt DIC and exhibiting a thrombotic clinical profile, the recommended intervention is prophylactic or therapeutic anticoagulation, such as heparin.

Despite the high incidence of coagulopathy and associated mortality in septic patients, targeted anticoagulant therapies have not yet demonstrated a clear survival benefit in clinical trials. Direct treatment approaches for SIC, such as the replacement of endogenous anticoagulants (APC, TFPI, ATIII, and TM), have also failed to consistently show a mortality benefit [68].

6.1 Tissue factor pathway inhibitor (TFPI)

Tissue Factor Pathway Inhibitor (TFPI) regulates the coagulation cascade by directly binding to the tissue factor-Factor VII/VIIa complex and factor Xa, modulating the overall coagulation process [89]. Given the central role of tissue factors in the development of sepsis-associated DIC, inhibiting this factor was believed to have a beneficial therapeutic effect. However, TFPI administration did not improve 28-day mortality in a large randomized controlled trial of patients with sepsis [90]. It resulted in an increased risk of bleeding, which consequently prevented its approval for use in sepsis or sepsis-related complications [91].

6.2 Activated protein C

Activated protein C (APC) is a natural anticoagulant that inactivates coagulation factors Va and VIIIa, thereby downregulating thrombin generation. The 2001 PROWESS study found that recombinant human-activated protein C in patients with severe sepsis was associated with a 19.4% relative reduction in the risk of death compared to placebo, with no significant increase in the risk of bleeding [92]. However, subsequent studies failed to confirm a survival benefit [93]. Similarly, the PROWESS SHOCK trial, a follow-up to the initial PROWESS study, found that the administration of APC did not significantly reduce mortality risk among sepsis patients. Additionally, the use of APC was associated with an elevated risk of bleeding complications [94], and the drug was ultimately withdrawn from the market due to safety concerns.

6.3 Thrombomodulin (TM)

Thrombomodulin is an endothelial anticoagulant cofactor promoting the thrombin-mediated activation of protein C [95]. Recombinant thrombomodulin was developed and approved for clinical use in Japan in 2008 for treating DIC [96]. However, the evidence regarding the efficacy of recombinant human soluble thrombomodulin as a treatment for sepsis-associated DIC is mixed. The SCARLET trial in 2019 investigated the use of recombinant thrombomodulin in a cohort of sepsis patients with coagulopathy and organ dysfunction (cardiovascular and/or respiratory failure, platelet count 30 to 150 × 109/L or > 30%-decrease within 24 h, and PT/INR > 1.4 (SIC score > 4) [97]. Although the study did not demonstrate a statistically significant improvement in 28-day all-cause mortality [97], a post-hoc analysis indicated potential benefit in the subgroup of patients meeting the criteria for sepsis-induced coagulopathy [98].

6.4 Transfusion of blood products

The British guidelines for the diagnosis and management of disseminated intravascular coagulation recommend the administration of platelet (trigger <50 × 109/L) and/or fresh-frozen plasma transfusions for patients with DIC who are experiencing active bleeding or require invasive procedures [87]. The clinical response and laboratory parameters, including platelet count and coagulation measures, should be closely monitored following the administration of blood component therapy. A recent prospective, open-label, randomized controlled trial involving children with severe sepsis or septic shock found that early administration of a combination therapy comprising fresh-frozen plasma, low-dose heparin, and tranexamic acid was associated with improved survival outcomes and a reduced risk of progression to overt sepsis-associated DIC, without an increased incidence of bleeding complications [99]. In summary, the efficacy of targeted anticoagulant interventions has remained inconclusive. The considered use of blood component therapy, combined with the prompt management of the underlying infectious source, may represent a reasonable therapeutic approach for improving clinical outcomes in this high-risk patient population.

7. Conclusion

SIC is a complication of sepsis that develops through the link between dysregulated coagulation and innate immune activation, and it is directly involved in the pathogenesis of organ injury and a high risk of death. The pathogenesis of SIC is multifactorial. The dysregulated coagulation activation, the disruption of the body's natural anticoagulant systems, and the impairment of fibrinolysis represent a basic pathogenic process for coagulopathy in sepsis. The development of these processes leads to multiple coagulation pathways, but the role of anticoagulants is unclear. Time to treatment is a critical factor, and delayed treatment is associated with increased mortality. Blood component therapy, combined with early measures to eliminate the focus of infection, may improve the outcomes in high-risk patients.

Author details

Abdelrahman Balal[1*], Ahmad M. Obeidat[1], Khalid Y. Fadul[2], Wala Sati[2], Sara M.I. Ahmed[2], Mohamed Elgassim[2] and Seema Nahid[3]

1 Department of Anesthesia, ICU and Perioperative Medicine, Surgical Intensive Care Unit, Hamad Medical Corporation, Doha, Qatar

2 Department of Emergency Medicine, ICU and Perioperative Medicine, Surgical Intensive Care Unit, Hamad Medical Corporation, Doha, Qatar

3 Department of Anesthesia, Hamad Medical Corporation, Doha, Qatar

*Address all correspondence to: abd.fa466@gmail.com

References

[1] Singer M et al. The third international consensus definitions for sepsis and septic shock (Sepsis-3). JAMA. 2016;**315**(8):801. DOI: 10.1001/jama.2016.0287

[2] Zhao H et al. Comparison between sepsis-induced coagulopathy and sepsis-associated coagulopathy criteria in identifying sepsis-associated disseminated intravascular coagulation. World Journal of Emergency Medicine. 2024;**15**(3):190-196. DOI: 10.5847/wjem.j.1920-8642.2024.041

[3] Schmoch T et al. The prevalence of sepsis-induced coagulopathy in patients with sepsis—A secondary analysis of two German multicenter randomized controlled trials. Annals of Intensive Care. 2023;**13**(1):3. DOI: 10.1186/s13613-022-01093-7

[4] van der Poll T, Herwald H. The coagulation system and its function in early immune defense. Thrombosis and Haemostasis. 2014;**112**(4):640-648. DOI: 10.1160/TH14-01-0053

[5] Semeraro N, Ammollo CT, Semeraro F, Colucci M. Sepsis, thrombosis and organ dysfunction. Thrombosis Research. 2012;**129**(3):290-295. DOI: 10.1016/j.thromres.2011.10.013

[6] Gando S et al. A multicenter, prospective validation of disseminated intravascular coagulation diagnostic criteria for critically ill patients: Comparing current criteria. Critical Care Medicine. 2006;**34**(3):625-631. DOI: 10.1097/01.ccm.0000202209.42491.38

[7] Levi M, Schultz M, Van Der Poll T. Sepsis and thrombosis. Seminars in Thrombosis and Hemostasis. 2013;**39**(05):559-566. DOI: 10.1055/s-0033-1343894

[8] Saito S et al. Epidemiology of disseminated intravascular coagulation in sepsis and validation of scoring systems. Journal of Critical Care. 2019;**50**:23-30. DOI: 10.1016/j.jcrc.2018.11.009

[9] Liufu R et al. Sepsis-induced coagulopathy: The different prognosis in severe pneumonia and bacteremia infection patients. Clinical and Applied Thrombosis. 2023;**29**:10760296231219249. DOI: 10.1177/10760296231219249

[10] Levi M. The coagulant response in sepsis. Clinics in Chest Medicine. 2008;**29**(4):627-642. DOI: 10.1016/j.ccm.2008.06.006

[11] Levi M, van der Poll T. Coagulation in patients with severe sepsis. Seminars in Thrombosis and Hemostasis. 2015;**41**(1):9-15. DOI: 10.1055/s-0034-1398376

[12] Sharma B, Sharma M, Majumder M, Steier W, Sangal A, Kalawar M. Thrombocytopenia in septic shock patients—A prospective observational study of incidence, risk factors and correlation with clinical outcome. Anaesthesia and Intensive Care. 2007;**35**(6):874-880. DOI: 10.1177/0310057X0703500604

[13] Cecconi M, Evans L, Levy M, Rhodes A. Sepsis and septic shock. The Lancet. 2018;**392**(10141):75-87. DOI: 10.1016/S0140-6736(18)30696-2

[14] Lyons PG, Micek ST, Hampton N, Kollef MH. Sepsis-associated coagulopathy severity predicts hospital mortality*. Critical Care Medicine.

2018;**46**(5):736-742. DOI: 10.1097/CCM.0000000000002997

[15] Nasa P, Juneja D, Singh O. Severe sepsis and septic shock in the elderly: An overview. World Journal of Critical Care Medicine. 2012;**1**(1):23-30. DOI: 10.5492/wjccm.v1.i1.23

[16] Rinaldi I, Sudaryo MK, Prihartono NA. Disseminated intravascular coagulation in sepsis and associated factors. Journal of Clinical Medicine. 2022;**11**(21):6480. DOI: 10.3390/jcm11216480

[17] Angus DC, van der Poll T. Severe sepsis and septic shock. The New England Journal of Medicine. 2013;**369**(9):840-851. DOI: 10.1056/NEJMra1208623

[18] Iba T, Arakawa M, Mochizuki K, Nishida O, Wada H, Levy JH. Usefulness of measuring changes in SOFA score for the prediction of 28-day mortality in patients with sepsis-associated disseminated intravascular coagulation. Clinical and applied thrombosis: Official Journal of the International Academy of Clinical and Applied Thrombosis. 2019;**25**:1076029618824044. DOI: 10.1177/1076029618824044

[19] Cangemi R et al. Low-grade endotoxemia and clotting activation in the early phase of pneumonia. Respirology. 2016;**21**(8):1465-1471. DOI: 10.1111/resp.12854

[20] Li Y, Zhang L, Gao M, Zhang C, Zhang D. Risk factors and incidence of sepsis-induced coagulopathy in patients with sepsis: A single-center retrospective cohort study. Research Square. 2023. DOI: 21203/10rs.3.rs-3302770/v1

[21] Schupp T et al. Diagnostic and prognostic significance of the prothrombin time/international normalized ratio in sepsis and septic shock. Clinical and applied thrombosis: Official Journal of the International Academy of Clinical and Applied Thrombosis. 2022;**28**:10760296221137893. DOI: 10.1177/10760296221137893

[22] Kreger BE, Craven DE, McCabe WR. Gram-negative bacteremia. IV. Re-evaluation of clinical features and treatment in 612 patients. The American Journal of Medicine. 1980;**68**(3):344-355. DOI: 10.1016/0002-9343(80)90102-3

[23] Semeraro N, Ammollo CT, Semeraro F, Colucci M. Sepsis-associated disseminated intravascular coagulation and thromboembolic disease. Mediterranean Journal of Hematology and Infectious Diseases. 2010;**2**(3):e2010024. DOI: 10.4084/MJHID.2010.024

[24] Goeijenbier M et al. Review: Viral infections and mechanisms of thrombosis and bleeding. Journal of Medical Virology. 2012;**84**(10):1680-1696. DOI: 10.1002/jmv.23354

[25] Bunce PE, High SM, Nadjafi M, Stanley K, Liles WC, Christian MD. Pandemic H1N1 influenza infection and vascular thrombosis. Clinical Infectious Diseases: An Official Publication of the Infectious Diseases Society of America. 2011;**52**(2):e14-e17. DOI: 10.1093/cid/ciq125

[26] Akiyama R, Komori I, Hiramoto R, Isonishi A, Matsumoto M, Fujimura Y. H1N1 influenza (swine flu)-associated thrombotic microangiopathy with a markedly high plasma ratio of von Willebrand factor to ADAMTS13. Internal Medicine Tokyo Japan. 2011;**50**(6):643-647. DOI: 10.2169/internalmedicine.50.4620

[27] Connors JM, Levy JH. COVID-19 and its implications for thrombosis

and anticoagulation. Blood. 2020;**135**(23):2033-2040. DOI: 10.1182/blood.2020006000

[28] Görlinger K, Dirkmann D, Gandhi A, Simioni P. COVID-19-associated coagulopathy and inflammatory response: What do we know already and what are the knowledge gaps? Anesthesia & Analgesia. 2020;**131**(5):1324-1333. DOI: 10.1213/ANE.0000000000005147

[29] Zhang L et al. D-dimer levels on admission to predict in-hospital mortality in patients with Covid-19. Journal of Thrombosis and Haemostasis. 2020;**18**(6):1324-1329. DOI: 10.1111/jth.14859

[30] Tsantes AG et al. Sepsis-induced coagulopathy: An update on pathophysiology, biomarkers, and current guidelines. Life. 2023;**13**(2):350. DOI: 10.3390/life13020350

[31] Chang JC. Sepsis and septic shock: Endothelial molecular pathogenesis associated with vascular microthrombotic disease. Thrombosis Journal. 2019;**17**:10. DOI: 10.1186/s12959-019-0198-4

[32] Samavedam S. Sepsis induced coagulopathy: Bringing science to the bedside. Indian Journal of Critical Care Medicine: Peer-reviewed, Official Publication of Indian Society of Critical Care Medicine. 2023;**27**(9):611-612. DOI: 10.5005/jp-journals-10071-24537

[33] Tsao C-M, Ho S-T, Wu C-C. Coagulation abnormalities in sepsis. Acta Anaesthesiologica Taiwanica. 2015;**53**(1):16-22. DOI: 10.1016/j.aat.2014.11.002

[34] Genga KR, Russell JA. Coagulation abnormalities in sepsis. In: Ronco C, Bellomo R, Kellum JA, Ricci Z, editors. Critical Care Nephrology. 3rd ed. Philadelphia: Elsevier; 2019. pp. 508-517.e3. DOI: 10.1016/B978-0-323-44942-7.00088-1

[35] Giustozzi M et al. Coagulopathy and sepsis: Pathophysiology, clinical manifestations and treatment. Blood Reviews. 2021;**50**:100864. DOI: 10.1016/j.blre.2021.100864

[36] Levi M, Van Der Poll T. Coagulation and sepsis. Thrombosis Research. 2017;**149**:38-44. DOI: 10.1016/j.thromres.2016.11.007

[37] Levi M, van der Poll T, Büller HR. Bidirectional relation between inflammation and coagulation. Circulation. 2004;**109**(22):2698-2704. DOI: 10.1161/01.CIR.0000131660.51520.9A

[38] Levi M, van der Poll T. Inflammation and coagulation. Critical Care Medicine. 2010;**38**(Suppl. 2):S26-S34. DOI: 10.1097/CCM.0b013e3181c98d21

[39] Abraham E et al. Efficacy and safety of monoclonal antibody to human tumor necrosis factor alpha in patients with sepsis syndrome. A randomized, controlled, double-blind, multicenter clinical trial. TNF-alpha MAb sepsis study group. JAMA. 1995;**273**(12):934-941

[40] Tang H et al. Sepsis-induced coagulation in the baboon lung is associated with decreased tissue factor pathway inhibitor. The American Journal of Pathology. 2007;**171**(3):1066-1077. DOI: 10.2353/ajpath.2007.070104

[41] van der Poll T et al. Elimination of interleukin 6 attenuates coagulation activation in experimental endotoxemia in chimpanzees. Journal of Experimental Medicine. 1994;**179**(4):1253-1259. DOI: 10.1084/jem.179.4.1253

[42] Iba T, Helms J, Connors JM, Levy JH. The pathophysiology, diagnosis, and management of sepsis-associated disseminated intravascular coagulation. Journal of Intensive Care. 2023;**11**(1):24. DOI: 10.1186/s40560-023-00672-5

[43] Joffre J, Hellman J, Ince C, Ait-Oufella H. Endothelial responses in sepsis. American Journal of Respiratory and Critical Care Medicine. 2020;**202**(3):361-370. DOI: 10.1164/rccm.201910-1911TR

[44] Assinger A, Schrottmaier WC, Salzmann M, Rayes J. Platelets in sepsis: An update on experimental models and clinical data. Frontiers in Immunology. 2019;**10**:1687. DOI: 10.3389/fimmu.2019.01687

[45] Ito T, Kakuuchi M, Maruyama I. Endotheliopathy in septic conditions: Mechanistic insight into intravascular coagulation. Critical Care. 2021;**25**(1):95. DOI: 10.1186/s13054-021-03524-6

[46] Iyer JK et al. Inflammatory cytokine response to bacillus anthracis peptidoglycan requires phagocytosis and lysosomal trafficking. Infection and Immunity. 2010;**78**(6):2418-2428. DOI: 10.1128/IAI.00170-10

[47] Salomão R et al. TLR signaling pathway in patients with sepsis. Shock Augusta Ga. 2008;**30**(Suppl. 1):73-77. DOI: 10.1097/SHK.0b013e318181af2a

[48] Pawlinski R, Mackman N. Cellular sources of tissue factor in endotoxemia and sepsis. Thrombosis Research. 2010;**125S1**:S70-S73. DOI: 10.1016/j.thromres.2010.01.042

[49] Aird WC. Endothelium as an organ system. Critical Care Medicine. 2004;**32**(Suppl. 5):S271-S279. DOI: 10.1097/01.ccm.0000129669.21649.40

[50] O'Brien M. The reciprocal relationship between inflammation and coagulation. Topics in Companion Animal Medicine. 2012;**27**(2):46-52. DOI: 10.1053/j.tcam.2012.06.003

[51] Mohammed BAB. Hemostatic aspect of sepsis. In: Infectious Process and Sepsis. London, UK: IntechOpen; 2020. DOI: 10.5772/intechopen.90800

[52] Hoffman M, Monroe D. A cell-based model of hemostasis. Thrombosis and Haemostasis. 2001;**85**(06):958-965. DOI: 10.1055/s-0037-1615947

[53] Simmons J, Pittet J-F. The coagulopathy of acute sepsis. Current Opinion in Anaesthesiology. 2015;**28**(2):227-236. DOI: 10.1097/ACO.0000000000000163

[54] Reyes Gil M. Overview of the coagulation system. In: Shaz BH, Hillyer CD, Reyes Gil M, editors. Transfusion Medicine and Hemostasis. 3rd ed. Amsterdam, Netherlands: Elsevier; 2019. pp. 559-564. DOI: 10.1016/B978-0-12-813726-0.00091-X

[55] Chu AJ. Role of tissue factor in thrombosis. Coagulation-inflammation-thrombosis circuit. Frontiers in Bioscience: A Journal and Virtual Library. 2006;**11**:256-271. DOI: 10.2741/1796

[56] Lupu F, Keshari RS, Lambris JD, Coggeshall KM. Crosstalk between the coagulation and complement systems in sepsis. Thrombosis Research. 2014;**133**(Suppl. 1):S28-S31. DOI: 10.1016/j.thromres.2014.03.014

[57] Saracco P, Vitale P, Scolfaro C, Pollio B, Pagliarino M, Timeus F. The coagulopathy in sepsis: Significance and implications for treatment. Pediatric Reports. 2011;**3**(4):e30. DOI: 10.4081/pr.2011.e30

[58] Semeraro F et al. Platelet drop and fibrinolytic shutdown in patients with sepsis. Critical Care Medicine. 2018;**46**(3):e221-e228. DOI: 10.1097/CCM.0000000000002919

[59] Fcf S et al. Acute fibrinolysis shutdown occurs early in septic shock and is associated with increased morbidity and mortality: Results of an observational pilot study. Annals of Intensive Care. 2019;**9**(1):1-15. DOI: 10.1186/s13613-019-0499-6

[60] Maneta E et al. Endothelial dysfunction and immunothrombosis in sepsis. Frontiers in Immunology. 2023;**14**:1144229. DOI: 10.3389/fimmu.2023.1144229

[61] Iba T, Nisio MD, Levy JH, Kitamura N, Thachil J. New criteria for sepsis-induced coagulopathy (SIC) following the revised sepsis definition: A retrospective analysis of a nationwide survey. BMJ Open. 2017;7(9):e017046. DOI: 10.1136/bmjopen-2017-017046

[62] Yamakawa K, Yoshimura J, Ito T, Hayakawa M, Hamasaki T, Fujimi S. External validation of the two newly proposed criteria for assessing coagulopathy in sepsis. Thrombosis and Haemostasis. 2019;**119**(2):203-212. DOI: 10.1055/s-0038-1676610

[63] Asakura H. Classifying types of disseminated intravascular coagulation: Clinical and animal models. Journal of Intensive Care. 2014;**2**(1):20. DOI: 10.1186/2052-0492-2-20

[64] Iba T et al. A proposal of the modification of Japanese society on thrombosis and hemostasis (JSTH) disseminated intravascular coagulation (DIC) diagnostic criteria for sepsis-associated DIC. Clinical and Applied Thrombosis. 2018;**24**(3):439-445. DOI: 10.1177/1076029617720069

[65] Iba T, Levy JH, Warkentin TE, Thachil J, Van Der Poll T, Levi M. Diagnosis and management of sepsis-induced coagulopathy and disseminated intravascular coagulation. Journal of Thrombosis and Haemostasis. 2019;**17**(11):1989-1994. DOI: 10.1111/jth.14578

[66] Williams B, Zou L, Pittet J-F, Chao W. Sepsis-induced coagulopathy: A comprehensive narrative review of pathophysiology, clinical presentation, diagnosis, and management strategies. Anesthesia & Analgesia. 2024;**138**(4):696-711. DOI: 10.1213/ANE.0000000000006888

[67] Mori K, Tsujita Y, Yamane T, Eguchi Y. Decreasing plasma fibrinogen levels in the intensive care unit are associated with high mortality rates in patients with sepsis-induced coagulopathy. Clinical and Applied Thrombosis: Official Journal of the International Academy of Clinical and Applied Thrombosis. 2022;**28**:10760296221101386. DOI: 10.1177/10760296221101386

[68] Brittney W, Lin Z, Jean-Francois P, Wei C. Sepsis-induced coagulopathy: A comprehensive narrative review of pathophysiology, clinical presentation, diagnosis, and management strategies. Anesthesia & Analgesia. 2024;**138**(4):696-711. DOI: 10.1213/ANE.0000000000006888

[69] Wada H, Matsumoto T, Yamashita Y. Diagnosis and treatment of disseminated intravascular coagulation (DIC) according to four DIC guidelines. Journal of Intensive Care. 2014;**2**(1):15. DOI: 10.1186/2052-0492-2-15

[70] Kamal AH, Tefferi A, Pruthi RK. How to interpret and pursue an abnormal prothrombin time, activated partial thromboplastin time, and

bleeding time in adults. Mayo Clinic Proceedings. 2007;**82**(7):864-873. DOI: 10.4065/82.7.864

[71] Scarlatescu E, Juffermans NP, Thachil J. The current status of viscoelastic testing in septic coagulopathy. Thrombosis Research. 2019;**183**:146-152. DOI: 10.1016/j.thromres.2019.09.029

[72] Gonzalez DA, Kumar R, Asif S, Bali A, Dang AK. Sepsis and thrombocytopenia: A nowadays problem. Cureus. 2022;**14**(5):e25421. DOI: 10.7759/cureus.25421

[73] Venkata C, Kashyap R, Farmer JC, Afessa B. Thrombocytopenia in adult patients with sepsis: Incidence, risk factors, and its association with clinical outcome. Journal of Intensive Care. 2013;**1**(1):9. DOI: 10.1186/2052-0492-1-9

[74] Semeraro F et al. Low D-dimer levels in sepsis: Good or bad? Thrombosis Research. 2019;**174**:13-15. DOI: 10.1016/j.thromres.2018.12.003

[75] Semeraro F et al. D-dimer corrected for thrombin and plasmin generation is a strong predictor of mortality in patients with sepsis. Blood transfusion = Trasfusione del sangue. 2020;**18**(4):304-311. DOI: 10.2450/2019.0175-19

[76] Adelborg K, Larsen JB, Hvas A-M. Disseminated intravascular coagulation: Epidemiology, biomarkers, and management. British Journal of Haematology. 2021;**192**(5):803-818. DOI: 10.1111/bjh.17172

[77] Görlinger K et al. The role of evidence-based algorithms for rotational thromboelastometry-guided bleeding management. Korean Journal of Anesthesiology. 2019;**72**(4):297-322. DOI: 10.4097/kja.19169

[78] Müller MC, Meijers JC, Vroom MB, Juffermans NP. Utility of thromboelastography and/or thromboelastometry in adults with sepsis: A systematic review. Critical Care. 2014;**18**(1):R30. DOI: 10.1186/cc13721

[79] Adamik B, Gozdzik W, Jakubczyk D, Welna M, Kübler A. Coagulation abnormalities identified by thromboelastometry in patients with severe sepsis: The relationship to endotoxemia and mortality. Blood Coagulation & Fibrinolysis. 2017;**28**(2):163-170. DOI: 10.1097/MBC.0000000000000572

[80] Scarlatescu E, Lancé MD, White NJ, Tomescu DR. Thromboelastometric prediction of mortality using the kinetics of clot growth in critically ill septic patients. Blood Coagulation & Fibrinolysis. 2018;**29**(6):533. DOI: 10.1097/MBC.0000000000000757

[81] Czempik PF, Wiórek A. Management strategies in septic coagulopathy: A review of the current literature. Healthcare (Basel, Switzerland). 2023;**11**(2):227. DOI: 10.3390/healthcare11020227

[82] Davies GR et al. The effect of sepsis and septic shock on the viscoelastic properties of clot quality and mass using rotational thromboelastometry: A prospective observational study. Journal of Critical Care. 2018;**44**:7-11. DOI: 10.1016/j.jcrc.2017.09.183

[83] Sivula M, Pettilä V, Niemi TT, Varpula M, Kuitunen AH. Thromboelastometry in patients with severe sepsis and disseminated intravascular coagulation. Blood Coagulation & Fibrinolysis: An International Journal in Haemostasis and Thrombosis. 2009;**20**(6):419-426. DOI: 10.1097/MBC.0b013e32832a76e1

[84] Boscolo A et al. Are thromboelastometric and thromboelastographic parameters associated with mortality in septic patients? A systematic review and meta-analysis. Journal of Critical Care. 2021;**61**:5-13. DOI: 10.1016/j.jcrc.2020.09.034

[85] Yoon S et al. Thromboelastographic evaluation in patients with severe sepsis or septic shock: A preliminary analysis. Journal of Acute Care Surgery. 2020;**10**(2):47-52. DOI: 10.17479/jacs.2020.10.2.47

[86] Rhodes A et al. Surviving sepsis campaign: International guidelines for Management of Sepsis and Septic Shock: 2016. Intensive Care Medicine. 2017;**43**(3):304-377. DOI: 10.1007/s00134-017-4683-6

[87] Levi M, Toh CH, Thachil J, Watson HG. Guidelines for the diagnosis and management of disseminated intravascular coagulation. British Committee for Standards in Haematology. British Journal of Haematology. 2009;**145**(1):24-33. DOI: 10.1111/j.1365-2141.2009.07600.x

[88] Evans L et al. Surviving sepsis campaign: International guidelines for management of sepsis and septic shock 2021. Intensive Care Medicine. 2021;**47**(11):1181-1247. DOI: 10.1007/s00134-021-06506-y

[89] Lwaleed BA, Bass PS. Tissue factor pathway inhibitor: Structure, biology and involvement in disease. Journal of Pathology. 2006;**208**(3):327-339. DOI: 10.1002/path.1871

[90] Efficacy and safety of Tifacogin (recombinant tissue factor pathway inhibitor) in severe sepsis: A randomized controlled trial. Critical Care Medicine | JAMA | JAMA Network. Available from: https://jamanetwork.com/journals/jama/fullarticle/196870. [Accessed: August 23, 2024]

[91] Abraham E. et al. Efficacy and Safety of Tifacogin (Recombinant Tissue Factor Pathway Inhibitor) in Severe Sepsis. Available from: https://jamanetwork.com/journals/jama/fullarticle/196870 [Accessed: September 9, 2024]

[92] Bernard GR et al. Efficacy and safety of recombinant human activated protein C for severe sepsis. The New England Journal of Medicine. 2001;**344**(10):699-709. DOI: 10.1056/NEJM200103083441001

[93] Abraham E et al. Drotrecogin alfa (activated) for adults with severe sepsis and a low risk of death. The New England Journal of Medicine. 2005;**353**(13):1332-1341. DOI: 10.1056/NEJMoa050935

[94] Ranieri VM, Thompson BT, Barie PS, Dhainaut JF, Douglas IS, Finfer S, et al. Drotrecogin Alfa (activated) in adults with septic shock. The New England Journal of Medicine. 2012;**366**(22):2055-2064. DOI: 10.1056/NEJMoa1202290

[95] Iba T, Levi M, Levy JH. Sepsis-induced coagulopathy and disseminated intravascular coagulation. Seminars in Thrombosis and Hemostasis. 2020;**46**(1):89-95. DOI: 10.1055/s-0039-1694995

[96] Murata A, Okamoto K, Mayumi T, Muramatsu K, Matsuda S. Recent change in treatment of disseminated intravascular coagulation in Japan: An epidemiological study based on a national administrative database. Clinical and applied thrombosis: Official Journal of the International Academy of Clinical and Applied Thrombosis. 2016;**22**(1):21-27. DOI: 10.1177/1076029615575072

[97] Vincent J-L et al. Effect of a recombinant human soluble

thrombomodulin on mortality in patients with sepsis-associated coagulopathy: The SCARLET randomized clinical trial. JAMA. 2019;**321**(20):1993-2002. DOI: 10.1001/jama.2019.5358

[98] François B et al. Efficacy and safety of human soluble thrombomodulin (ART-123) for treatment of patients in France with sepsis-associated coagulopathy: Post hoc analysis of SCARLET. Annals of Intensive Care. 2021;**11**:53. DOI: 10.1186/s13613-021-00842-4

[99] El-Nawawy AA et al. Outcome of early hemostatic intervention in children with sepsis and non-overt disseminated intravascular coagulation admitted to PICU: A randomized controlled trial. Pediatric Critical Care Medicine Journal of the Society of Critical Care Medicine and the World Federation of Pediatric Intensive and Critical Care. 2021;**22**(3):e168-e177. DOI: 10.1097/PCC.0000000000002578

Chapter 10

Sepsis Associated Acute Kidney Injury

Sohel Mohamed Gamal Ahmed, Ebtihal Mahmoud, Malek Abusannuga, Zakaria Attique and Jawdat Alali

Abstract

Acute kidney injury (AKI) associated with sepsis is a critical medical condition characterised by a sudden decrease of renal function as a result of an infection, particularly severe sepsis. Sepsis is a potentially fatal condition that arises from the immune system's reaction to an infection, which involves the release of chemicals into the circulation in an effort to combat the infection; this results in extensive inflammation throughout the body. This inflammation may occasionally hinder optimal blood flow to the kidneys, resulting in AKI. AKI can develop rapidly in the context of sepsis and necessitates immediate medical attention. Laboratory tests are frequently used to assess kidney function, while radiological imaging is used to detect any abnormalities. Antibiotics are commonly prescribed to treat the underlying infection, while supportive care is implemented to maintain kidney function. Patients with severe conditions might require renal replacement modalities to assist in the removal of metabolites and excess fluids from the bloodstream until renal function recovers. Early diagnosis and treatment of sepsis, in addition to implementing strategies to minimise complications are essential for preventing and treating sepsis-associated AKI.

Keywords: sepsis, acute kidney injury, pathophysiology, management, renal replacement therapies

1. Introduction

Sepsis, a severe and often perilous condition, arises from a malfunctioning host response to infection, culminating in profound and life-threatening organ dysfunction. Among the array of complications that can ensue, acute kidney injury (AKI) is particularly common, with sepsis being implicated in 45–70 percent of AKI cases within critically ill patients. The intersection between sepsis and AKI results in a significantly graver prognosis than either condition alone. Mortality rates for septic AKI can range from 30–60%, depending on illness severity. However, no study to date has precisely determined the contribution of sepsis to AKI-related mortality. This interplay, known as Sepsis-Associated AKI (SA-AKI), is linked to prolonged stays in intensive care units and hospitals, escalated mortality rates, and a higher likelihood of enduring long-term disability. Both adult and paediatric populations are affected, with SA-AKI contributing to a marked decline in quality of life [1].

IntechOpen

2. Definition

Sepsis represents a severe clinical condition characterised by a dysregulated systemic inflammatory response to infection, leading to critical organ dysfunction, commonly involving the kidneys. It is a major contributor to severe illness in critically ill patients, posing a considerable threat in intensive care environments due to its high morbidity and mortality rates [2].

The diagnosis of sepsis is mainly based on the established Sepsis-3 criteria. In intensive care settings, sepsis often coexists with other severe conditions, such as acute kidney injury (AKI). AKI is characterised by a complex clinical syndrome involving the accumulation of nitrogenous and other metabolic waste products in the body, resulting from impaired renal function [2]. AKI typically manifests as reduced urine output "oliguria," though non-oliguric forms can also occur [2].

Acute kidney injury (AKI) is defined as an increase in serum creatinine of at least 0.3 mg/dL within 48 hours or an increase to 1.5 times the baseline level, which is either confirmed or assumed to have occurred within the last 7 days. Furthermore, AKI can be identified by a decrease in urine output to less than 0.5 mL/kg/h for a duration of 6 hours [2].

Until recently, a standardised definition of SA-AKI was lacking. The 28th Acute Disease Quality Initiative (ADQI-28) has established that *SA-AKI is defined as acute kidney injury occurring within 7 days of the onset of sepsis*. In this context, SA-AKI identified within 48 hours from the start of sepsis is termed early SA-AKI. Conversely, SA-AKI that develops between 48 hours and 7 days after sepsis begins is termed late SA-AKI [2].

Sepsis-induced acute kidney injury (SI-AKI) falls under the broader category of sepsis-associated acute kidney injury (SA-AKI) and specifically involves renal dysfunction directly linked to the pathophysiological processes of sepsis. SI-AKI exclusively encompasses renal damage that originates directly from sepsis, distinct from kidney injuries that arise from indirect consequences of sepsis or its management, such as nephrotoxicity induced by antimicrobial treatments or from conditions like abdominal compartment syndrome [1, 2].

Importantly, mechanisms that underlie cellular and organ injury in ischaemic AKI or nephrotoxic AKI, such as microcirculation failure, inflammation and mitochondrial injury, might also contribute to SI-AKI [1].

The rationale for defining SA-AKI within a 7-day window is grounded in observations that acute kidney injury (AKI) typically occurs within a few days of sepsis onset. It is generally agreed that AKI occurring beyond this period is less likely to be directly attributable to the initial septic insult.

The distinction between early and late SA-AKI hinges on evidence that AKI occurring later in the course of sepsis is associated with worse clinical outcomes and increased mortality rates compared to early SA-AKI. This distinction may enhance the precision of phenotyping, allowing for more targeted assessments and management strategies. Specifically, early SA-AKI is more likely to be associated with sepsis-induced mechanisms, whereas late SA-AKI may involve additional factors influenced by subsequent sepsis-related interventions [1].

3. Disease burden

Disease burden is a critical measure of population health. In the context of acute kidney injury (AKI) associated with sepsis, the disease burden can be assessed through several dimensions. The incidence and prevalence of AKI in septic patients, while the resulting health loss—both fatal and non-fatal—can be quantified through disability-adjusted life years (DALYs). Furthermore, the financial costs of AKI in sepsis include both direct healthcare expenditures, such as those related to hospitalisation and renal replacement therapy (RRT), and indirect costs, which may encompass lost productivity and long-term care needs. Thus, the burden of AKI in sepsis is significant, impacting both patient outcomes and healthcare systems [3].

The incidence of acute kidney injury (AKI) among hospitalised patients is rising, reflecting an ageing population, with estimates ranging from 1.6–20% of all inpatients. Severe cases of AKI may necessitate renal replacement therapy (RRT) in up to 7% of critically ill patients [4].

The mortality rate associated with acute kidney injury (AKI) in patients with sepsis is 9.1%, whereas septic shock is associated with a significantly higher mortality rate for AKI compared to sepsis alone [5].

The high costs associated with RRT, coupled with AKI's potential to impair other organ systems, often result in additional diagnostic and therapeutic interventions. Consequently, AKI may lead to increased healthcare resource utilisation and extended length of stay (LOS), thereby escalating direct hospital costs over time. A study showed that when AKI was present, an increase in costs of 70% was estimated in patients with sepsis [4].

4. Risk factors

It is crucial to assess patients for the risk of developing acute kidney injury (AKI) to enable early diagnosis and timely intervention for high-risk individuals. Early identification of AKI in hospitalised patients has been demonstrated to reduce the necessity for dialysis [6].

The incidence of acute kidney injury (AKI) is highest in the context of septic shock. Several other key risk factors, including essential hypertension, diabetes mellitus, and abdominal infections, significantly influence the development of AKI in sepsis. Additional factors contributing to AKI include the use of vasopressors and vasoactive drugs, mechanical ventilation—where hypoxaemia, hypercapnia, and excessive positive end-expiratory pressure (PEEP) are notable risk factors—positive blood culture results, and a history of smoking. Other relevant risk factors encompass cardiovascular diseases, male sex, coronary artery disease, liver disease, infections of unknown aetiology, and the use of diuretics, which can exacerbate AKI risk through mechanisms such as stimulating the renin-angiotensin-aldosterone system (RAAS). The use of angiotensin-converting enzyme inhibitors (ACEI) or angiotensin receptor blockers (ARB) is also associated with increased AKI risk. Moreover, infections caused by gram-negative bacteria, particularly *Escherichia coli*, and a history of organ transplantation further heighten the risk of AKI patients with sepsis (**Table 1**) [7].

5. Pathophysiology

The pathophysiological mechanisms underlying S-AKI remain insufficiently understood. Efforts to address this gap include obtaining renal biopsies from patients with acute kidney injury (AKI) to enhance the understanding needed [8].

Risk factors for AKI in sepsis	Details
Septic shock	Major contributing factor to AKI incidence.
Hypertension	Common underlying condition in AKI development.
Diabetes mellitus	Increases susceptibility to AKI.
Abdominal infections	Higher risk in patients with infections, especially abdominal.
Vasopressors and vasoactive drugs	Medications used in sepsis treatment can increase AKI risk.
Mechanical ventilation	Risk enhanced by hypoxemia, hypercapnia, and excessive PEEP (positive end-expiratory pressure).
Positive blood cultures	Indicator of infection severity, associated with AKI risk.
Smoking	History of smoking contributes to higher risk.
Cardiovascular diseases	Increased AKI susceptibility in patients with heart conditions.
Male sex	Males are at higher risk compared to females.
Coronary artery disease and liver disease	Underlying diseases that exacerbate AKI risk.
Infections of unknown aetiology	Presence of unidentified infections elevates AKI likelihood.
Diuretic use	Can worsen AKI risk by stimulating RAAS (renin-angiotensin-aldosterone system).
ACE inhibitors and ARBs	Use of these medications is linked with increased AKI risk.
Gram-negative bacterial infections	Infections, especially with Escherichia coli, contribute to AKI development.
History of organ transplantation	Further increases AKI risk in septic patients.

Table 1.
Risk factors for AKI in sepsis.

Historically, ischaemia and reduced renal perfusion were believed to be the primary causes of AKI in sepsis. While ischaemic injury does contribute to cellular apoptosis and tubular necrosis, it is now recognised that ischaemia is not the sole mechanism of AKI, which can also occur with increased renal blood flow [8].

In sepsis, organ damage, including renal injury, occurs through different mechanisms: systemic and renal inflammation, microcirculatory dysfunction, complement system activation, dysregulation of the renin-angiotensin-aldosterone system (RAAS), mitochondrial dysfunction, metabolic reprogramming, and macrocirculatory abnormalities [1, 8]. The revised definition of sepsis posits that a dysregulated inflammatory response may underlie organ dysfunction and adverse outcomes. During sepsis, inflammatory mediators such as cytokines and chemokines are released into the bloodstream. Renal tubular epithelial cells (TECs) express Toll-like receptors, notably TLR2 and TLR4. Exposure of these receptors to inflammatory mediators filtered through the glomerulus or present in adjacent peritubular capillaries leads to increased oxidative stress, elevated production of reactive oxygen species, and mitochondrial damage in proximal TECs. Additionally, TECs may engage in paracrine signalling, which can lead to the suppression of neighbouring cells' function in an effort to reduce cell death, thereby compromising overall cellular function [8].

Early events involve the activation of innate immunity through the recognition of danger-associated molecular patterns (DAMPs), which are normally intracellular molecules released from dying or damaged cells or pathogen-associated molecular patterns (PAMPs). An initial hyperinflammatory response, often described as a "cytokine storm," can lead to circulatory collapse, lactic acidosis, and hypercatabolism, contributing to early mortality. The extent of the inflammatory response and associated early deaths are influenced by factors such as patient comorbidities, genetic predispositions, and the virulence of the pathogen and bacterial load. Subsequently, mitochondrial dysfunction, apoptosis, and other regulated cell death mechanisms, including ferroptosis, necroptosis, and pyroptosis, are observed [2].

The interplay of various disease mechanisms can lead to diverse disease endotypes. SA-AKI encompasses both direct and indirect forms of kidney injury. In some cases, SA-AKI arises directly from the renal injury induced by the sepsis response itself. In other cases, additional sepsis-related factors, such as therapeutic interventions, can indirectly contribute to kidney damage. For instance, high doses of norepinephrine may reduce microvascular blood flow and worsen the microcirculatory dysfunction caused by sepsis. Several tissue-protective mechanisms, such as the activation of heme oxygenase 1 or mitochondrial autophagy (mitophagy), can help safeguard cells and tissues from damage inflicted by PAMPs and DAMPs [1].

The main factor implicated in SA-AKI was historically considered to be widespread arterial vasodilation, resulting in a reduction in systemic vascular resistance. Systematic analyses have revealed that in three human studies on sepsis renal blood flow (RBF) was increased. In the remaining 38% of these studies, the RBF showed no change or an increase. These findings emphasise the role of injury mechanisms that persist despite maintained RBF, highlighting the critical importance of microcirculatory dysfunction [2].

Microvascular function Has a significant impact on the microcirculation, and alterations in microcirculatory flow may result in impaired kidney tissue perfusion despite maintained renal blood flow (RBF). Wu et al., using intravital video microscopy, revealed that peritubular capillary flow was markedly diminished in lipopolysaccharide (LPS)-induced sepsis. Peritubular capillary flow decreased by 88%, while intermittent flow increased by 400%, and absence of flow increased by approximately 300%. In addition, multiparametric photoacoustic microscopy indicated that sepsis led to a significant and acute decrease in peritubular capillary oxygen saturation of haemoglobin, which was associated with a significant reduction in renal ATP levels [2].

The development of SA-AKI can result in various clinical phenotypes and subphenotypes, contingent upon the interplay between genetic predispositions and environmental exposures. This variability creates challenges in evaluating the therapeutic effectiveness of sepsis interventions in clinical trials, as different therapies may be effective only for specific disease endotypes. It is crucial to acknowledge that multiple pathophysiological mechanisms may simultaneously contribute to the manifestation of AKI in an individual patient with sepsis. Thus, recognising specific SA-AKI endotypes is crucial for advancing the development of targeted and effective therapies [1].

The release of PAMPs, including lipopolysaccharides and DAMPs from injured cells and tissues, can cause the aberrant activation of the immune system, which is characteristic of sepsis. Susceptibility to tissue and organ damage differs among individuals as a result of both non-adjustable factors—such as comorbidities, lifestyle decisions (e.g., smoking), genetic variants (e.g., single nucleotide polymorphisms), comorbidities, and medication use (e.g., renin-angiotensin-aldosterone system (RAAS) inhibitors for blood pressure management)—and adjustable factors, comprising the use of vasopressors, mechanical ventilation, or the presence of bacteraemia [1].

The pathways activated in response to sepsis are affected by this underlying susceptibility and determine the endotype-specific pathophysiological mechanisms leading to AKI in patients with sepsis [1].

6. Clinical diagnosis

6.1 The RIFLE criteria

Three distinct impairment categories—risk, injury, and failure—are crucial for understanding renal health and were adopted by the RIFLE criteria (Risk, Injury, Failure, Loss and End Stage Renal Disease) as in **Table 2**. Additionally, recognising the long-term outcomes of loss and end-stage renal disease (ESRD) is essential for effective patient care.

The primary criterion for impairment is used for categorisation. If the baseline creatinine (Cr) is not provided, a GFR of 75–100 mL/min is assumed, or the baseline Cr can be estimated using the MDRD equation [9].

6.2 Clinical presentation and work-up

SA-AKI is caused by the direct impact of sepsis on the kidneys. Additionally, sepsis can indirectly lead to AKI through factors such as hypotension or certain therapies used during resuscitation, such as antibiotics, fluids, or high-dose vasopressors.

Recent evidence has called into question the long-standing belief that sepsis-induced renal ischaemia is primarily a result of hypotension and vasoconstriction.

1. AKI can occur in septic patients even without haemodynamic instability.

2. Laboratory studies have revealed that plasma from septic patients can lead to cellular changes that suggest the presence of AKI.

3. Both animal and human studies have shown an increase in renal blood flow (RBF) rather than a decrease, which contradicts previous assumptions [10].

More than 10 years back, the Kidney Disease Improving Global Outcomes (KDIGO) guideline established a uniform definition for acute kidney injury (AKI) and included severity levels. AKI is now defined as an increase in serum creatinine

Criteria	Cr	GFR	Urine output	Time
Risk	↑of1.5x baseline	↓25%	<0.5 mL/kg/h	For 6 hours
Injury	↑ of 2x baseline	↓50%	<0.5 mL/kg/h	For 12 hours
Failure	↑ of 3x baseline	↓75%	<0.5 mL/kg/h	For 12 hours
Loss		Loss of kidney function		For over 4 weeks
ESRD		Loss of kidney function		for over 3 months

**ESRD = end stage renal disease.*

Table 2.
RIFLE criteria.

of 0.3 mg/dL or more within 48 hours., or 1.5 times the baseline level within 7 days, or a reduction in urine volume below 0.5 mL/kg/h for 6 hours. KDIGO has adopted a three-stage classification based on disease severity, utilising increased serum creatinine and reduced urine output.

The severity of acute kidney injury (AKI), as indicated by levels of creatinine and urine output, is linked to an increased risk of mortality.

6.3 Early detection of AKI

Sepsis and AKI are associated with high mortality, morbidity and length of stay. The length of hospital stay can be influenced by various factors, including the severity of the condition, the effectiveness of treatment, and the patient's overall health. For conditions such as Acute Kidney Injury (AKI), early detection and intervention can significantly reduce the length of hospital stay. By implementing strategies for timely diagnosis and management, healthcare professionals aim to mitigate the impact of AKI and potentially shorten the duration of hospitalisation.

Based on the current diagnostic criteria for AKI, the diagnosis is primarily made based on increased serum creatinine or decreases in urine output. While these measures are useful, their limitations highlight the need for newer and more effective methods to detect AKI and SA-AKI. Considering the limitations of serum creatinine and urine output, the initial limitation of a definition that relies on a change in serum creatinine is establishing a baseline serum creatinine [11].

6.4 Prevention of SA-AKI

Most treatment strategies for SA-AKI are symptoms-specific and primarily targeted to prevent secondary injuries such as pre-renal injury, venous congestion, and nephrotoxin exposure. Although there have been attempts to protocolise the treatment, SA-AKI is still managed according to a clinician's individualised approach [12].

On the other part of the spectrum, the challenge of pinpointing the exact timing of injury has made developing preventive therapies for patients with new-onset sepsis extremely difficult. This is because the majority of patients already present with AKI when they seek medical attention [12]. This challenge is compounded by the limitations of conventional biomarkers used to identify AKI, as outlined by the Kidney Disease: Improving Global Outcomes (KDIGO) criteria. These biomarkers often fail to detect AKI early enough, resulting in a significant number of cases going unrecognised at the time of development [9]. Consequently, by the time AKI is diagnosed, the opportunity for early intervention has often passed, making prevention efforts largely ineffective. However, preventive strategies might still be beneficial for hospitalised patients if a timely diagnosis can be made.

6.5 The timing of detection of AKI varies with definitions

The median time for detecting AKI based on urine output criteria was 13 hours across all three definitions (RIFLE IQR 7–22 hours, AKIN IQR 7–23 hours, KDIGO IQR 7–23 hours).

Regarding AKI based on serum creatinine criteria, the timing and incidence were similar for RIFLE, AKIN, and KDIGO within the first 48 hours of admission. AKI was identified after a median of 24 hours (IQR 24–48) using the serum creatinine criteria for RIFLE, AKIN, or KDIGO definitions.

7. SA-AKI in obese patients

The rising prevalence of obesity is reflected in ICU statistics, where over 20% of patients are obese. Some researchers propose that obesity, despite its negative aspects, might provide certain clinical advantages for individuals with chronic heart failure, dialysis patients, and those critically ill. This potential benefit is attributed to the greater nutritional reserves in obese individuals, which may support better survival outcomes. Elevated fat and cholesterol levels can aid in the removal of harmful substances like endotoxins and contribute to steroid production during sepsis. Conversely, adipocytes in obesity release various adipokines, promoting cytokine production and inducing low-grade systemic inflammation. This inflammation exacerbates insulin resistance and chronic sympathetic nervous system activation, which leads to high blood pressure and increases the risk of cardiovascular issues and stroke.

Acute kidney infection is linked to poor clinical outcomes, especially in critical care environments, as supported by numerous studies. The association between obesity and acute kidney injury (AKI) is well-established, particularly in ICU settings. However, the impact of obesity on SA-AKI remains insufficiently studied. SA-AKI is divided into two phases: the early phase, which involves sepsis-induced kidney damage, and the late phase, which is related to complications from sepsis treatment. Both phases are associated with increased mortality and prolonged hospitalisations.

The effect of obesity on these outcomes is debated. Some studies suggest that obesity may have a beneficial effect on clinical outcomes in ICU patients with SA-AKI, whereas other research indicates no significant relationship.

A recent multicenter, prospective cohort study, which was published in February 2024, involved over 4000 patients and investigated the relationship between high body mass index (BMI) and SA-AKI in intensive care units. The findings indicate that obesity is associated with a higher risk of developing early SA-AKI. Additionally, SA-AKI is linked to increased mortality rates across all BMI levels. While a higher BMI generally appeared to provide some survival advantages and improved recovery for patients without SA-AKI, these benefits were less pronounced for those with SA-AKI. Obesity impacts kidney function through mechanisms such as hormonal imbalances and increased inflammation. Furthermore, patients with obesity in the ICU are at a higher risk of intra-abdominal hypertension, which may contribute to kidney dysfunction through a combination of venous congestion and poor arterial perfusion. Therefore, timely identification and management of SA-AKI are essential for enhancing outcomes in obese patients [12].

8. SA-AKI in ICU patients

The incidence of AKI among sepsis patients in the ICU is notably high, ranging from 40–50%, with varying rates reported across different studies and regions. For instance, a prospective cohort study including 1177 patients with sepsis across 198 ICUs in 24 European countries identified a 51% incidence of AKI with a substantial ICU mortality rate of 41%, while a retrospective study across China including 146,148 patients reported a 47.1% incidence in sepsis cases. Furthermore, a multicenter randomised controlled trial on septic shock showed that AKI was present in over half of patients at enrolment, with additional cases developing within the following week.

The prevalence of AKI is not confined to severe sepsis or shock; even patients with less severe infections, such as non-severe community-acquired pneumonia, exhibit a significant rate of AKI development (34%). This underscores the broad impact of AKI in various clinical contexts.

The semantic challenge in defining sepsis—characterised as infection-associated organ dysfunction—complicates the accurate assessment of AKI in this setting. Current sepsis guidelines utilise the Sepsis-related Organ Failure Assessment (SOFA) score to evaluate organ dysfunction, including renal impairment. However, the SOFA score has limitations, such as not distinguishing between AKI and chronic kidney disease (CKD) or accounting for baseline creatinine variations across different demographics. This can lead to inaccuracies in evaluating infection-associated kidney dysfunction.

SA-AKI is linked with adverse clinical outcomes. It is associated with an increased risk of in-hospital mortality, with patients experiencing SA-AKI having a higher likelihood of death compared to those with AKI from other causes. Moreover, the requirement for renal replacement therapy (RRT) is strongly associated with poor survival rates. Despite these challenges, patients who recover from SA-AKI, especially those who regain kidney function within 24 hours, demonstrate markedly improved survival rates. However, relapse of AKI post-recovery is not uncommon.

Long-term outcomes for patients with SA-AKI are influenced by the severity of the AKI and the recovery status at hospital discharge. Patients who recover, even partially, tend to have a prognosis similar to those without AKI. Conversely, those who do not recover from SA-AKI face the worst outcomes, including higher mortality rates. Recovery from AKI does not eliminate the risk of developing chronic kidney disease (CKD) or end-stage renal disease, as a significant proportion of patients with AKI reversal eventually progress to CKD. Thus, the severity of AKI, the need for RRT, and recovery status are crucial determinants of both immediate and long-term renal outcomes.

In summary, AKI remains a critical issue in the management of sepsis, with significant implications for both short-term and long-term patient outcomes. Accurate assessment and management of AKI, alongside effective strategies for recovery and monitoring for chronic complications, are essential for improving patient prognosis [8].

9. SA-AKI: The paediatric perspective

The reliance on Sepsis-3 criteria for defining sepsis in adults does not fully address the unique aspects of SA-AKI in neonates and children. While significant progress has been made in understanding and predicting SA-AKI in paediatric populations—such as through modifications to the renal angina index and the use of prognostic biomarkers—gaps remain in aligning these advancements with clinical practice.

Recent recommendations from the 26th Acute Disease Quality Initiative (ADQI) focus on the role of developmental factors in paediatric AKI and highlight the differences in fluid management practices between adults and children. For instance, balanced crystalloids are preferred for children, reflecting a distinct approach to fluid therapy compared to adults. The inclusion of paediatric populations in studies of evidence-based practices (EBP) therapies, such as selective cytopheretic devices, is a positive step forward but does not yet resolve the lack of a precise paediatric SA-AKI definition.

Ongoing efforts, including those by the Society of Critical Care Medicine (SCCM) task force, aim to develop a more accurate and applicable definition of paediatric sepsis. However, until such definitions are established, the management of SA-AKI in children may continue to be guided by less tailored, adult-centric protocols. Future research and clinical guidelines should strive to align paediatric sepsis definitions with SA-AKI management strategies to improve care and outcomes for younger patients [1, 13, 14].

10. SA-AKI and COVID-19

Early reports of severe COVID-19 initially suggested that kidney injury was rare, which was surprising given the extensive involvement of other organs such as the heart, brain, and gastrointestinal tract. Early observations also indicated significant systemic inflammation, similar to that seen in sepsis, although data from initial studies did not fully support the term "cytokine storm" used by the media. Standardised tests for inflammation, like C-reactive protein and ferritin, did show severe inflammation in the most critically ill patients, indicating that hyper-inflammation is indeed a characteristic of severe COVID-19.

However, by late March 2020, it became clear that acute kidney injury (AKI) was a significant issue in severe COVID-19 cases. By mid-April 2020, the term "second surge" was used to describe the increased prevalence of renal failure associated with COVID-19.

Much of the early contradictory information on AKI in COVID-19 resulted from the rush to publish findings, with many studies not thoroughly tracking secondary outcomes like AKI. As research progressed, it became evident that AKI affects about 25–35% of hospitalised COVID-19 patients, with rates nearly doubling in those admitted to intensive care units. These rates are consistent with what is seen in bacterial pneumonia, prompting two key questions: (i) How does AKI in COVID-19 differ from AKI in other types of sepsis? and (ii) Can we apply the existing evidence on sepsis-associated AKI to COVID-19 patients?

It is crucial to address these questions because overlooking differences could lead to applying recommendations without validating them specifically for COVID-19. For instance, while caution is advised for vancomycin use in bacterial sepsis due to its nephrotoxic potential, this caution should similarly apply to COVID-19 patients, as there is no evidence suggesting they are less vulnerable to this drug's toxicity.

Although COVID-19 sepsis shares many similarities with bacterial sepsis, including the development of AKI, there are notable differences that may impact treatment approaches (**Table 3**). Despite these differences, most recommendations for managing sepsis-associated AKI can also apply to COVID-19-related AKI. Nevertheless, uncertainties remain in the management of sepsis-associated AKI, such as the timing for initiating extracorporeal kidney support and the use of other blood purification therapies. Additional questions specific to COVID-19 include the effects of low-dose corticosteroids and anticoagulation on AKI, as well as the potential protective effects of antivirals against kidney damage from the virus.

While our standard approaches for managing sepsis-associated AKI—such as careful fluid and haemodynamic management, cautious use of nephrotoxic agents, and personalised extracorporeal kidney support—should be maintained, it is important to adapt these strategies based on emerging evidence specific to COVID-19 [16].

Aetiology/mechanism	Bacterial sepsis	COVID-19 sepsis	Comments
Systemic inflammation affecting multiple organs	+++	++	Corticosteroids have been shown to improve survival in COVID-19, whereas the effect in bacterial sepsis is only on reversal of shock.
DAMPS released from injured tissue	+++	+++	Injured lung and also remote organs (e.g., muscle) may contribute DAMPs.
PAMPs released from microorganisms	+++	?	Extensive involvement of the GI tract in some patients raises concern for translocation of bacteria/bacterial products.
TMA	+	++	The TMA in COVID-19 appears to be unique from DIC, TTP, and HUS.
Nephrotoxic drugs	+++	+++	Different agents are used in the 2 syndromes.
Direct viral infection of tubular epithelial cells	n/a	±	The full extent of this pathobiologic mechanism is still unknown.
Cardiac dysfunction and/or reduced preload	+	++	COVID-19 may directly affect the heart and high PEEP ± volume depletion may impair venous return.
Macrophage activation syndrome	+	+	Generally more common in viral infection and in children.

+, weak evidence/involvement; ++, moderate evidence/involvement; +++, strong evidence/involvement; ±, evidence/ involvement is equivocal,? unknown; COVID-19, coronavirus disease 2019; DAMPs, danger-associated molecular patterns; DIC, disseminated intravascular coagulation; GI, gastrointestinal; HUS, hemolytic uremic syndrome; n/a, not available; PAMPs, pathogen-associated molecular patterns; PEEP, positive end-expiratory pressure; TMA, thrombotic microangiopathy; TTP, thrombocytopenic purpura [15].

Table 3.
Comparison of bacterial and COVID-19 sepsis.

11. Fluid resuscitation

Ensuring appropriate fluid management is imperative in managing acute kidney injury (AKI). Both hypovolemia and hypervolemia are associated with adverse outcomes, making careful monitoring and adjustment of fluid levels crucial [17]. Hypovolemia can lead to decreased renal perfusion, exacerbating kidney injury, while hypervolemia can cause fluid overload, resulting in increased venous congestion, which causes further damage to the kidneys [18, 19]. Moreover, this balancing act of managing fluids is usually based on trial and error, as the means of assessing fluid status inwards, such as urine output (UOP), central venous pressure (CVP), heart rate and blood pressure, are unable to adequately determine fluid status[17], and more dynamic measurements, such as stroke volume variations and passive leg raises, are rarely performed even in critical care settings. Thus, it becomes imperative to manage patients on an individual basis and to closely monitor clinical response after every intervention.

One of the classic ways of conceptualising fluid therapy is to divide it into four phases: rescue, optimisation, stabilisation, and deescalation [17]. Rescue implies the administration of fluid boluses to *rescue* patients from tissue hypo-perfusion. Surviving sepsis guidelines of 2021 suggest a bolus of 30 ml/kg (of ideal body weight) for initial resuscitation within the first 3 hours of onset of sepsis [18]. This concept is supported by observational studies that suggest that failure to give a 30 ml/kg fluid bolus within 3 hours increases the odds of in-hospital mortality, irrespective of comorbidities [20]. Moreover, several recent trials and reviews indicate that fluid boluses of 30 ml/kg are not harmful in patients with comorbidities that make them prone to developing volume overload [21, 22].

Optimisation refers to the "adjustment of fluid type, rate, and amount based upon context to achieve optimisation of tissue perfusion." Fluid optimisation is usually goal-directed, i.e., fluid challenges guided by dynamic haemodynamic measurements such as stroke volume variation. A typical practice is to administer 250 ml of fluid and to observe if this challenge increases the cardiac output or stroke volume by 10–15% [23].

Stabilisation seeks to maintain a neutral or slightly negative fluid balance to support organ function. *De-escalation* involves reducing fluid intake and mobilising excess fluid to optimise balance. During these phases, clinicians should aim for a neutral fluid balance initially, followed by a negative balance if there is fluid overload. Diuretics, such as loop diuretics, can be used, and if indicated, renal replacement therapy could also be initiated [24].

11.1 Choice of fluids

It has long been established that colloids, such as hydroxyethyl starch and gelatin-based solutions, increase the risk of developing AKI when used in critically ill patients. Numerous randomised control trials have shown that colloids not only increase the risk of requiring renal replacement therapies but also increase the overall mortality [25–27].

On the other hand, the use of albumin-based colloids has been found not to be associated with such worse outcomes. 'The Saline Versus Albumin Fluid Evaluation (SAFE) trial,' encompassing 6997 critically ill patients, demonstrated that fluid resuscitation with either saline or albumin yielded similar relative risks of mortality. Moreover, no significant differences were observed in the incidence of new single-organ or multiple-organ failure or the duration of kidney replacement therapy (KRT) [28]. A common clinical practice, thus, is to consider using albumin when volume resuscitation requires large quantities of crystalloids.

The choice of crystalloids also seems to influence renal outcomes in patients. Growing evidence suggests that isotonic crystalloid fluid preparations differ in their side effects and physiological profiles. Although they are isotonic, normal saline (NS) has a higher chloride content compared to plasma. In both human and animal models, large infusions of hyperchloremic solutions have been shown to cause debilitating changes in renal physiology that could result in exacerbation of diminishing renal function [29, 30]. This has further been proved by various randomised control trials that have shown that when compared with balanced crystalloids, patients receiving hyperchloremic solutions such as normal saline are at higher risk of developing adverse renal outcomes [31, 32].

There have been concerns about using physiologically balanced solutions that more closely resemble serum, such as lactated Ringer's (LR), due to their higher potassium content and the perceived risk of hyperkalaemia. However, evidence indicates that these balanced solutions are generally safe, even in situations with a potentially higher risk of hyperkalaemia, such as in AKI, provided that appropriate monitoring is in place [33].

11.2 Use of diuretics

The preventive use of diuretics in patients at high risk of AKI has proven ineffective in critically ill individuals. Likewise, diuretics do not mitigate AKI after it has developed. As a result, diuretics are not advised for either the prevention or treatment of sepsis-associated AKI [34].

Despite this, diuretics are often used to treat volume overload in the optimisation and elimination phase of fluid therapy.

12. Role of vasopressors

There is no agreement on the optimal use of vasopressors to prevent AKI or prevent further kidney function decline. Surviving sepsis guidelines recommend starting vasopressors after initial fluid resuscitation with 30 mL/kg of crystalloids and adding albumin in patients needing large volumes of crystalloids to maintain sufficient mean arterial pressure (MAP). Vasopressors should then be used to achieve a MAP above 65 mm Hg[19].

Noradrenaline is recommended as the first drug of choice, but increasing evidence suggests that angiotensin II and vasopressin may enhance better glomerular flow through various mechanisms [35, 36].

13. Renal replacement therapy in AKI

Renal replacement therapy (RRT) has been vital in treating AKI since the 1960s. However, the timing of RRT initiation remains debated. The ELAIN trial suggested early RRT reduces mortality and hospital stay [37], while the AKIKI trial showed delayed RRT could avoid RRT for 49% of patients and reduce complications [38]. Other studies, including IDEAL-ICU and STARRT-AKI, support delayed RRT, with many patients recovering renal function without RRT [39, 40]. Delayed RRT avoids unnecessary iatrogenic complications and allows potential spontaneous recovery. Nonetheless, delaying RRT excessively can result in poor outcomes, such as preventable complications and death.

In SA-AKI settings, large clinical trials fail to demonstrate any significant clinical outcomes on whether intermittent or continuous RRT is more beneficial [41, 42]. However, it may be worthwhile to consider Continuous Renal Replacement Therapy (CRRT) for haemodynamically unstable patients.

The ADQI suggests RRT should be based on kidney demand-capacity mismatch rather than just AKI severity. This involves assessing the kidney's ability to meet the body's needs and initiating RRT accordingly [34].

14. Dialysis disequilibrium syndrome

In SA-AKI, one of the complications is the accumulation of nitrogen-containing compounds. Paradoxically, when these compounds are rapidly cleared, they can trigger a rare condition known as dialysis disequilibrium syndrome (DDS). This syndrome is characterised by nausea, vomiting, headaches, encephalopathy, and seizures.

The underlying cause is thought to be the faster reduction of urea levels in the blood compared to the brain during dialysis. This delay, called the "reverse urea effect," creates an osmotic gradient that causes water to shift from the bloodstream into the brain, leading to cerebral oedema and its related symptoms [43].

DDS most commonly occurs after the first hemodialysis (HD) session. Although the exact incidence is unknown, it appears to have decreased since the early days of dialysis. This is likely because modern patients begin dialysis with much lower urea concentrations than in the past. Despite being recognised for over 50 years and the long history of hemodialysis treatment, this syndrome remains poorly understood (2).

Most cases of DDS tend to be mild and self-limiting. Patients may experience symptoms such as headaches, nausea, blurred vision, and other central nervous system issues like restlessness and confusion. These symptoms typically start soon after dialysis begins and usually resolve within a few hours. Some additional signs, like dizziness and muscle cramps that appear toward the end of dialysis, are also considered part of DDS. In rare cases, DDS can manifest as increased intraocular pressure. In severe instances, the condition can escalate to seizures, excessive drowsiness, stupor, or coma, which can be life-threatening [44].

The treatment of DDS mainly depends upon prevention strategies. Since the primary cause of DDS is the creation of an osmotic gradient that draws water into the brain, preventing this gradient can help avoid the syndrome. The simplest approach is to use hemofiltration instead of dialysis. Along with the slow removal of urea, another method is to introduce an osmotic agent into the bloodstream. This helps prevent the formation of a blood-brain osmotic gradient and, in turn, cerebral oedema. The easiest osmotic agent to add is sodium, though other agents like mannitol and glucose have also been used effectively [43].

Dialysis disequilibrium syndrome (DDS) may occur in patients with sepsis or septic shock, even after multiple hemodialysis (HD) sessions [45].

Two cases of acute kidney injury (AKI) were reported in Qatar, highlighting the development of dialysis disequilibrium syndrome (DDS) after a few sessions of hemodialysis (HD) in septic patients requiring prolonged HD and mechanical ventilation. Both cases featured young males with severe injuries and septic shock, who suffered sudden clinical deterioration, becoming unresponsive after several HD sessions, ultimately resulting in death [45].

15. Conclusion

In summary, SA-AKI is a significant complication in critically ill patients, leading to increased morbidity and mortality. The complicated dynamics of inflammatory processes, microcirculatory dysfunction, and cellular injury emphasise the need for a nuanced understanding of SA-AKI's pathophysiology. Considering the high incidence of AKI in septic patients and its significant consequences for patient outcomes, early recognition and targeted intervention strategies are essential. While current management remains largely supportive and symptom-focused, additional research into the mechanisms of SA-AKI may yield new preventive and therapeutic approaches. Ultimately, improving awareness and clinical protocols surrounding SA-AKI will be pivotal in enhancing patient care, reducing hospital stays, and enhancing the overall quality of life for those affected by this devastating condition.

Author details

Sohel Mohamed Gamal Ahmed[1*], Ebtihal Mahmoud[2], Malek Abusannuga[2], Zakaria Attique[2] and Jawdat Alali[2]

1 Qatar University College of Medicine, Qatar

2 Department of Anaesthesia, ICU and Perioperative Medicine, Hamad Medical Corporation, Qatar

*Address all correspondence to: sohelm@yahoo.com

References

[1] Zarbock A, Nadim MK, Pickkers P, et al. Sepsis-associated acute kidney injury: Consensus report of the 28th acute disease quality initiative workgroup. Nature Reviews Nephrology. 2023;**19**(6):401-417. DOI: 10.1038/s41581-023-00683-3

[2] Kuwabara S, Goggins E, Okusa MD. The pathophysiology of sepsis-associated AKI. Clinical Journal of the American Society of Nephrology. 2022;**17**(7):1050-1069. DOI: 10.2215/cjn.00850122

[3] Udompap P, Kim D, Kim WR. Current and future burden of chronic nonmalignant liver disease. Clinical Gastroenterology and Hepatology. 2015;**13**(12):2031-2041. DOI: 10.1016/j.cgh.2015.08.015

[4] Monard C, Rimmelé T, Blanc E, Goguillot M, Bénard S, Textoris J. Economic burden of in-hospital AKI: A one-year analysis of the nationwide French hospital discharge database. BMC Nephrology. 2023;**24**(1):343. DOI: 10.1186/s12882-023-03396-8

[5] Jia HM, Jiang YJ, Zheng X, et al. The attributable mortality of sepsis for acute kidney injury: A propensity-matched analysis based on multicenter prospective cohort study. Renal Failure. 2023;**45**(1):2162415. DOI: 10.1080/0886022x.2022.2162415

[6] Chen JJ, Kuo G, Hung CC, et al. Risk factors and prognosis assessment for acute kidney injury: The 2020 consensus of the Taiwan AKI task force. Journal of the Formosan Medical Association. 2021;**120**(7):1424-1433. DOI: 10.1016/j.jfma.2021.02.013

[7] Liu J, Xie H, Ye Z, Li F, Wang L. Rates, predictors, and mortality of sepsis-associated acute kidney injury: A systematic review and meta-analysis. BMC Nephrology. 2020;**21**(1):318. DOI: 10.1186/s12882-020-01974-8

[8] Peerapornratana S, Manrique-Caballero CL, Gómez H, Kellum JA. Acute kidney injury from sepsis: Current concepts, epidemiology, pathophysiology, prevention and treatment. Kidney International. 2019;**96**(5):1083-1099. DOI: 10.1016/j.kint.2019.05.026

[9] Goyal A, Daneshpajouhnejad P, Hashmi MF, et al. Acute kidney injury. In: StatPearls [Internet]. Treasure Island (FL): StatPearls Publishing; 2023, Jan 2025 [Updated: Nov 25, 2023]

[10] Brenner M, Schaer GL, Mallory DL, Suffredini AF, Parrillo JE. Detection of renal blood flow abnormalities in septic and critically ill patients using a newly designed indwelling thermodilution renal vein catheter. Chest. 1990;**98**(1):170-179. DOI: 10.1378/chest.98.1.170

[11] Alobaidi R, Basu RK, Goldstein SL, Bagshaw SM. Sepsis-associated acute kidney injury. Seminars in Nephrology. 2015;**35**(1):2-11. DOI: 10.1016/j.semnephrol.2015.01.002

[12] Ahn YH, Yoon SM, Lee J, et al. Early sepsis-associated acute kidney injury and obesity. JAMA Network Open. 2024;**7**(2):e2354923-e2354923. DOI: 10.1001/jamanetworkopen.2023.54923

[13] Stanski NL, Stenson EK, Cvijanovich NZ, et al. PERSEVERE biomarkers predict severe acute kidney injury and renal recovery in pediatric septic shock. American Journal of Respiratory and Critical Care Medicine.

2020;**201**(7):848-855. DOI: 10.1164/rccm.201911-2187OC

[14] Weiss SL, Fitzgerald JC, Pappachan J, et al. Global epidemiology of pediatric severe sepsis: The sepsis prevalence, outcomes, and therapies study. American Journal of Respiratory and Critical Care Medicine. 2015;**191**(10):1147-1157. DOI: 10.1164/rccm.201412-2323OC

[15] Jalil BA, Cavallazzi R. Predicting fluid responsiveness: A review of literature and a guide for the clinician. The American Journal of Emergency Medicine. 2018;**36**(11):2093-2102. DOI: 10.1016/j.ajem.2018.08.037

[16] Kellum JA, Nadim MK, Forni LG. Sepsis-associated acute kidney injury: Is COVID-19 different? Kidney International. 2020;**98**(6):1370-1372. DOI: 10.1016/j.kint.2020.08.009

[17] Hoste EA, Maitland K, Brudney CS, et al. Four phases of intravenous fluid therapy: A conceptual model. British Journal of Anaesthesia. 2014;**113**(5):740-747. DOI: 10.1093/bja/aeu300

[18] Evans L, Rhodes A, Alhazzani W, et al. Surviving sepsis campaign: International guidelines for management of sepsis and septic shock 2021. Critical Care Medicine. 2021;**49**(11):e1063-e1143. DOI: 10.1097/ccm.0000000000005337

[19] Patil VP, Salunke BG. Fluid overload and acute kidney injury. Indian Journal of Critical Care Medicine. 2020;**24**(Suppl. 3):S94-s97. DOI: 10.5005/jp-journals-10071-23401

[20] Kuttab HI, Lykins JD, Hughes MD, et al. Evaluation and predictors of fluid resuscitation in patients with severe sepsis and septic shock. Critical Care Medicine. 2019;**47**(11):1582-1590. DOI: 10.1097/ccm.0000000000003960

[21] Haley M, Foroutan NK, Gronquist JM, Reddy R, Wusirika R, Khan A. Fluid resuscitation and sepsis management in patients with chronic kidney disease or end-stage renal disease: Scoping review. American Journal of Critical Care. 2024;**33**(1):45-53. DOI: 10.4037/ajcc2024756

[22] Khan RA, Khan NA, Bauer SR, et al. Association between volume of fluid resuscitation and intubation in high-risk patients with sepsis, heart failure, end-stage renal disease, and cirrhosis. Chest. 2020;**157**(2):286-292. DOI: 10.1016/j.chest.2019.09.029

[23] Martin GS, Kaufman DA, Marik PE, et al. Perioperative quality initiative (POQI) consensus statement on fundamental concepts in perioperative fluid management: Fluid responsiveness and venous capacitance. Perioperative Medicine (London). 2020;**9**:12. DOI: 10.1186/s13741-020-00142-8

[24] Vincent JL. Fluid management in the critically ill. Kidney International. 2019;**96**(1):52-57. DOI: 10.1016/j.kint.2018.11.047

[25] Perner A, Haase N, Guttormsen Anne B, et al. Hydroxyethyl starch 130/0.42 versus Ringer's acetate in severe sepsis. New England Journal of Medicine. Jul 2012;**367**(2):124-134. DOI: 10.1056/NEJMoa1204242

[26] Myburgh John A, Finfer S, Bellomo R, et al. Hydroxyethyl starch or saline for fluid resuscitation in intensive care. New England Journal of Medicine. 2012;**367**(20):1901-1911. DOI: 10.1056/NEJMoa1209759

[27] Zarychanski R, Abou-Setta AM, Turgeon AF, et al. Association of hydroxyethyl starch administration with mortality and acute kidney injury in critically ill patients requiring volume

resuscitation: A systematic review and meta-analysis. Journal of the American Medical Association. 2013;**309**(7):678-688. DOI: 10.1001/jama.2013.430

[28] Finfer S, Bellomo R, Boyce N, French J, Myburgh J, Norton R, et al. A comparison of albumin and saline for fluid resuscitation in the intensive care unit. New England Journal of Medicine. 2004;**350**(22):2247-2256. DOI: 10.1056/NEJMoa040232

[29] Kotchen TA, Luke RG, Ott CE, Galla JH, Whitescarver S. Effect of chloride on renin and blood pressure responses to sodium chloride. Annals of Internal Medicine. 1983;**98**(5 Pt 2):817-822. DOI: 10.7326/0003-4819-98-5-817

[30] Wilcox CS. Regulation of renal blood flow by plasma chloride. The Journal of Clinical Investigation. 1983;**71**(3):726-735. DOI: 10.1172/jci110820

[31] Yunos NM, Bellomo R, Hegarty C, Story D, Ho L, Bailey M. Association between a chloride-liberal vs chloride-restrictive intravenous fluid administration strategy and kidney injury in critically ill adults. Journal of the American Medical Association. 2012;**308**(15):1566-1572. DOI: 10.1001/jama.2012.13356

[32] Semler MW, Self WH, Wanderer JP, et al. Balanced crystalloids versus saline in critically ill adults. The New England Journal of Medicine. 2018;**378**(9):829-839. DOI: 10.1056/NEJMoa1711584

[33] Rajasekaran A, Bade N, Cutter GR, Rizk DV, Zarjou A. Lactated Ringer's solution and risk of hyperkalemia in patients with reduced kidney function. The American Journal of the Medical Sciences. 2022;**364**(4):433-443. DOI: 10.1016/j.amjms.2022.04.024

[34] Zarbock A, Koyner JL, Gomez H, Pickkers P, Forni L. The acute disease quality initiative g. sepsis-associated acute kidney injury—Treatment standard. Nephrology Dialysis Transplantation. 2024;**39**(1):26-35. DOI: 10.1093/ndt/gfad142

[35] Tumlin JA, Murugan R, Deane AM, et al. Outcomes in patients with vasodilatory shock and renal replacement therapy treated with intravenous angiotensin II. Critical Care Medicine. 2018;**46**(6):949-957

[36] Bellomo R, Forni LG, Busse LW, et al. Renin and survival in patients given angiotensin II for catecholamine-resistant vasodilatory shock. A clinical trial. American Journal of Respiratory and Critical Care Medicine. 2020;**202**(9):1253-1261. DOI: 10.1164/rccm.201911-2172OC

[37] Zarbock A, Kellum JA, Schmidt C, et al. Effect of early vs delayed initiation of renal replacement therapy on mortality in critically ill patients with acute kidney injury: The ELAIN randomized clinical trial. Journal of the American Medical Association. 2016;**315**(20):2190-2199. DOI: 10.1001/jama.2016.5828

[38] Gaudry S, Hajage D, Schortgen F, et al. Initiation strategies for renal-replacement therapy in the intensive care unit. New England Journal of Medicine. Oct 2018;**375**(2):122-133. DOI: 10.1056/NEJMoa1603017

[39] Barbar SD, Clere-Jehl R, Bourredjem A, et al. Timing of renal-replacement therapy in patients with acute kidney injury and sepsis. New England Journal of Medicine. 2018;**379**(15):1431-1442. DOI: 10.1056/NEJMoa1803213

[40] Gaudry S, Hajage D, Schortgen F, Martin-Lefevre L, Pons B, Boulet E, et al. Timing of initiation of renal-replacement

therapy in acute kidney injury. The New England Journal of Medicine. 2016;**375**(2):122-133. DOI: 10.1056/NEJMoa1603017

[41] Schefold JC, Sv H, Pschowski R, et al. The effect of continuous versus intermittent renal replacement therapy on the outcome of critically ill patients with acute renal failure (CONVINT): A prospective randomized controlled trial. Critical Care. 2014;**18**(1):R11. DOI: 10.1186/cc13188

[42] Bagshaw SM, Berthiaume LR, Delaney A, Bellomo R. Continuous versus intermittent renal replacement therapy for critically ill patients with acute kidney injury: A meta-analysis. Critical Care Medicine. 2008;**36**(2):610-617

[43] Saha M, Allon M. Diagnosis, treatment, and prevention of hemodialysis emergencies. Clinical Journal of the American Society of Nephrology. 2017;**12**(2):357-369. DOI: 10.2215/cjn.05260516

[44] Zepeda-Orozco D, Quigley R. Dialysis disequilibrium syndrome. Pediatric Nephrology. 2012;**27**(12):2205-2211. DOI: 10.1007/s00467-012-2199-4

[45] Shaikh N, Louon A, Hanssens Y. Fatal dialysis disequilibrium syndrome: A tale of two patients. Journal of Emergencies, Trauma, and Shock. 2010;**3**:300

Chapter 11

Septic Shock and Myocardial Dysfunction

Hossam Algallie, Siddhartha Banerjee, Ashish Kumar, Um I. Rubab, Anil Kumar Agarwal, Seema Nahid, Nissar Shaikh and Mohammad Ataur Rahman

Abstract

Cardiac dysfunction in sepsis is strongly linked to increased mortality. The pathophysiology of sepsis-induced Myocardial dysfunction is multifaceted, involving impaired myocardial circulation, direct myocardial depression, and mitochondrial dysfunction. Recent studies have emphasized that mitochondrial dysfunction plays a crucial role in sepsis-induced Myocardial dysfunction. Various medications have been utilized to treat sepsis, aiming to prevent and address sepsis-induced cardiomyopathy. Nevertheless, these treatments have not significantly improved patient outcomes. This underscores the need for new therapeutic strategies that target the specific mechanisms of sepsis-induced myocardial dysfunction. Monitoring sepsis-induced cardiac dysfunction is essential, as it significantly impacts the prognosis. To effectively monitor this condition, clinicians use a combination of clinical assessments, hemodynamic monitoring, and echocardiography and biomarkers. Integrating these methods allows for a comprehensive understanding of cardiac function, enabling timely adjustments to treatment plans. Patients with this condition will benefit from established sepsis and septic shock treatments. However, apart from general management with vasopressors, inotropes, and fluid resuscitation, there is limited data and a lack of evidence regarding more specific treatments. This chapter provides an overview of the current understanding of the pathophysiological processes involved in sepsis-related cardiac dysfunction and the impact of monitoring and current management in sepsis-induced Myocardial dysfunction.

Keywords: sepsis, septic shock, myocardial dysfunction, mitochondrial dysfunction, septic cardiomyopathy

1. Introduction

Sepsis-induced Myocardial dysfunction encompasses a range of acute myocardial impairments resulting from sepsis [1]. Sepsis is commonly recognized as a systemic inflammatory response syndrome triggered by an infection, resulting from a dysregulated immune response to pathogens. Over the past 50 years, myocardial dysfunction in sepsis has been extensively studied. This condition is associated with a significantly elevated mortality rate of 20–50% [2, 3].

Cardiac dysfunction associated with sepsis has been referred to by several names, including septic cardiomyopathy, sepsis-induced cardiomyopathy (SIC), and sepsis-induced myocardial dysfunction (SIMD) [4].

Despite considerable research into its clinical manifestations, pathophysiological mechanisms, and diagnostic methods, septic cardiomyopathy remains a challenging medical issue. Our understanding of it is still incomplete, and there are no definitive treatment options available. Recent studies have attempted to clarify the classification of myocardial function alterations in sepsis and elucidate its underlying mechanisms. Nevertheless, established evidence links sepsis-induced cardiovascular impairment with a compromised immune response to invading microorganisms. This leads to an inflammatory reaction, exacerbated by inflammatory mediators released into the bloodstream, causing hemodynamic changes that impair cardiac function [5, 6]. Although numerous biochemical mediators and pathways have been extensively studied, the exact cause of myocardial depression in sepsis is still not fully understood. Both clinicians and researchers have faced significant challenges in fully elucidating the pathophysiology of sepsis-induced Myocardial dysfunction. This review seeks to clarify the current knowledge on myocardial dysfunction in sepsis by summarizing the existing insights into the underlying pathophysiological mechanisms and the clinical manifestations of SICM and then focusing on monitoring and the current therapeutic strategies.

2. Clinical manifestations of sepsis-induced myocardial dysfunction

Contractile dysfunction is a key feature of cardiac impairment in sepsis, characterized by biventricular dilatation, a reversible reduction in ejection fraction, a diminished blood pressure response to intravenous fluid resuscitation, and an inability to enhance cardiac output despite elevated levels of circulating catecholamines [1]. Clinically, myocardial dysfunction can present as one or more of the following: left ventricular (LV) systolic dysfunction, LV diastolic dysfunction, right ventricular (RV) impairment, and dilation of both ventricles. Research has linked pump failure to significant afterload reduction associated with decreased systemic vascular resistance (SVR) and reduced cardiac output/cardiac index, which leads to regional or even global contractile impairment.LV and RV dilation, often resulting from increased compliance, is generally considered an adaptive response. However, RV dysfunction negatively affects LV function by reducing LV ejection fraction, decreasing LV filling pressure, and causing mechanical compromise from LV septum shift [7, 8]. Previously, cardiac dysfunction was believed to occur only during the hypodynamic phase of shock, marked by increased SVR, tissue hypoperfusion, cold skin, and eventual organ failure. However, it is now recognized that myocardial impairment can also manifest during hyperdynamic septic shock, which features increased cardiac output, decreased SVR, and warm, well-perfused skin [9]. In hyperdynamic septic shock, LV dilation is seen as an adaptive mechanism that helps maintain cardiac output through the Starling mechanism, and this adaptation is associated with lower mortality and better prognosis in sepsis patients. The pathophysiology of left ventricular (LV) systolic dysfunction in septic patients has been found to encompass a spectrum that includes isolated diastolic dysfunction as well as a combination of both systolic and diastolic abnormalities. Septic patients were observed to have a decreased left ventricular (LV) ejection fraction and acute LV dilation, which was indicated by an increased LV end-diastolic volume index compared to controls [10–12].

Type of cardiac dysfunction	Results/Consequences
Reduced Cardiac Output	Leads to tissue hypoperfusion and organ dysfunction.
Impaired Myocardial Contractility	Results in lower ejection fraction, reduced stroke volume, and impaired blood flow to organs.
Hypotension	This may lead to inadequate blood flow to vital organs, requiring vasopressor support.
Heart Failure	Can manifest as symptoms of volume overload or poor perfusion.
Arrhythmias	May exacerbate cardiac dysfunction and contribute to hemodynamic instability.
Diastolic Dysfunction	Results in elevated filling pressures and symptoms of heart failure.
Ventricular Dilatation	Can compromise cardiac function and lead to congestive heart failure.
Increased Myocardial Oxygen Demand	Risk of myocardial ischemia, especially in patients with coronary disease.
Impaired Coronary Perfusion	Increased risk of myocardial ischemia and infarction.

Table 1.
Cardiac dysfunctions in septic patients.

Right ventricular (RV) systolic dysfunction is characterized by a reduced RV ejection fraction and RV dilation. Given that RV dysfunction occurs independently of changes in peripheral vascular resistance and pulmonary arterial pressure, some studies suggest that increased RV afterload may not be the primary cause of RV depression in septic shock. While sepsis-related RV dilation can lead to septal displacement, which in turn reduces left ventricular (LV) compliance, preload, and overall performance, it is important to note that this finding is not frequently observed [13]. Despite the structural and functional differences between the ventricles, recent evidence indicates that sepsis-induced right ventricular (RV) dysfunction is generally similar to left ventricular (LV) dysfunction.

3. Types of cardiac dysfunctions in septic patients

The cardiac dysfunctions commonly observed in sepsis summarized in (**Table 1**).

4. Risk factors for sepsis-induced myocardial dysfunction

In the context of sepsis, several risk factors can contribute to the development of myocardial dysfunction:

1. *Severity of sepsis*: The more severe the sepsis (e.g., septic shock), the higher the risk of myocardial dysfunction. Severe infections and widespread inflammation can significantly impact heart function.

2. *Preexisting cardiovascular disease*: Individuals with preexisting heart conditions, such as heart failure, coronary artery disease, or hypertension, are more susceptible to myocardial dysfunction when they develop sepsis. These conditions can compromise the heart's ability to cope with the additional stress imposed by sepsis.

3. *Comorbid conditions*: Conditions such as diabetes mellitus or chronic obstructive pulmonary disease (COPD) can increase the risk due to their impact on overall health and inflammatory response.

4. *High levels of inflammatory markers*: Elevated levels of inflammatory markers, such as cytokines, can contribute to cardiac dysfunction. High levels of these markers often correlate with more severe cases of sepsis.

5. *High acute illness severity*: Patients who present with severe organ dysfunction, and high Sequential Organ Failure Assessment (SOFA) scores are at greater risk for myocardial dysfunction.

6. *Nutritional status*: Malnutrition or poor nutritional status can impair immune function and contribute to increased susceptibility to severe sepsis and myocardial dysfunction.

7. *Inadequate or delayed treatment*: Delays in treating sepsis or inadequate management of sepsis can lead to more severe systemic effects, including cardiac dysfunction.

8. *High lactic acid*: Elevated lactic acid levels greater than 4.0 mmol/L at ICU admission are independently at higher risk for developing septic cardiomyopathy [14–16].

Addressing these risk factors through early intervention, appropriate treatment, and supportive care is essential for managing and mitigating the impact of sepsis-induced myocardial dysfunction.

5. Pathophysiology of sepsis-induced myocardial dysfunction

Our understanding of sepsis-induced Myocardial dysfunction is closely tied to our knowledge of sepsis itself. The pathophysiology of sepsis involves an uncontrolled inflammatory response due to defective interactions between the immune system and invading pathogens. Typically, the host immune system detects pathogenic invasions through pattern recognition receptors (PRRs), which bind to pathogen-associated molecular patterns (PAMPs). PRRs, including Toll-like receptors (TLRs), are found on the surface of immune cells, while PAMPs, such as lipopolysaccharide (LPS) and lipoteichoic acid, are components of the invading microorganisms. In addition to initiating immune responses against pathogens, PRRs also recognize and bind to danger-associated molecular patterns (DAMPs) released during inflammation, thereby activating the innate immune system [17].

Ca5, Complement a5; DAMPs, damage-associated molecular patterns; NO, nitric oxide; PAMPs, pathogen-associated molecular patterns; ROS, reactive oxygen species.

Despite decades of research, the pathophysiology of septic cardiomyopathy remains incompletely understood. Recently, cytokines have been identified as primary mediators of myocardial depression in sepsis, as their release is triggered by the body's response to surgical, traumatic, ischemic, or septic insults [18]. However, septic cardiomyopathy can also be influenced by various other factors, highlighting the need to investigate specific contributing mechanisms to develop effective therapeutic targets (**Figure 1**).

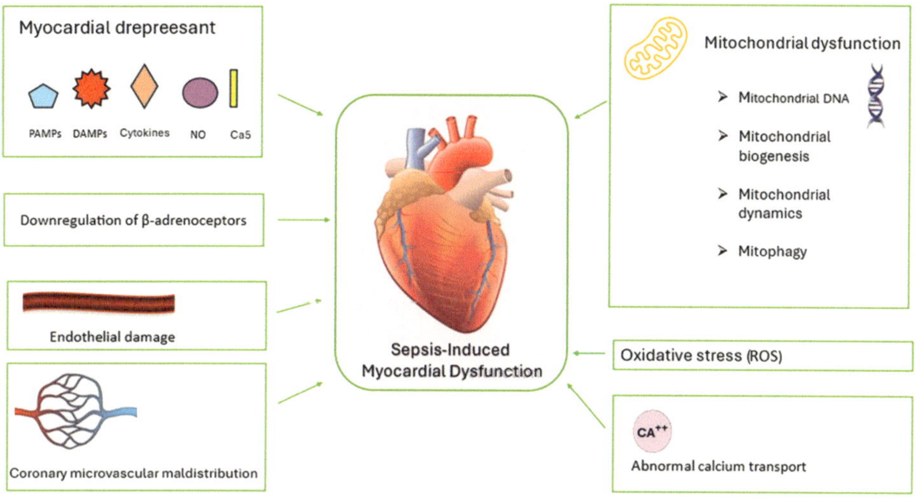

Figure 1.
Pathophysiology of sepsis-induced myocardial dysfunction.

5.1 Impaired myocardial circulation

Decreased blood flow to the myocardium is a key mechanism underlying sepsis-induced Myocardial dysfunction. The reversible nature of myocardial depression in sepsis has been linked to the concept of myocardial hibernation, an adaptive response to ischemia and hypoxia. This phenomenon is considered a common manifestation of myocardial dysfunction in sepsis [19].

Despite this protective mechanism, ischemia of the cardiac muscle can significantly worsen septic myocardial dysfunction in patients with severe sepsis. Cardiac function is heavily influenced by intravascular fluid status. The loss of vascular tone due to arterial vasodilation is a major contributor to hemodynamic instability in septic patients. Recently identified physiological factors include cardiac contractility, end-systolic ventricular elastance (Ees), arterial elastance (Ea), and left ventricular (LV) systolic performance. Additionally, ventriculo-arterial coupling, which is the ratio of Ea to Ees, is a crucial factor in assessing the efficiency of the cardiovascular system.

While the endothelium plays a significant role in sepsis, the effects of sepsis-associated endothelial dysfunction are not well understood. A previous study found that, despite maintaining or even increasing microcirculatory coronary blood flow in patients with septic shock, optimal coronary flow did not prevent myocardial dysfunction. This was attributed to septic endothelial damage, which led to blood flow maldistribution. This finding supports the notion that septic cardiomyopathy involves multiple contributing factors [20]. Although these results highlight significant changes in coronary flow and myocardial metabolism, there is still limited evidence to suggest that myocardial ischemia alone is the primary cause of myocardial dysfunction in sepsis.

5.2 Mitochondrial metabolism dysfunction

Although the mechanisms behind mitochondrial dysfunction in sepsis are not fully understood, multiple studies have established that mitochondrial dysfunction is a critical factor in septic cardiomyopathy, primarily through energy depletion. The heart's high mitochondrial content explains why mitochondrial dysfunction is closely linked to sepsis-induced cardiac dysfunction and its prognosis. The heart is particularly susceptible to sepsis-induced mitochondrial dysfunction due to its high reliance on adenosine triphosphate (ATP) for maintaining contraction and diastolic function. To restore mitochondrial function, various mechanisms have been investigated, notably mitochondrial uncoupling proteins located in the inner mitochondrial membrane. These proteins facilitate proton leakage across the membrane, which is crucial for regulating mitochondrial membrane potential and generating reactive oxygen species (ROS) and ATP. Other relevant biochemical pathways include oxidative stress, mitochondrial Ca^{2+} flux, mitochondrial DNA (mtDNA) in sepsis, mitochondrial dynamics, mitochondrial biogenesis, and mitochondrial autophagy [21–23].

5.2.1 Mitochondrial oxidative stress and injury

In sepsis, mitochondrial dysfunction leads to elevated levels of reactive oxygen species (ROS), such as superoxide, which contributes to oxidative injury and ongoing damage to cells and organs [24]. An imbalance in ROS and reactive nitrogen species disrupts oxidative phosphorylation in the septic myocardium, directly inhibiting mitochondrial respiration and damaging several subcellular components, including mitochondrial proteins, often resulting in mitochondrial apoptosis. This oxidative stress is closely linked to mitochondrial dysfunction and organ failure in sepsis models and has been observed in septic patients [25, 26]. Additionally, oxidative stress depletes the antioxidant capacity due to reduced levels of antioxidants like vitamins C and E, unconjugated bilirubin, and uric acid. Therefore, oxidative stress plays a crucial role in septic myocardial dysfunction, suggesting that antioxidants may offer a potential therapeutic avenue in the future [27–29].

5.2.2 Abnormal mitochondrial calcium transport

A critical step in ATP production is the establishment of a proton gradient, which relies on the inner mitochondrial membrane's impermeability and is primarily regulated by Ca2+ [30, 31]. During sepsis, the release of inflammatory mediators, such as cytokines, elevates mitochondrial Ca2+ levels by promoting its leakage from the sarcoplasmic reticulum and reducing its uptake [32]. This Ca2+ overload leads to the opening of mitochondrial permeability transition pores (mPTPs) and initiates a series of pathological changes, including caspase activation, which causes irreversible mitochondrial damage and ultimately impairs cardiomyocyte contractile function [33, 34]. When cytoplasmic Ca2+ levels decrease, smooth muscle relaxation and subsequent vasodilation occur. In cardiac cells, this reduction in Ca2+ levels results in diminished myocyte contraction and compromised myocardial function [35].

Given the essential role of Ca2+ in myocardial contraction, research has identified several pathways involved in septic myocardial depression, including impaired Ca^{2+} uptake, disrupted Ca2+ release from the sarcoplasmic reticulum, and diminished sensitivity of Ca2+ channels [36]. Thus, abnormal Ca2+ transport is a significant factor influencing heart function.

5.2.3 Mitochondrial DNA

Mitochondrial dysfunction during sepsis is also linked to damage to mitochondrial DNA (mtDNA), Mitochondrial DNA (mtDNA) is involved in the immune system and can serve as a biomarker for predicting mortality rates in septic patients, as its levels increase in plasma. During sepsis, elevated ROS production, reduced mitochondrial membrane potential (MMP), and the opening of the mitochondrial permeability transition pore (mPTP) can cause mtDNA to leak into the cytosol.

As mtDNA acts as a Damage-Associated Molecular Pattern (DAMP), its release can trigger Toll-like receptors, resulting in the secretion of IL-1β and IL-18, which in turn induces cell death. Mitochondrial DNA (mtDNA) is more susceptible to damage during sepsis. This damage disrupts oxidative phosphorylation, initiates calcium-dependent stress signaling, induces apoptosis, and activates inflammatory responses. Studies involving intensive care unit patients have shown that circulating mtDNA levels are notably higher in non-survivors compared to survivors. These findings suggest that elevated mtDNA concentrations are linked to poorer outcomes in sepsis patients [37–39].

5.2.4 Mitochondrial dynamics

Mitochondria constantly undergo cycles of fission and fusion to regulate their morphology, number, and size. Under normal physiological conditions, this balance between mitochondrial fusion and fission is crucial for maintaining mitochondrial and cellular homeostasis, including regulating cell division, proliferation, and the elimination of damaged mitochondria. Mitochondrial fusion involves proteins such as mitofusin-1 (encoded by MFN1) and mitofusin-2 (MFN2), while mitochondrial fission is mediated by the dynamin-like GTPase (encoded by OPA1) [40].

These proteins are linked to changes in mitochondrial membrane potential and decreased oxygen consumption. In response to stress, the rates of fission and fusion increase, playing vital roles in clearing damaged mitochondria and supporting repair processes. Despite their importance, the precise roles of these proteins in fission and fusion are not fully understood. During sepsis, mitochondrial dysfunction leads to increased fission and reduced fusion, resulting in fragmented and dysfunctional mitochondria, which contribute to organ failure. Pharmacological interventions that either enhance mitochondrial biogenesis or autophagy or reduce excessive mitochondrial fission have been shown to improve mitochondrial function and mitigate organ failure in septic models [41–43].

5.2.5 Mitochondrial biogenesis

Mitochondrial biogenesis refers to the generation of mitochondrial proteins, which are encoded either by nuclear DNA and subsequently imported and integrated into the mitochondria or by mitochondrial DNA (mtDNA), which encodes proteins primarily involved in the oxidative phosphorylation pathway. This process helps replace damaged proteins and enhances the mitochondria's ability to produce energy, particularly when energy demands rise [44]. Thus, mitochondrial biogenesis plays a crucial role in fulfilling the energy requirements of cellular metabolism.

5.2.6 Mitophagy

Mitophagy, a form of selective autophagy, is responsible for the removal and degradation of dysfunctional mitochondria. It regulates mitochondrial repair and renewal by recycling components from old mitochondria. This process also protects the heart from cell death by preserving energy substrates, eliminating damaged mitochondria that could lead to excessive ATP production, and reducing oxidative stress. Consequently, inhibiting mitophagy can result in reduced mitochondrial mass, accumulation of dysfunctional mitochondria, and worsening outcomes in sepsis [37, 45, 46]. Mitophagy is being explored as a potential therapeutic target to enhance heart function.

5.3 Direct myocardial depression

The first biochemical mechanism behind direct myocardial depression involves a reduction in β-adrenergic receptor components, which disrupts the adrenergic response at the cardiomyocyte level. This effect is mediated by various pro-inflammatory substances, primarily cytokines and nitric oxide (NO). The second mechanism involves cardiomyocyte injury and/or death induced by toxins, complements, DAMPs, and other myocardial depressants [47]. Thirdly, cardiomyocyte apoptosis is one of the primary contributors to myocardial depression and sepsis-related multiple-organ dysfunction. If not addressed promptly, myocardial dysfunction can advance to cardiomyocyte apoptosis, which leads to the downregulation of β-adrenoceptors and impairs myofibril function due to disrupted calcium release.

5.3.1 Cytokines

Cytokines are peptides produced locally by both somatic cells (such as endothelial, epithelial, and fibroblast cells) and immune cells (including neutrophils, lymphocytes, and macrophages) in response to stress or challenges like surgical procedures, trauma, ischemia, or sepsis. These signals facilitate communication among cells affected by these stressors [48]. Cytokines also stimulate the release of other inflammatory factors, including prostanoids and nitric oxide (NO), which further contribute to myocardial dysfunction.

Tumor necrosis factor (TNF)-α and interleukin (IL)-1β are among the most prominent pro-inflammatory cytokines, produced by macrophages during sepsis, these cytokines have been shown to significantly depress cardiac contractility in vitro [49]. While TNF-α and IL-1β are recognized as key drivers of the inflammatory response, nitric oxide (NO) and oxygen-free radicals are considered secondary contributors to septic myocardial depression [50, 51]. Synthesized in response to TNF-α, IL-1 reduces cardiac contractility by stimulating nitric oxide synthase (NOS). Consequently, IL-1 inhibitors, such as IL-1 receptor antagonists, could be a promising option to reduce morbidity and improve survival in patients with septic cardiomyopathy. However, there is currently insufficient evidence to fully support this approach [52, 53].

Elevated cytokine levels trigger the release of additional cytokines and other chemical mediators, which exacerbates and complicates myocardial dysfunction. Additionally, the heart itself can produce cytokines during inflammatory responses, further aggravating myocardial depression and impairing cardiac function. This was particularly evident when IL-6 was produced in the heart due to stimulation of myocardial α- and β-adrenoreceptors and excessive catecholamine use. Elevated serum levels of IL-6 have been correlated with greater illness severity and higher vasopressor requirements in patients with septic shock [54, 55].

5.3.2 Nitric oxide

NO, produced in the vascular endothelium, is a potential mediator of septic cardiomyopathy and exerts a broad spectrum of physiological effects on the cardiovascular system. NO is synthesized by different isoforms of nitric oxide synthase (NOS) located in subcellular compartments, serving as a second messenger within these components. NOS isoforms 1 and 3 have been implicated in early septic cardiomyopathy, whereas NOS isoform 2 has been identified as a potential contributor to contractile depression during late sepsis [56, 57].

Several studies have linked nitric oxide (NO) to the severity of Myocardial dysfunction and an increased mortality rate. This association arises from NO's impact on various sites, including the β-adrenergic receptors in the heart and mitochondrial function. At the mitochondrial level, NO impairs mitochondrial function, which is a significant pathway in the development of sepsis-induced cardiomyopathy [58].

5.3.3 Endothelin-1

Elevated levels of endothelin-1 (ET-1) have been shown to stimulate the release of inflammatory cytokines. In a porcine endotoxic model, endothelin-receptor blockade with bosentan enhanced cardiac performance [59]. However, the involvement of ET-1 in septic myocardial dysfunction is not well-established, highlighting the need for further research to elucidate its mechanism of action.

5.3.4 Intracellular adhesion molecules

In mice, stimulation with LPS and TNF-α led to elevated expression of intercellular adhesion molecule-1 (ICAM-1) and vascular cell adhesion molecule-1 (VCAM-1) in the coronary endothelium and cardiomyocytes. Blocking VCAM-1 prevented myocardial dysfunction and reduced neutrophil accumulation in the myocardium [60, 61]. Additionally, both ICAM-1 knockout and antibody blockade improved myocardial function during endotoxemia, though they did not affect neutrophil accumulation. Despite the resolution of contractile dysfunction with antibody blockade of ICAM-1 or VCAM-1, further investigation is needed to understand how these adhesion molecules influence calcium homeostasis and the production of oxygen-free radicals.

5.3.5 Prostanoids

In septic patients, serum levels of thromboxane, prostacyclin, and other prostanoids are elevated. These prostanoids have been shown to potentially disrupt coronary endothelial function; however, their impact can be lessened by cyclooxygenase inhibitors like indomethacin. The use of nonsteroidal anti-inflammatory drugs (NSAIDs) such as ibuprofen and lornoxicam to inhibit prostanoids has been suggested as a treatment strategy, but clinical trials have shown that neither drug significantly improves survival rates [62].

5.3.6 Histones and high mobility group box 1 (HMGB1)

Extracellular histones act as endogenous damage-associated molecular patterns (DAMPs) that may interact with TLR2 and TLR4 on various cell types, including cardiomyocytes. This interaction can lead to reduced mitochondrial membrane potential and ATP levels, resulting in cell damage, and organ dysfunction—including in the heart. Alhamdi et al. found that elevated levels of circulating histones correlate with increased cardiac troponin T (cTnT) levels in sepsis patients, which probably contributes to septic cardiac dysfunction and mortality [47, 63]. The pro-inflammatory mediator HMGB1 has a significant role in the development of cardiac dysfunction. Zhang et al. demonstrated that one mechanism by which HMGB1 induces cardiac dysfunction involves the increase in intracellular ROS levels caused by HMGB1–TLR4 interaction. This interaction leads to greater oxidative stress [64]. Additionally, HMGB1 disrupts cardiac excitation-contraction (EC) coupling. Consequently, systolic $Ca2^{+}$ transients and myocyte contractility are diminished. In summary, circulating damage-associated molecular patterns (DAMPs) like histone and/or HMGB1 either directly damage myocytes or are released by injured myocytes, leading to cardiac dysfunction.

5.3.7 Complement system

In sepsis, the complement system is activated, and complement component 5 (C5a) is strongly associated with multiorgan failure. C5a's involvement in septic myocardial dysfunction can be attributed to the alteration of calcium and ROS levels in cardiomyocytes, causing cardiac dysfunction [65]. Furthermore, C5a receptor (C5aR) expression in cardiomyocytes mediates C5a-induced cardiodepression [66].

5.3.8 Other mediators

The evidence for additional myocardial depressant substances is still developing, with various new endogenous compounds emerging as potential contributors to septic myocardial depression. These include histamine, prostaglandins, leukocyte lysozyme, and estrogenic compounds. However, certain newly identified substances, such as endotoxin and natriuretic peptides, require further investigation. Both B-type natriuretic peptide and atrial natriuretic peptide were significantly higher in septic patients compared to controls. Caspase-3 activation has been linked to reduced sensitivity of myofilaments to calcium and structural breakdown of sarcomeres, though further research is needed to fully clarify these effects. Additionally, emerging data suggest that cyclooxygenase products, platelet-activating factor, lipoteichoic acid, leukotrienes, and protein kinase C may also play a role in septic myocardial depression [67–69].

6. Monitoring of sepsis-induced myocardial dysfunction

Monitoring sepsis-induced cardiac dysfunction involves a multifaceted approach to accurately assess the impact on cardiac function. Key elements include:

1. *Hemodynamic monitoring*: Continuous assessment of vital signs, including heart rate, blood pressure, and central venous pressure, helps gauge the overall cardiovascular status.

   Advanced hemodynamic monitoring devices, such as pulmonary artery catheters and transpulmonary thermodilution method, provide detailed information on cardiac output, global ejection fraction, preload, and afterload and help determine the adequacy of perfusion and the effectiveness of fluid resuscitation.

   Hemodynamic monitoring devices

   Measuring cardiac output (CO) and other hemodynamic parameters is crucial in sepsis-induced myocardial dysfunction. While the pulmonary artery catheter (PAC) was once commonly used for hemodynamic monitoring in critically ill patients, its use has declined due to the lack of evidence showing it improves patient mortality. As an alternative, the transpulmonary thermodilution method has been proposed for assessing CO and cardiac performance metrics such as the cardiac function index (CFI) and global ejection fraction (GEF). Reports indicate that low CFI and GEF values from transpulmonary thermodilution can identify cardiac dysfunction in septic patients. Additionally, pulse contour analysis has been found reliable for continuous CO measurement in sepsis. However, the efficacy of these methods for diagnosing septic cardiomyopathy still requires further validation [70–72].

Non-invasive hemodynamic methods, including pulse contour analysis, pulse pressure variation, stroke volume variation, inferior vena cava collapse, passive straight leg raise, and end-expiratory occlusion, are supported by evidence for assessing fluid responsiveness in patients with septic shock. However, these techniques do have certain limitations. After the initial resuscitation phase, careful fluid management is essential. This should be guided by dynamic measures of fluid responsiveness.

2. *Echocardiography*: This imaging technique evaluates cardiac structure and function in real time. It helps detect changes in ejection fraction, ventricular size, and wall motion abnormalities, which are indicative of sepsis-induced cardiomyopathy. Echocardiographic findings in sepsis-induced Myocardial dysfunction are listed in (**Table 2**). Also, ECG monitoring is crucial for detecting arrhythmias or ischemic changes that may arise from sepsis-induced cardiac dysfunction.

Parameter		**Values suggestive of septic cardiomyopathy**	**Pros**	**Limitations**
LV systolic dysfunction	LVEF	LVEF <40–50%	Easy to obtain, Physician familiarity	LVEF depends on loading conditions, quantification varies by "eyeballing"
	MAPSE	MAPSE <11.65 mm	Easy to obtain.	Preload and angle-dependent, varies due to cardiac size, fails to detect regional myocardial abnormalities
	GLS	GLS < −18–20%	More sensitive and less varied, Independent of loading conditions and angle	Lack of consensus on thresholds for abnormal values and low feasibility.
LV diastolic dysfunction		E/e′ > 14 e′ < 7 cm/s (septal) or < 10 cm/s(lateral)	Easy to obtain	May be affected by patients' age and regional wall motion abnormalities.
RV dysfunction		TAPSE <17 mm	Easy to obtain	May be affected by LV dysfunction and tricuspid regurgitation

LVEF, left ventricular ejection fraction; MAPSE, mitral annular plane systolic excursion; GLS, global longitudinal strain; E, transmittal early filling velocity; e′, early mitral annular velocity; TAPSE, tricuspid annular systolic excursion.

Table 2.
Echocardiography parameters of septic cardiomyopathy.

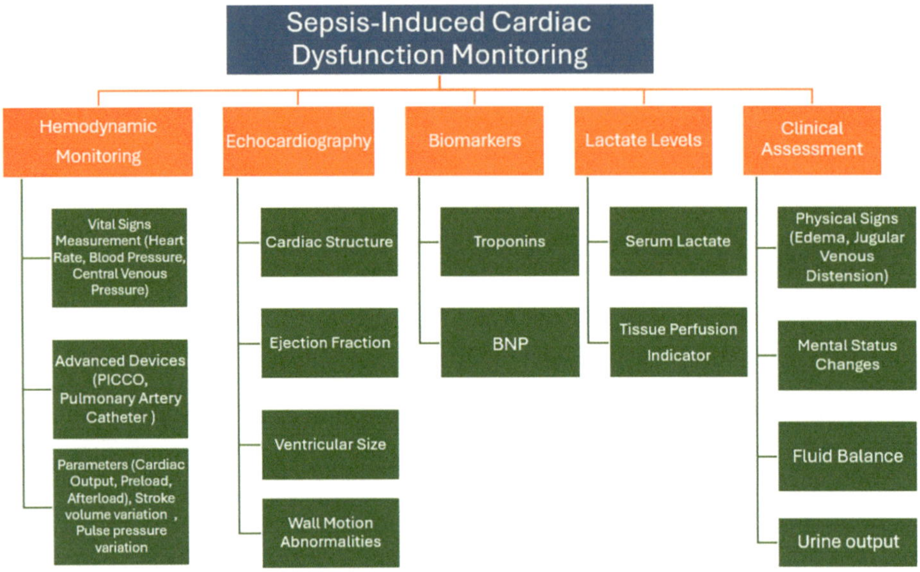

Figure 2.
Monitoring during sepsis-induced myocardial dysfunction.

3. *Blood biomarkers:* Measurement of biomarkers such as B-type natriuretic peptide (BNP) and troponins helps gauge myocardial stress and injury. Elevated levels of these markers can indicate cardiac dysfunction and guide treatment decisions.

4. *Lactate levels*: Monitoring lactate levels helps assess tissue perfusion and oxygenation. Elevated lactate can indicate inadequate cardiac output and assist in adjusting treatment strategies.

5. *Clinical assessment*: Regular evaluation of clinical signs such as edema, jugular venous distension, and altered mental status can provide clues about worsening cardiac function and fluid balance.

Effective monitoring requires integrating these data points to provide a comprehensive view of cardiac function and guide appropriate management strategies in patients with sepsis. Monitoring of Septic cardiac dysfunction is summarized in (**Figure 2**).

7. Management of sepsis-induced myocardial dysfunction

The management of sepsis-induced Myocardial dysfunction should target the underlying infection along with supportive measures such as fluid replacement, oxygen therapy, and medications to improve heart function. Initial sepsis treatment emphasizes early recognition, infection control, and the optimization of hemodynamic status through fluid resuscitation and vasopressor therapy. This approach is considered the standard care for septic cardiomyopathy.

Treatment strategies for sepsis-induced Myocardial dysfunction are summarized in (**Table 3**).

Therapy	Mechanism of action	Benefits	Limitations
Vasopressors (noradrenaline first Choice, Vasopressin second line)	Vasoconstriction induced by the stimulation of alpha- or beta-adrenergic receptors, vasopressin receptors, or dopamine receptors.	Familiar to physicians. Well-studied in septic shock. May reverse hypotension due to the vasoconstrictive effects. Beta and dopamine activity will increase contractility.	Beta-adrenergic and dopamine activity can elevate myocardial demand, which might exacerbate cardiomyopathy and/or lead to arrhythmias. An excessive rise in afterload may result in cardiac dysfunction, particularly with the use of phenylephrine and vasopressin.
Fluids	Increase preload, thereby enhancing stroke volume through the Frank–Starling mechanism	Familiar, well-studied treatment in septic shock. Augment cardiac output by increasing stroke volume.	Excessive fluid may lead to worsening organ failure and higher mortality. Excessive preload may produce exacerbation of right ventricular dysfunction, leading to low cardiac output.
Dobutamine	Beta-adrenergic agent	Well-known. Increased cardiac output, SvO2, oxygen delivery	Risk of tachycardia. Impact on outcome is ambiguous. Elevated myocardial demand and vasodilation may impair hemodynamics.
Milrinone	Phosphodiesterase inhibitor increases cAMP	Increased contractility without adrenergic activity. No trials for SIDM.	Can cause vasodilation and is limited by renal dysfunction. Risk of arrhythmias.
Levosimendan	Calcium sensitizer	Increases myocardial contractility, may improve cardiac output and hemodynamic parameters	Vasodilation, no evidence of survival benefit
Beta-Blockers	Beta-adrenergic blockade	Controlled heart rate and decreased myocardial demand	Negative inotropic effects may aggravate hemodynamic instability.
Methylene Blue	Nitric oxide metabolism	Treats vasoplegia. Improved cardiac contractility, reduced requirement of vasopressors	No difference in outcomes. Risk of serotonin syndrome. Interference with pulse oximetry. Contraindicated in patients with G6PD deficiency, Renal dysfunction
Mechanical Support	Types of mechanical support include the intra-aortic balloon pump, venoarterial extracorporeal membrane oxygenation (VA ECMO), and Impella	Provides aggressive supportive care until reversibility occurs. May have a mortality benefit	Invasive, may cause severe complications include bleeding, thrombosis, and exacerbation of infection

CO, cardiac output; cAMP, cyclic adenosine monophosphate; SIMD, sepsis-induced Myocardial dysfunction; G6PD, glucose-6-phosphate dehydrogenase.

Table 3.
Treatment strategies for sepsis-induced myocardial dysfunction.

Fluid resuscitation is an essential strategy to improve septic hypoperfusion, oxygen delivery, and organ function by raising cardiac output. However, excessive fluid volumes after initial resuscitation can lead to an increase in cardiac filling pressure and tissue edema, which are linked to higher mortality rates [73, 74].

Current international guidelines for sepsis treatment recommend "hemodynamic monitoring." Therefore, the hemodynamics status should be continuously monitored to assess the fluid responsiveness and guide fluid therapy. Approaches to determine fluid responsiveness include pulse pressure variation and systolic pressure variation measured by arterial waveform, stroke volume variation by pulse contour analysis, LV end-diastolic area by echocardiography, global end-diastolic volume by a transpulmonary thermodilution, and central venous pressure by central venous catheter [73, 75].

Norepinephrine, which acts as both an alpha and beta agonist, is the preferred vasopressor for treating patients with sepsis. Current guidelines support the use of dobutamine in the presence of myocardial dysfunction, such as elevated filling pressures and low cardiac output or signs of sustained hypoperfusion [73], but convincing evidence of benefit is lacking.

Levosimendan, an inotropic calcium sensitizer, has been shown to increase cardiac output and systemic hemodynamics with minimal increase on oxygen consumption in sepsis and septic cardiomyopathy [76]. However, Liu et al. [77] demonstrated in their meta-analysis that the use of levosimendan had no effect on mortality.

Beta-blockers can be effective when it is difficult to maintain blood pressure and systemic circulation due to tachycardia. However, a recent study evaluating the effects of landiolol in patients with sepsis and tachycardia, in conjunction with norepinephrine, did not demonstrate an improvement in the SOFA (Sequential Organ Failure Assessment) score or 28-day mortality [6, 78].

Cardiogenic shock caused by sepsis, if unresponsive to conservative treatment, is considered an indication for mechanical support, such as an intra-aortic balloon pump (IABP), venoarterial ECMO (VA-ECMO), or an Impella device, which can aid cardiac output [79]. However, they are all invasive and can cause severe complications, Further research is needed to better assess their value in septic myocardial dysfunction.

Various medications have been employed to treat sepsis with the aim of preventing sepsis-induced cardiomyopathy or multiorgan dysfunction. However, these treatments have not improved outcomes significantly. This highlights the necessity for new therapeutic strategies that focus on specific mechanisms of sepsis-induced myocardial dysfunction.

8. Conclusions

The pathophysiology of sepsis-induced cardiac dysfunction and its mechanisms are not yet fully understood. Despite extensive research over many years, treating sepsis-induced cardiac dysfunction remains a complex challenge. Apart from general management of sepsis with infection control, antibiotics, vasopressors, inotropes, fluid resuscitation, and hemodynamic monitoring, there is limited data and a lack of evidence regarding more specific treatments. Numerous clinical and experimental studies have explored treatment options for both sepsis and its cardiac manifestations, but many have reported ineffective or inconclusive results during validation. Therefore, a more precise understanding of the pathophysiology of sepsis-induced cardiac dysfunction is crucial for developing more effective treatment strategies.

Author details

Hossam Algallie[1*], Siddhartha Banerjee[1], Ashish Kumar[1], Um I. Rubab[1], Anil Kumar Agarwal[1], Seema Nahid[2], Nissar Shaikh[1] and Mohammad Ataur Rahman[1]

1 Surgical Intensive Care, Hamad Medical Corporation, Doha, Qatar

2 Anesthesiology and Perioperative Medicine, Hamad Medical Corporation, Doha, Qatar

*Address all correspondence to: hossam.algallie@gmail.com

References

[1] Vieillard-Baron A. Septic cardiomyopathy. Annals of Intensive Care. 2011;**1**:6

[2] Hotchkiss RS, Karl IE. Pathophysiology and treatment of sepsis. The New England Journal of Medicine. 2003;**348**:138-150

[3] Geri G, Vignon P, Aubry A, Fedou AL, Charron C, Silva S, et al. Cardiovascular clusters in septic shock combining clinical and echocardiographic parameters: A post hoc analysis. Intensive Care Medicine. 2019;**45**:657-667

[4] Wasyluk W, Nowicka-Stążka P, Zwolak A. Heart metabolism in sepsis-induced cardiomyopathy—Unusual metabolic dysfunction of the heart. International Journal of Environmental Research and Public Health. 2021;**18**(14):7598

[5] Fernandes CJ Jr, de Assuncao MS. Myocardial dysfunction in sepsis: A large, unsolved puzzle. Critical Care Research and Practice. 2012;**2012**:896430

[6] L'Heureux M, Sternberg M, Brath L, Turlington J, Kashiouris MG. Sepsis-induced cardiomyopathy: A comprehensive review. Current Cardiology Reports. 2020;**22**:35

[7] Pulido JN, Afessa B, Masaki M, Yuasa T, Gillespie S, Herasevich V, et al. Clinical spectrum, frequency, and significance of myocardial dysfunction in severe sepsis and septic shock. Mayo Clinic Proceedings. 2012;**87**:620-628

[8] Muller-Werdan U, Buerke M, Ebelt H, Heinroth KM, Herklotz A, Loppnow H, et al. Septic cardiomyopathy: A not yet discovered cardiomyopathy? Experimental and Clinical Cardiology. 2006;**11**:226-236

[9] Hoesel LM, Niederbichler AD, Ward PA. Complement-related molecular events in sepsis leading to heart failure. Molecular Immunology. 2007;**44**:95-102

[10] Parker MM, Suffredini AF, Natanson C, Ognibene FP, Shelhamer JH, Parrillo JE. Responses of left ventricular function in survivors and nonsurvivors of septic shock. Journal of Critical Care. 1989;**4**:19-25

[11] Poelaert J, Declerck C, Vogelaers D, Colardyn F, Visser CA. Left ventricular systolic and diastolic function in septic shock. Intensive Care Medicine. 1997;**23**:553-560

[12] Parker MM, Shelhamer JH, Bacharach SL, Green MV, Natanson C, Frederick TM, et al. Profound but reversible myocardial depression in patients with septic shock. Annals of Internal Medicine. 1984;**100**:483-490

[13] Parker MM, McCarthy KE, Ognibene FP, Parrillo JE. Right ventricular dysfunction and dilatation, similar to left ventricular changes, characterize the cardiac depression of septic shock in humans. Chest. 1990;**97**:126-131

[14] Li Y, Li H. Analysis of incidence and risk factors of septic cardiomyopathy. Zhonghua jizhen yixue zazhi. 2019;**28**(7):836-840

[15] Sato R, Kuriyama A, Takada T, Nasu M, Luthe SK. Prevalence, and risk factors of sepsis-induced cardiomyopathy: A retrospective cohort study. Medicine. 2016;**95**:e5031

[16] Jeong HS, Lee TH, Bang CH, Kim J-H HSJ. Risk factors and outcomes of sepsis-induced myocardial dysfunction and stress induced cardiomyopathy in sepsis or septic shock: A comparative retrospective study. Medicine. 2018;**97**:e0263

[17] Akira S, Uematsu S, Takeuchi O. Pathogen recognition and innate immunity. Cell. 2006;**124**:783-801

[18] Raeburn CD, Sheppard F, Barsness KA, Arya J, Harken AH. Cytokines for surgeons. American Journal of Surgery. 2002;**183**:268-273

[19] Levy RJ, Piel DA, Acton PD, Zhou R, Ferrari VA, Karp JS, et al. Evidence of myocardial hibernation in the septic heart. Critical Care Medicine. 2005;**33**:2752-2756

[20] Antonucci E, Fiaccadori E, Donadello K, Taccone FS, Franchi F, Scolletta S. Myocardial depression in sepsis: From pathogenesis to clinical manifestations and treatment. Journal of Critical Care. 2014;**29**:500-511

[21] Jang DH, Greenwood JC, Spyres MB, Eckmann DM. Measurement of mitochondrial respiration and motility in acute care: Sepsis, trauma, and poisoning. Journal of Intensive Care Medicine. 2017;**32**:86-94

[22] Carré JE, Singer M. Cellular energetic metabolism in sepsis: The need for a systems approach. Biochimica et Biophysica Acta. 2008;**1777**:763-771

[23] Brealey D, Brand M, Hargreaves I, Heales S, Land J, Smolenski R, et al. Association between mitochondrial dysfunction and severity and outcome of septic shock. Lancet. 2002;**360**:219-223

[24] Potz BA, Sellke FW, Abid MR. Endothelial ROS and impaired myocardial oxygen consumption in sepsis-induced cardiac dysfunction. Journal of Intensive Critical Care. 2016;**2**:20

[25] Larsen FJ, Schiffer TA, Weitzberg E, Lundberg JO. Regulation of mitochondrial function and energetics by reactive nitrogen oxides. Free Radical Biology and Medicine. 2012;**53**:1919-1928

[26] Crouser ED. Mitochondrial dysfunction in septic shock and multiple organ dysfunction syndrome. Mitochondrion. 2004;**4**:729-741

[27] Lowes DA, Webster NR, Murphy MP, Galley HF. Antioxidants that protect mitochondria reduce interleukin-6 and oxidative stress, improve mitochondrial function, and reduce biochemical markers of organ dysfunction in a rat model of acute sepsis. British Journal of Anaesthesia. 2013;**110**:472-480

[28] Kayali R, Aydin S, Cakatay U. Effect of gender on main clinical chemistry parameters in aged rats. Current Aging Science. 2009;**2**(67):71

[29] Galley HF. Oxidative stress and mitochondrial dysfunction in sepsis. British Journal of Anaesthesia. 2011;**107**:57-64

[30] Bernardi P, Di Lisa F. The mitochondrial permeability transition pore: Molecular nature and role as a target in cardioprotection. Journal of Molecular and Cellular Cardiology. 2015;**78**:100-106

[31] Duncan DJ, Yang Z, Hopkins PM, Steele DS, Harrison SM. TNF alpha and IL-1beta increase Ca2+ leak from the sarcoplasmic reticulum and susceptibility to arrhythmia in rat ventricular myocytes. Cell Calcium. 2010;**47**:378-386

[32] Hassoun SM, Marechal X, Montaigne D, Bouazza Y, Decoster B, Lancel S, et al. Prevention of endotoxin-induced sarcoplasmic reticulum calcium leak improves mitochondrial and myocardial dysfunction. Critical Care Medicine. 2008;**36**:2590-2596

[33] Shanmuganathan S, Hausenloy DJ, Duchen MR, Yellon DM. Mitochondrial permeability transition pore as a target for cardioprotection in the human heart. American Journal of Physiology. Heart and Circulatory Physiology. 2005;**289**:H237-H242

[34] Smeding L, Plötz FB, Groeneveld AB, Kneyber MC. Structural changes of the heart during severe sepsis or septic shock. Shock. 2012;**37**:449-456

[35] Finkel MS, Oddis CV, Jacob TD, Watkins SC, Hattler BG, Simmons RL. Negative inotropic effects of cytokines on the heart mediated by nitric oxide. Science. 1992;**257**:387-389

[36] Wu LL, Ji Y, Dong LW, Liu MS. Calcium uptake by sarcoplasmic reticulum is impaired during the hypodynamic phase of sepsis in the rat heart. Shock. 2001;**15**:49-55

[37] Salami OM, Habimana O, Peng JF, Yi GH. Therapeutic strategies targeting mitochondrial dysfunction in sepsis-induced cardiomyopathy. Cardiovascular Drugs and Therapy. 2024;**38**(1):163-180

[38] Nunnari J, Suomalainen A. Mitochondria: In sickness and in health. Cell. 2012;**148**:1145-1159

[39] Nakahira K, Kyung SY, Rogers AJ, Gazourian L, Youn S, Massaro AF, et al. Circulating mitochondrial DNA in patients in the ICU as a marker of mortality: Derivation and validation. PLoS Medicine. 2013;**10**:e1001577

[40] Sánchez-Villamil JP, D'Annunzio V, Finocchietto P, Holod S, Rebagliati I, Pérez H, et al. Cardiac-specific overexpression of thioredoxin 1 attenuates mitochondrial and myocardial dysfunction in septic mice. The International Journal of Biochemistry and Cell Biology. 2016;**81**(Pt B):323-334

[41] Zhan M, Brooks C, Liu F, Sun L, Dong Z. Mitochondrial dynamics: Regulatory mechanisms and emerging role in renal pathophysiology. Kidney International. 2013;**83**:568-581

[42] Liesa M, Palacín M, Zorzano A. Mitochondrial dynamics in mammalian health and disease. Physiological Reviews. 2009;**89**:799-845

[43] Wu Y, Yao YM, Lu ZQ. Mitochondrial quality control mechanisms as potential therapeutic targets in sepsis-induced multiple organ failure. Journal of Molecular Medicine (Berlin, Germany). 2019;**97**:451-462

[44] Singer M. The role of mitochondrial dysfunction in sepsis-induced multi-organ failure. Virulence. 2014;**5**:66-72

[45] Gunst J, Derese I, Aertgeerts A, Ververs EJ, Wauters A, Van den Berghe G, et al. Insufficient autophagy contributes to mitochondrial dysfunction, organ failure, and adverse outcome in an animal model of critical illness. Critical Care Medicine. 2013;**41**:182-194

[46] Rocha M, Herance R, Rovira S, Hernández-Mijares A, Victor VM. Mitochondrial dysfunction and antioxidant therapy in sepsis. Infectious Disorders Drug Targets. 2012;**12**:161-178

[47] Kakihana Y, Ito T, Nakahara M, Yamaguchi K, Yasuda T. Sepsis-induced myocardial dysfunction: Pathophysiology

and management. Journal of Intensive Care. 2016;**4**:22

[48] Kumar A, Krieger A, Symeoneides S, Kumar A, Parrillo JE. Myocardial dysfunction in septic shock. Part II. Role of cytokines and nitric oxide. Journal of Cardiothoracic and Vascular Anesthesia. 2001;**15**:485-511

[49] Pathan N, Hemingway CA, Alizadeh AA, Stephens AC, Bold Rick JC, Oragui EE, et al. Role of interleukin 6 in myocardial dysfunction of meningococcal septic shock. Lancet. 2004;**363**:203-209

[50] Loppnow H, Werdan K, Reuter G, Flad HD. The interleukin-1 and interleukin-1 converting enzyme families in the cardiovascular system. European Cytokine Network. 1998;**9**:675-680

[51] Kelly RA, Balligand JL, Smith TW. Nitric oxide and cardiac function. Circulation Research. 1996;**79**:363-380

[52] Francis SE, Holden H, Holt CM, Duff GW. Interleukin-1 in myocardium and coronary arteries of patients with dilated cardiomyopathy. Journal of Molecular and Cellular Cardiology. 1998;**30**:215-223

[53] Opal SM, Fisher CJ Jr, Dhainaut JF, Vincent JL, Brase R, Lowry SF, et al. Confirmatory interleukin-1 receptor antagonist trial in severe sepsis: A phase III, randomized, double-blind, placebo-controlled, multicenter trial. The interleukin-1 receptor antagonist sepsis investigator group. Critical Care Medicine. 1997;**25**:1115-1124

[54] Müller-Werdan U, Werdan K. Immune modulation by catecholamines: A potential mechanism of cytokine release in heart failure? Herz. 2000;**25**:271-273

[55] Geppert A, Steiner A, Zorn G, Delle-Karth G, Koreny M, Haumer M, et al. Multiple organ failure in patients with cardiogenic shock is associated with high plasma levels of interleukin-6. Critical Care Medicine. 2002;**30**:1987-1994

[56] Rudiger A, Singer M. Mechanisms of sepsis-induced cardiac dysfunction. Critical Care Medicine. 2007;**35**:1599-1608

[57] Zanotti-Cavazzoni SL, Hollenberg SM. Cardiac dysfunction in severe sepsis and septic shock. Current Opinion in Critical Care. 2009;**15**:392-397

[58] Crouser ED, Julian MW, Huff JE, Joshi MS, Bauer JA, Gadd ME, et al. Abnormal permeability of inner and outer mitochondrial membranes contributes independently to mitochondrial dysfunction in the liver during acute endotoxemia. Critical Care Medicine. 2004;**32**:478-488

[59] Konrad D, Oldner A, Rossi P, Wanecek M, Rudehill A, Weitzberg E. Differentiated and dose-related cardiovascular effects of a dual endothelin receptor antagonist in endotoxin shock. Critical Care Medicine. 2004;**32**:1192-1199

[60] Raeburn CD, Calkins CM, Zimmerman MA, Song Y, Ao L, Banerjee A, et al. ICAM-1 and VCAM-1 mediate endotoxemic myocardial dysfunction independent of neutrophil accumulation. American Journal of Physiology. Regulatory, Integrative and Comparative Physiology. 2002;**283**:R47786

[61] Raeburn CD, Calkins CM, Zimmerman MA, Song Y, Ao L, Banerjee A, et al. Vascular cell adhesion molecule: 1 expression is obligatory for endotoxin-induced

myocardial neutrophil accumulation and contractile dysfunction. Surgery. 2001;**130**:319-325

[62] Memiş D, Karamanlioğlu B, Turan A, Koyuncu O, Pamukçu Z. Effects of lornoxicam on the physiology of severe sepsis. Critical Care. 2004;**8**:R474-R482

[63] Alhamdi Y, Abrams ST, Cheng Z, Jing S, Su D, Liu Z, et al. Circulating histones are major mediators of cardiac injury in patients with sepsis. Critical Care Medicine. 2015;**43**:2094-2103

[64] Zhang C, Mo M, Ding W, Liu W, Yan D, Deng J, et al. High-mobility group box 1 (HMGB1) impaired cardiac excitation-contraction coupling by enhancing the sarcoplasmic reticulum (SR) Ca (2+) leak through TLR4-ROS signaling in cardiomyocytes. Journal of Molecular and Cellular Cardiology. 2014;**74**:260-273

[65] Pei XB, Liu B. Research progress on the mechanism and management of septic cardiomyopathy: A comprehensive review. Emergency Medicine International. 2023;**2023**:8107336. DOI: 10.1155/2023/8107336

[66] Niederbichler AD, Hoesel LM, Westfall MV, Gao H, Ipaktchi KR, Sun L, et al. An essential role for complement C5a in the pathogenesis of septic cardiac dysfunction. The Journal of Experimental Medicine. 2006;**203**:53-61

[67] Court O, Kumar A, Parrillo JE, Kumar A. Clinical review: Myocardial depression in sepsis and septic shock. Critical Care. 2002;**6**:500-508

[68] Witthaut R, Busch C, Fraunberger P, Walli A, Seidel D, Pilz G, et al. Plasma atrial natriuretic peptide and brain natriuretic peptide are increased in septic shock: Impact of interleukin-6 and sepsis-associated left ventricular dysfunction. Intensive Care Medicine. 2003;**29**:1696-1702

[69] Grandel U, Hopf M, Buerke M, Hattar K, Heep M, Fink L, et al. Mechanisms of cardiac depression caused by lipoteichoic acids from *Staphylococcus aureus* in isolated rat hearts. Circulation. 2005;**112**:691-698

[70] Wiener RS, Welch HG. Trends in the use of the pulmonary artery catheter in the United States, 1993-2004. Journal of the American Medical Association. 2007;**298**(4):423-429

[71] Ritter S, Rudiger A, Maggiorini M. Transpulmonary thermodilution-derived cardiac function index identifies cardiac dysfunction in acute heart failure and septic patients: An observational study. Critical Care. 2009;**13**(4):R133

[72] Schuerholz T, Meyer MC, Friedrich L, Przemeck M, Sümpelmann R, Marx G. Reliability of continuous cardiac output determination by pulse-contour analysis in porcine septic shock. Acta Anaesthesiologica Scandinavica. 2006;**50**(4):407-413

[73] Rhodes A, Evans LE, Alhazzani W, et al. Surviving sepsis campaign: International guidelines for management of sepsis and septic shock: 2016. Critical Care Medicine. 2017;**45**:486-552

[74] Brown RM, Semler MW. Fluid management in sepsis. Journal of Intensive Care Medicine. 2019;**34**(5):364-373

[75] Marik PE, Monnet X, Teboul JL. Hemodynamic parameters to guide fluid therapy. Annals of Intensive Care. 2011;**1**:1. DOI: 10.1186/2110-5820-1-1

[76] Morelli A, De Castro S, Teboul JL, et al. Effects of levosimendan on systemic and regional hemodynamics in

septic myocardial depression. Intensive Care Medicine. 2005;**31**:638-644. DOI: 10.1007/s00134-005-2619-z

[77] Liu DH, Ning YL, Lei YY, Chen J, Liu YY, Lin XF, et al. Levosimendan versus dobutamine for sepsis-induced cardiac dysfunction: A systematic review and meta-analysis. Scientific Reports. 2021;**11**:20333

[78] Whitehouse T, Hossain A, Perkins GD, Gordon AC, Bion J, Young D, et al. Landiolol and organ failure in patients with septic shock: The STRESS-L randomized clinical trial. Journal of the American Medical Association. 2023;**330**:1641-1652

[79] Wada K, Bunya N, Kakizaki R, Kasai T, Uemura S, Harada K, et al. Successful use of venoarterial extracorporeal membrane oxygenation for septic cardiomyopathy in a patient with preexisting chronic heart failure. Acute Medicine and Surgery. 2019;**6**:301-304

Chapter 12

Septic Shock: Pathophysiology to Patient Care

Erum Saboohi, AbdulHadi Hassan Mallick and Yusra Shahid

Abstract

Septic shock is a serious, complex, and life-threatening complication of sepsis that is characterized by fluid resistant hypotension and involves organ dysfunction caused by a dysregulated response to infection. At the tissue level, sepsis triggers a catastrophic inflammatory response ending up in endothelial damage, vascular dysfunction, and organ failure. The clinical picture of septic shock may comprise tachycardia, tachypnea, fever or hypothermia/chills, oliguria or anuria, declining Glasgow coma scale (GCS), severe body aches, multi-organ dysfunction, delayed CRT, and rash/ecchymosis. SIRS, qSOFA, and SOFA are some of the clinical scores aiding in diagnosing septic shock. Septic shock can rapidly progress to respiratory failure, cardiovascular compromise, multiorgan failure, and death. Mortality rates are exceptionally high, and survivors present with multi-organ dysfunction and neurological impairment. Prompt recognition and early and individualized aggressive treatment (fluid resuscitation, vasopressor support, broad spectrum antibiotics) and meticulous monitoring are the cornerstones of management.

Keywords: sepsis, septic shock, multi-organ dysfunction, mortality, score

1. Introduction

Sepsis is a serious illness that affects all age groups. From data published in 2020, there were 48.9 million cases and 11 million sepsis-related deaths worldwide, representing 20% of all global deaths [1]. According to the Third International Consensus Definitions for Sepsis and Septic Shock (Sepsis-3), sepsis is defined as "life-threatening organ dysfunction caused by a dysregulated host response to infection." Septic shock is defined as a subset of sepsis in which the underlying circulatory and cellular/metabolic abnormalities profoundly increase the risk of mortality [2]. It is a condition in which sepsis is accompanied by cardiovascular dysfunction, cellular damage, and severe metabolic abnormality. The definition focuses on organ dysfunction associated with infection and assesses the progression of organ dysfunction in infectious diseases.

2. Pathophysiology of septic shock

Underlying mechanisms for septic shock are multifactorial and include:

1. Sepsis, usually bacterial, rarely viral or fungal triggers cascade.
2. Activation of immune system by the release of proinflammatory chemokines and cytokine (TNF-alpha, IL-1 beta, IL-6 etc.).
3. Increased permeability of capillary endothelium leading to 3rd space shift, impaired tissue perfusion, and hypotension.
4. Activation of anti and pro-coagulants causes thrombosis and disseminated intravascular coagulation (DIC).
5. Impaired ability to combat infection because of immunosuppression.
6. Dysfunctionality of mitochondria causing impaired ATP production at the cellular level.
7. Multi-organ dysfunction like:

    a. Acute respiratory distress syndrome (ARDS)

    b. Acute kidney injury (AKI)

    c. Hepatic dysfunction and failure

    d. Dysfunctionality of cardiomyocytes causing cardiac depression

8. Hypoperfusion leads to:

    a. Tissue hypoxia

    b. Anaerobic metabolism

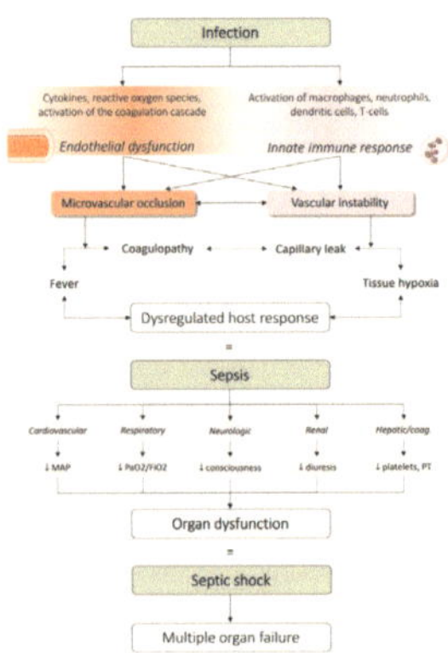

Figure 1.
Courtesy; Springer Link [3].

c. Lactic acidosis

d. Altered amino acid metabolism

9. Multiorgan failure

Better understanding of pathophysiology of septic shock is crucial in formulating effective treatment strategies (**Figure 1**).

3. Clinical features of septic shock

Host response to sepsis varies from patient to patient, and signs and symptoms depend upon the stage of the shock at the time of presentation. Clinical features include the following:

1. Fever/hypothermia

   a. It is a common symptom but may not be seen in old age and in immunocompromised patients. Only fever is not a strong clinical feature of septic shock; hypothermia in sepsis is a stronger predictor of morbidity and mortality.

2. Breathing difficulty

   a. Manifests as hyperventilation with respiratory alkalosis because of cytokines and endotoxin stimulation of the respiratory center in medulla.

3. Nausea and vomiting

4. Fatigue and malaise

5. Confusion and or anxiety

   a. These are early symptoms of metabolic encephalopathy seen commonly in elderly.

6. Site of infection

   a. Head and neck:

      i. Severe headache

      ii. Neck stiffness

      iii. Altered mentation

      iv. Sore throat

      v. Earache

      vi. Sinus pain or tenderness

      vii. Submandibular lymphadenopathy

b. Chest and lungs

i. Cough

ii. Chest pain (pleuritic)

iii. Dyspnea

iv. Dull percussion notes

v. Bronchial breathing

vi. Localized wheeze

c. Heart

i. New or changing murmurs especially in IV drug addicts

d. Gastrointestinal

i. Acute abdomen

ii. Diarrhea

iii. Distended abdomen

e. Genitourinary and pelvis:

i. Flank of pelvis pain/tenderness

ii. Adnexal mass or tenderness

iii. Vaginal or urethral discharge

iv. Urinary urgency, frequency, dysuria

f. Bone and soft tissues

i. Focal limb pain/tenderness

ii. Limb edema

iii. Arthritis

iv. Joint effusion or crepitus

g. Skin

i. Boils

ii. Petechiae

iii. Purpura

iv. Erythema

v. Ulcers

7. Clinical examination

Subclinical septic cascade at the cellular level is already happening before the overt clinical picture is evident.

i. General impression

a. Ill-looking, flushed, or toxic

ii. Airway, breathing, circulation (ABC)

a. Tachypnea is an indicator of pulmonary dysfunction and occurs because of endotoxins and chemokines stimulating the respiratory center.

b. Tachycardia indicate a systemic response to stress. Tachycardia and narrow pulse pressure are the early signs of shock.

c. Signs of hypoperfusion or delayed capillary refill time (CRT).

iii. Temperature

a. Rectal temperature is a preferred option

b. Hypothermia carries grave prognosis

iv. Head to toe examination to localize infection

a. Pale, gray, or mottled skin favors septic shock

b. Warm skin, warm extremities, and normal CRT indicates "warm shock"

c. Cold and clammy skin, cold extremities. and prolonged CRT represent "cold shock," followed by oliguria and cyanosis

d. Petechiae and purpura are indicative of disseminated intravascular coagulation (DIC)

e. Cerebral dysfunction in septic shock can range from mild disorientation and anxiety to overt obtundation and coma, caused though poorly understood, related to brain hypoperfusion and altered amino-acid metabolism.

f. Localization of the possible source of infection is crucial to tailored management.

8. Complications

Multiorgan failure precedes the development of septic shock.

a. Acute Respirator Distress Syndrome (ARDS)

i. Septic shock leads to moderate to severe ARDS [4]. Intrapulmonary shunting causes severe hypoxemi, leading to acute respiratory failure.

b. Acute Kidney Injury (AKI)

i. Risk of mortality with acute renal failure increases when urosepsis accompanies sepsis and septic shock [5].

c. Disseminated Intravascular Coagulation (DIC)

i. Coagulation disorders in septic shock play a significant role in multiorgan dysfunction.

9. Scoring systems

a. Systemic Inflammatory Response score (SIRS) [6]

Meet two or more of the following in **Table 1**:

b. Early warming scores (EWS)

This automated early warning score helps to identify subtle signs of deterioration that precede a potential life-threatening condition [8]. It's also termed as NEW score (**Table 2**).

Interpretation (**Table 3**)

c. Quick Sequential Organ Failure Assessment (qSOFA) score (**Table 4**) [9]

If the score is ≥2, there is high risk of mortality.

d. Mortality in emergency department score (MEDS) (**Table 5**) [10]

e. Risk-stratification of ED suspected Sepsis (REDS) score (**Table 6**) [11]

10. Laboratory workup

a. Prompt recognition and quick stabilization are the key steps to septic shock. Diagnostic laboratory workup includes:

i. Blood test

- Complete blood count with differential count (**Table 7**)

Temperature	>38°C or <36°C
Heart rate	90 beats/minute
Respiratory rate	>20 or $PaCO_2$ < 32 mmHg
White blood cells WBCs	>12,000/mm^3 or >10% bands

Table 1.
Criteria for SIRS [7].

Physiological parameters:
1. Respiratory rate 2. Oxygen saturation 3. Any supplemental oxygen 4. Temperature 5. Systolic BP 6. Heart rate 7. Level of consciousness

Table 2.
New early warning score (NEWS).

NEWS score	Clinical risk
0(1–4)	Low
5–6	Medium
7 or more	High

Table 3.
Interpretation of NEWS.

Respiratory rate	>22 breaths/min
Systolic blood pressure (SBP)	≤100 mmHg
Mental function	Altered

Table 4.
qSOFA score.

- Prothrombin time
- Activated Partial thromboplastin time
- Fibrinogen levels
- Fibrin degradation products
- Blood chemistries
    - Serum levels of:
        - Calcium: deranged
        - Phosphates: deranged
        - Magnesium: deranged
        - Glucose: hyperglycemia correlates with increase mortality

Variables	Points
Terminal illness	6
Tachypnea or hypoxemia	3
Septic shock	3
Platelet count <150,000 cell/mm^3	3
Bands >5%	3
Age > 65 years	3
Lower respiratory tract infection	2
Nursing home resident	2
Altered mental status	2

Table 5.
Mortality in emergency department score (MEDS).

Variables	Score
Age	1
Altered mental status	1
Systolic BP	1
Respiratory rate	1
Lactate <2 mmol/l	0
2.1–3.9 mmol/l	1
>4 mmol/l	3
Albumin	1
INR	1
No refractory hypotension	0
Refractory hypotension and lactate ≤2 mmol/l	2
Refractory hypotension and lactate >2 mmol/l	3
Total	12

Table 6.
Risk-stratification of ED suspected sepsis score (REDS).

HB	<7 gm/dl carries bad prognosis
WBCs	>15,000/ul with neutrophil band >1500/ul
Platelets	Decreases with sepsis and DIC

Table 7.
Complete blood count with differential count.

- Sodium and chloride: decreased in severe dehydration
- Bicarbonate: indicator of tissue perfusion. Levels
- Lactate >2.5 mmol/l is associated with higher mortality
- pH: acidosis carries guarded prognosis

o Blood chemistry in kidney involvement (renal failure)

- Blood urea nitrogen (BUN)
- Serum creatinine

o Blood chemistry in hepatic involvement (hepatic dysfunction)

- Serum bilirubin
- Alanine aminotransferase (ALT)
- Serum albumin
- Aspartate aminotransferase (AST)

o Blood test in adrenal insufficiency:

- Delta cortisol or total random cortisol

o Blood cultures: at least two blood culture collections are recommended by Surviving Sepsis Campaign before administering antibiotics; though blood cultures are positive in <50% of cases. Both aerobic and anaerobic cultures are done.

- Urinalysis and urine culture points to urosepsis as the potential cause of septic shock.
- Gram-staining and culture of secretions and tissues
- Cerebrospinal fluid (CSF), intraabdominal secretions

ii. Diagnostic imaging

- Plain radiographs

a. X-ray chest: useful in detecting ARDS (**Figure 2**).

b. X-ray abdomen: obtain plain X-ray abdomen when there is clinical evidence of bowel obstruction or perforation (**Figure 3**).

c. X-ray of extremities: helpful in osteomyelitis and necrotizing fasciitis.

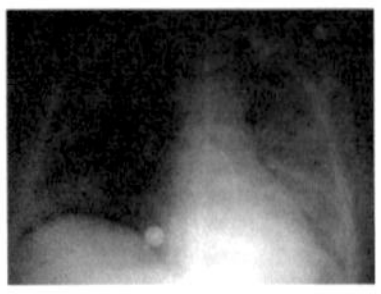

Figure 2.
ARDS in a patient who developed septic shock secondary to toxic shock syndrome (TSS). Courtesy: Medscape [12].

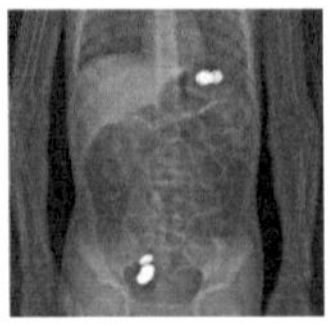

Figure 3.
A complicated case of small bowel obstruction in sepsis and methamphetamine toxicity [12].

- Ultrasonography: ultrasound abdomen aids in diagnosing acute cholecystitis and ascending cholangitis.

    a. Endoscopic retrograde cholangiopancreatography (ERCP) for ascending cholangitis.

- Echocardiography:

It provides a comprehensive and valuable cardiac evaluation in septic shock patients presenting with myocardial infarction, right heart failure, cardiac tamponade, and left ventricular obstruction.

- CT scan and MRI:

    - CT scan is the preferred modality of choice for intraabdominal abscesses and perforation.

    - MRI is more sensitive for osteomyelitis than plain X-ray.

iii. Interventional procedures

- Lumbar puncture: this invasive procedure for CSF analysis and culture is indicated when there is clinical suspicion of meningitis or encephalitis.

- Central venous catheter insertion: CVP monitoring helps guide fluid resuscitation vasopressor dose adjustment and indicates right atrial pressure and early detection of fluid overload and cardiac dysfunction.

11. Management and patient care [13–15]:

    a. Prompt recognition and robust management is the cornerstone of managing a septic shock patient.

    b. Emergency room management involves:

i. Fluid resuscitation (20 ml/kg of crystalloids or colloids)

ii. Vasopressor support (nor-epinephrine) for hypotension

iii. Oxygen therapy and ventilation if needed

iv. Early and correct institution of broad-spectrum intravenous antibiotics

c. In intensive care unit (fluid therapy refractive patients or clinical deterioration)

i. Cardiovascular support

- Titration of vasopressor by mean arterial pressure (MAP); goal ≥65 mmHg
- Inotropes if indicated
- Fluid monitoring and titration

ii. Respiratory support

- Oxygen therapy
- Mechanical ventilation if indicated

a. Adjustment of respiratory rate and depth

b. FiO2 and PEEP titration

iii. Renal and hepatic support

- Judicious fluid therapy
- Use of diuretics when indicated
- Renal replacement therapy if indicated
- Lactulose, N-acetylcysteine use for hepatic support

iv. Infectious disease management

- Administration of antibiotics and their de-escalation
- Control of source of infection
- Surgical intervention for abscess or large collections
- Antifungal or antiviral therapy when indicated

v. Monitoring and re-assessment

- Regular assessment of patient's clinical status, vitals, and treatment response for an accordingly tailored treatment
- Use of laboratory and imaging studies and interventional procedures when indicated

vi. Supportive care

- Pain and sedation
- Nutritional support
- Decubitus ulcer prophylaxis
- Deep venous thrombosis (DVT) prophylaxis

Management principles, based on the current literature, include the following:

- Early recognition
- Source control
- Early and adequate antibiotic therapy
- Early hemodynamic resuscitation and continued support
- Proper ventilator management with low tidal volume in patients with acute respiratory distress syndrome (ARDS).

Challenges in managing sepsis and septic shock:

- Antimicrobial resistance
    - According to 2019 data, approximately 49.5 million deaths are associated with antimicrobial resistance [16].
- Heterogeneity due to age, gender, comorbidities, site of infection, pathogen involved, and immune response of patients [17].

4. Conclusion

Septic shock is a life-threatening complication of sepsis and requires prompt diagnosis, timely management, and a multidisciplinary approach to optimize patient survival.

Acknowledgements

The author acknowledges the use of AI tools - meta AI- for language polishing of the manuscript.

Authorship

Erum Saboohi contributed to the conception of work, drafting, approval, and accountability.
Abdul Hadi Hassan Mallick contributed to the acquisition of data, revision, and accountability.
Yusra Shahid contributed to the interpretation of data, drafting, and accountability.

- All Authors critically revised the manuscript.

All authors agreed to be accountable for all aspects of the work in ensuring that questions related to the accuracy or integrity of any part of the work are appropriately investigated and resolved.

Conflict of interest

No conflicting interest.

Author details

Erum Saboohi[1*], AbdulHadi Hassan Mallick[2] and Yusra Shahid[3]

1 Sir Syed College of Medical Sciences for Girls, Karachi, Pakistan

2 Civil Hospital Karachi, Pakistan

3 Liaquat National Hospital, Karachi, Pakistan

*Address all correspondence to: erumsaboohi@gmail.com

References

[1] Sepsis. Available from: https://www.who.int/news-room/fact-sheets/detail/sepsis [Accessed: November 6, 2024]

[2] Singer M, Deutschman CS, Seymour CW, Shankar-Hari M, Annane D, Bauer M, et al. The third international consensus definitions for sepsis and septic shock (Sepsis-3). Journal of the American Medical Association. 2016;**315**(8):801-810. DOI: 10.1001/jama.2016.0287

[3] Rozencwajg S, Montravers P. Septic shock. In: Coccolini F, Catena F, editors. Textbook of Emergency General Surgery. Cham: Springer; 2023. DOI: 10.1007/978-3-031-22599-4_10

[4] Ranieri VM, Rubenfeld GD, Thompson BT, Ferguson ND, Caldwell E, Fan E, et al. Acute respiratory distress syndrome: The Berlin definition. Journal of the American Medical Association. 2012;**307**(23):2526-2533

[5] Dennen P, Douglas IS, Anderson R. Acute kidney injury in the intensive care unit: An update and primer for the intensivist. Critical Care Medicine. 2010;**38**(1):261-275

[6] Bone RC, Balk RA, Cerra FB, et al. Definitions for sepsis and organ failure and guidelines for the use of innovative therapies in sepsis. Chest. 1992;**101**(6):1644-1655. DOI: 10.1378/chest.101.6.1644

[7] Leadership Members of ACCP/Society of Critical Care Medicine (SCCM). American College of Chest Physicians/Society of Critical Care Medicine consensus conference: Definitions for sepsis and organ failure and guidelines for the use of innovative therapies in sepsis. Critical Care Medicine. 1992;**20**(6):864-874. DOI: 10.1097/00003246-199206000-00025

[8] Smith GB, Prytherch DR, Meredith P, et al. The ability of the National Early Warning Score (NEWS) to discriminate patients at risk of early cardiac arrest, unanticipated intensive care unit admission, and death. Resuscitation. 2013;**84**(4):465-470. DOI: 10.1016/j.resuscitation.2012.12.016

[9] Seymour CW, Liu VX, Iwashyna TJ, et al. Assessment of clinical criteria for sepsis: For the third international consensus definitions for sepsis and septic shock (Sepsis-3). Journal of the American Medical Association. 2016;**315**(8):762-774. DOI: 10.1001/jama.2016.0288

[10] Shapiro NI, Wolfe RE, Moore RB, et al. Mortality in emergency department sepsis (MEDS) score: A prospectively derived and validated clinical prediction rule. Critical Care Medicine. 2003;**31**(3):670-675. DOI: 10.1097/01.CCM.0000054867.01688.D1

[11] Sivayoham N, Hussain AN, Sheerin T, Dwivedi P, Curpanen D, Rhodes A. Prognostic performance of the REDS score, SOFA score, NEWS2 score, and the red-flag, NICE high-risk, and SIRS criteria to predict survival at 180 days, in emergency department patients admitted with suspected sepsis – An observational cohort study. Frontiers in Medicine. 2023;**10**:985444. DOI: 10.3389/fmed.2023.985444

[12] Stevens C, Ton E, Jones P, et al. A complicated case of bowel obstruction with sepsis and methamphetamine toxicity in a child with pica. Forensic Science, Medicine, and Pathology. 2019;**15**:598-602. DOI: 10.1007/s12024-019-00143-0

[13] NIH Press Release. Sepsis Study Comparing Three Treatment Methods shows Same Survival Rate. United States: National Institutes of Health; 2014. Available from: https://www.nih.gov/news/health/mar2014/nigms-18.htm [Accessed: June 5, 2024]

[14] ProCESS Investigators; Yealy DM, Kellum JA, Huang DT, Barnato AE, Weissfeld LA, et al. A randomized trial of protocol-based care for early septic shock. The New England Journal of Medicine. 1 May 2014;**370**(18):1683-1693. DOI: 10.1056/NEJMoa1401602. Epub 2014 Mar 18. PMID: 24635773; PMCID: PMC4101700

[15] Khanna A, English SW, Wang XS, et al. Angiotensin II for the treatment of vasodilatory shock. The New England Journal of Medicine. 2017;**377**(5):419-430

[16] Antimicrobial Resistance Collaborators. Global burden of bacterial antimicrobial resistance in 2019: A systematic analysis. Lancet. 2022;**399**(10325):629-655. DOI: 10.1016/S0140-6736(21)02724-0

[17] Santacroce E, D'Angerio M, Ciobanu AL, Masini L, Lo Tartaro D, Coloretti I, et al. Advances and challenges in sepsis management: Modern tools and future directions. Cells. 2024;**13**:439. DOI: 10.3390/cells13050439

Chapter 13

Experimental Animal Models of Septic Shock and Sepsis: An Overview

Alper B. Iskit

Abstract

Sepsis is usually the result of an inflammatory response to several illnesses. It still presents a picture of a complex and varied disease that kills millions of people worldwide and frequently causes the onset of many organ dysfunctions. The purpose of this study is to give the most widely used experimental sepsis models ever developed in order to explain the pathogenetic causes of the disease, its clinical and paraclinical characteristics, as well as opportunities for its therapeutic management. "Non-surgical" models involve the parenteral administration of endotoxins or pathogenic bacteria; "surgical" models refer to an operative intervention that precedes and aims to induce peritonitis, such as puncturing the cecum and then ligating it, inserting a stent in the wall of the ascending colon, implanting bacterial cultures, or using pathogens that are part of the composition of various carriers. The pros and downsides of the models under consideration are discussed, as well as the extent to which they resemble clinical sepsis in all of its forms. Sepsis is a complicated, diverse, and dynamic illness, and no model has been able to accurately capture it. Any of them, however, can supply credible information on specific septic process processes.

Keywords: sepsis, septic shock, experimental, animal, lipopolysaccharide, cecal ligation, puncture

1. Introduction

Research on animals aims to clarify the pathophysiology of different diseases, evaluate novel therapy strategies and pharmaceuticals for future clinical trial advancement, and better comprehend complex physiological processes. Research on animals is being used more and more to improve veterinary and human health. The use of animal models in the study of trauma, shock, and sepsis has been acknowledged, much like in other medical specializations, and *in vivo* findings have produced a number of important advances in those fields. However, there are times when errors are made, poor investigative methods are used, and standards are lacking in animal-based research [1]. Erroneous data resulting from these defects can lead to false conclusions and, ultimately, misguided judgments regarding the transfer from animals to people, including whether or not to start phase 1 clinical trials.

Large mammals like sheep and pigs have been used in sepsis research to enable interventions that more closely match with the clinical critical care situation and are therefore thought to be beneficial for proof-of-concept studies prior to human investigations. These include high-volume fluid resuscitation to mimic the hyperdynamic state of the circulatory system and the invasive monitoring of multiple physiological parameters, which can be technically challenging in smaller species [2]. Rats are the most often used species in preclinical research. This is due to the ease of genetic modification, large litter sizes, quick generation periods, and minimal housing and upkeep needs [3].

The well-researched nature of the species, the similarities in gene expression patterns observed during inflammation between humans and rodents, the similarities between the physiological, genetic, and biochemical traits of humans and rodents, and the low cost, ease of use, and ethical complexity of rodent experiments make it impossible to avoid conducting rodent experiments. Furthermore, a large panel of genetically modified rodents with modified immune system components provides further opportunities to investigate the molecular processes underlying the pathogenesis of sepsis. Expanding the use of humanized rodent strains is essential to more widely imitate sepsis experimentally, as the disease progression in humans is more faithfully mirrored in such models. But it's important to keep in mind that humanization has a significant impact on immune system components [4].

2. Experimental septic shock models

With a fatality rate ranging from 30 to 90%, septic shock remains an important clinical entity, despite the many treatment regimens that employ novel pharmaceuticals, antibiotics, or immunomodulatory drugs. Preclinical research employing animal models of septic shock yields valuable data for clinical trials, while there is ongoing disagreement on the appropriateness of these experimental models [5]. Given that multiple models can be used with different animal species, there is no universal experimental model. All clinical aspects of this intricate condition cannot be sufficiently represented by a single animal model. The other reasons for the differences are the lack of studies using Gram-positive bacteria as opposed to Gram-negative bacteria and the differences in endotoxin response between studies conducted on laboratory animals and human clinical subjects. Combining existing methods can significantly improve analysis [6].

2.1 Live pathogen administration through intravenous or intraperitoneal route

Bacteria, especially an *Escherichia coli* strain, could be infused or injected once to simulate septic shock. Intraperitoneal inoculation is another method for treating septic shock. It entails making an abdominal midline incision and then injecting gelatin capsules containing bacteria or fecal material (inoculum). The abdomens of the animals in the control group are filled with sterile gelatin capsules.

After intravenous delivery of 10^8–10^9–10^{10} colony-forming units (CFUs) per kilogram, the hyperdynamic phase of septic shock is reached in roughly two hours. A model that includes vasoactive support or fluid resuscitation for the improvement of hemodynamic status in larger experimental animal species will be considered clinically acceptable. A rapidly lethal model, intraperitoneal injection (*E. coli*, *Klebsiella pneumoniae*, or *Bacteroides fragilis*) had a 100% mortality rate within 24 hours.

Osmotic minipumps that are implanted intraperitoneally are utilized to control bacterial discharge and postpone early mortality. An 18–20-day controlled bacterial release model study has been conducted.

Models that involve the administration of a live pathogen lack clinical correlation since animals are gradually exposed to high bacterial loads. In certain studies, the bacterial burden is adjusted by adding agarose or excrement [7].

It is important to remember that sepsis is usually brought on by a polymicrobial infection, even if single bacterial strains are commonly employed. Researchers and laboratory personnel should consider the risk of contamination.

2.2 Intravenous or intraperitoneal lipopolysaccharide administration

Lipopolysaccharide (LPS) is one of the complex pathogen-associated molecular patterns that an organism releases. For use in septic shock studies, LPS, a glycolipid molecule, is isolated from the cell wall of Gram-negative bacteria. LPS is sold commercially as lyophilized powder. The manufacturer performs the lyophilization chemical process that includes extracting phenol, trichloroacetic acid (TCA), and phenol-chloroform ether. Although many Gram-negative bacterial species, such as *E. coli, Salmonella typhimurium, K. pneumoniae, Pseudomonas aeruginosa*, and others, can produce LPS, it is most frequently employed in septic shock experimental models. The serotypes of various *E. coli* strains vary. Even when endotoxin and LPS administration are combined, metabolic, immunological, physiological, toxicological, and pharmacological data are collected in septic models produced with LPS treatment [8–12]. Despite the fact that endotoxin and lipoprotein (LPS) are sometimes used interchangeably, their molecular structures are different. Lipid A is the dangerous part of LPS, which is a chain of pure glycolipids. In addition to the lipopolysaccharide chain, endotoxins also contain lipids, lipoproteins, cell wall proteins, and polysaccharides.

Dissolved LPS is administered intravenously or intraperitoneally as a single dose or as a component of an infusion. The LPS dosage might vary from 1 to 80 mg/kg based on the objectives of the investigation. Higher dosages are preferred for studies on septic shock survival [5]. Another important consideration for choosing a dose is the bacterial strain from which LPS is produced. The clinical profile changes depending on the bacterial strain or LPS dosage.

The best laboratory animal to use for this model is still up for debate. The following is a list of the selection-influencing factors:

a. Cost.

b. The researchers' prior experiences.

c. Accessibility.

d. Compliance with the study's purpose and premise.

Because mice, rats, and guinea pigs are more widely available, less expensive, and require less maintenance before and after research, they perform better in scientific settings for LPS investigations than dogs, pigs, and sheep. Particularly small species are selected for studies on survival. Designing an *in vitro* or perfusion method experiment with smaller species to evaluate isolated organ functions is more straightforward and efficient [3]. The same is true for examinations using histology. It might be difficult to manage the hemodynamics of smaller laboratory animals when providing supportive care, such as fluid resuscitation, intubation, or mechanical breathing [2].

Septic shock models with LPS delivery have the following drawbacks:

1. There is inconsistency in the results of LPS investigations conducted utilizing different extraction procedures or serotypes. When planning an experimental inquiry, it is crucial to consider the bacterial strain, LPS serotype, and extraction method because the purity of the various products varies.

2. The levels of plasma endotoxins, clinical or microbiological outcomes, or prognosis do not seem to be associated with each other. In this paradigm, patients who receive a single injection or infusion and have increased endotoxin levels are not clinically linked to sepsis. LPS dosages that produce similar effects in humans are different from those in rats due to a much greater LD_{50} (median lethal dose) for LPS in rats.

3. Models containing the endotoxin of single bacteria cannot replace human septic shock due of its microbial diversity. Numerous studies favor the "Cecal ligation and puncture" technique due to its microbiological variety [13].

4. The hyperdynamic phase of sepsis is characterized by compensatory mechanisms that include an increase in cardiac output and a decrease in systemic vascular resistance. Low systemic vascular resistance—a prognostic indicator—persists while cardiac output progressively declines. In animal models, high dosages of lipopolysaccharide (LPS) result in decreased cardiac output and increased vascular resistance. The model uses the hyperdynamic phase to mimic the compensated stage of true sepsis, which is induced by modest doses of LPS.

Septic shock models with LPS delivery have the following benefits:

1. The model is easy to use because it only requires a single intravenous or intraperitoneal injection.

2. Compared to live pathogens, LPS is less contaminated and easier to preserve due to the stability and purity of its lyophilized condition.

Instead, these controlled reproducible models mimic some features of endotoxemia or the acute phase of Gram-negative sepsis, such as the lack of an infection focus, the emergence of a hypodynamic stage without an earlier hyperdynamic stage, lactic acidosis, the short-term and abundant production of pro-inflammatory cytokines, the increased expression of damage-associated molecular patterns (DAMPs) (like high mobility group box-1 (HMBG-1)), and strong activation. These features greatly simplify the multistage clinical picture of sepsis development.

2.3 Cecal ligation and puncture (CLP)

In the currently available therapeutically most appropriate models, the gut integrity is impaired, allowing microbiota components to reach the peritoneal cavity and mimicking polymicrobial peritonitis. The model also includes other features associated with sepsis, such as the induction of pro- and anti-inflammatory immune responses. Sepsis progresses quickly from its pro-inflammatory phase to an anti-inflammatory phase that compensates and often leads to immunosuppression. Higher cardiac output and lower systemic vascular resistance indicate a subsequent hypodynamic period; conversely, higher cardiac output and higher systemic vascular resistance indicate an early hyperdynamic phase. Because sepsis is also associated with increased coagulation, decreased fibrinolysis, multiple organ failure, and other pathological alterations, it is challenging to create an accurate animal model for the condition. This model included early hyperdynamic and late hypodynamic phases, multiple organ failure, hypothermia, metabolic alterations, DAMP production, and similar cytokine response kinetics [14, 15].

The procedure involves closing a portion of the cecum with a regular thread so as not to impede the digestive tract, and then using a standard-sized syringe needle to puncture the cecum once or twice (cecal colotomy). After the procedure, the animals' abdominal cavity is closed off and subcutaneous fluid is administered for resuscitation according to their weight [16]. This approach has been used to study mice and lambs; however, it has been primarily employed on rats.

According to this framework, there are three offenses: 1. Ischemic tissues of the ligated cecum; 2. surgical injury to tissues; and 3. polymicrobial sepsis from fecal leaks following needle punctures.

In addition to aiding in the spread of microorganisms, the ligated and ischemic cecal tissue exacerbates the immunological dysfunction that has been noted (**Figures 1** and **2**).

Cecal ligation and puncture have the following drawbacks:

There may be differences and contradictions in the conclusions of every study. The following are a few possible reasons for this situation:

1. Varying ligation lengths or anatomical levels in the cecum.

2. Blockage of the digestive passageway.

3. The number of cecal colotomies performed and the gauge (usually between 18 and 25 gauge) of the needle.

4. After a puncture, intestinal motility quickens.

5. As with other shock models, the outcomes in animals that are fed and deprived are contradictory [18].

6. Fluid resuscitation is necessary. If it is absent, the hyperdynamic phase will not begin, which will result in a surge in death rates.

It should be noted that the model is only repeatable when the experimental animal sample size is large enough. This is because the method is difficult to standardize due to the variation in surgery-related parameters, such as the type of anesthesia, the laparotomy technique, the length of the cecal ligation, the needle size, and the number of punctures, as well as the dependence on the mouse genetic strain, gender, age, microbiota composition, and rearing conditions.

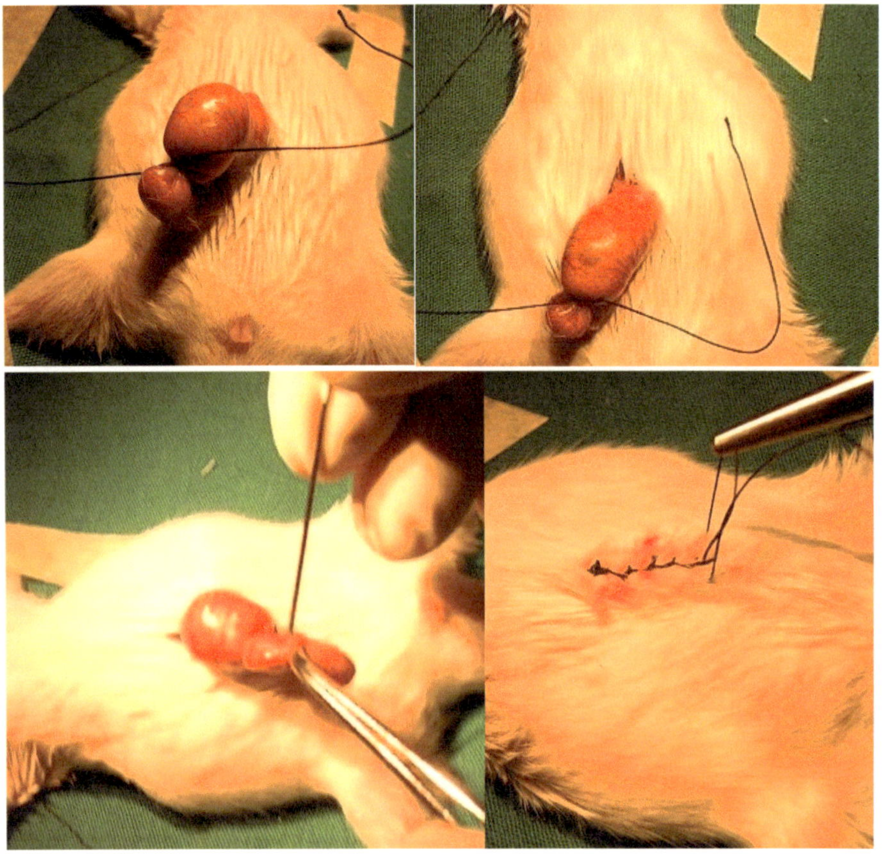

Figure 1.
Representation of cecal ligation and puncture method on rat [17].

Benefits of the cecal ligation and puncture technique:

1. The technique is easy to apply and reasonably priced. No need to give LPS or microorganisms.

2. Constant source of bacterial release.

3. In contrast to other models, this one is polymicrobial, meaning that distinct microbes are responsible for generating the septic shock profile in septic patients that is clinically acceptable.

4. A clinically similar pattern that causes septic shock is mirrored by cecal ligation and puncture (perforated appendicitis, diverticulitis, and colonic perforation).

Sepsis dynamics can be controlled by adjusting the size of the needle (18–25G), the number of punctures (to a lesser extent), the length of the cecal region to be ligated, the use of infusion therapy, the administration of antibiotics, or the simulation of an appendectomy by excising the necrotic cecal region through a subsequent operation.

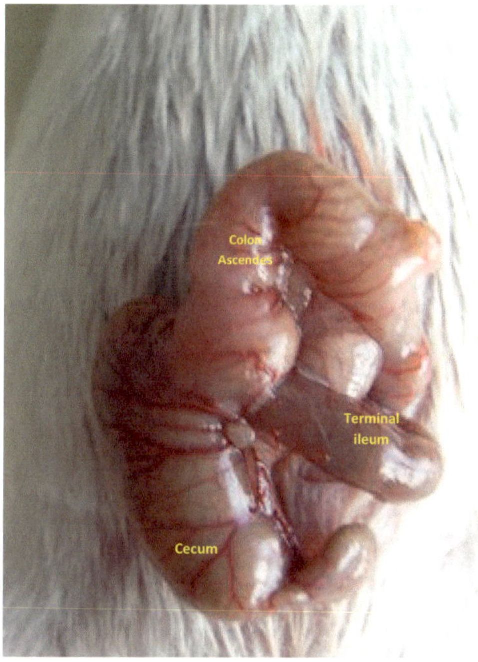

Figure 2.
Localization of cecum.

- *Colon ascendens stent peritonitis*

Similar to CLP, colon ascendens stent peritonitis requires surgery. The ascending colon in this model has a stent inserted between the abdominal cavity and the intestinal lumen. It is said to more closely resemble the pathophysiological alterations in human sepsis than the CLP model. The process is more challenging than the CLP model, though. It has also been shown that pro- and anti-inflammatory cytokine responses happen nearly concurrently in the immune system's reaction to sepsis [19].

- *Cecal ligation and incision*

A surgical technique called cecal ligation and incision is used to create a severe sepsis model that can satisfy global sepsis standards. In contrast to the CLP model, the said surgical technique generates a more acute-onset sepsis model. It is not yet as popular as the CLP model because the immunological, metabolic, and hemodynamic responses produced by this model have not been thoroughly studied [20].

- *Model of cecal slurry*

An alternative model of intra-abdominal sepsis is cecal slurry. The intraperitoneal injection of a specified and characterized volume of cecal contents serves as the foundation for this model. It's a model meant to mimic the human neonatal disease known as necrotizing enterocolitis, which typically affects premature babies and has a high death rate. Scholars who investigate newborn sepsis frequently like this paradigm. In fact, it is regarded as the gold standard by many researchers studying newborn sepsis. Because of their small bodies, newborn mice are challenging to perform the CLP operation on them. However, after the surgery, rodent moms have a propensity to become cannibals, which makes CLP undesirable. The Cecal Slurry approach does not require surgery, in contrast to the CLP method. Consequently, there is not any surgical tissue damage without any necrotized areas. The fact that it triggers a more potent but brief early inflammatory response is another significant distinction [21].

2.4 Syndrome of systemic inflammatory response and multiple organ failure caused by zymosan

Zymosan is present in the cell wall of the fungus *Saccharomyces cerevisiae*. It contains 73% polysaccharides, 15% protein, 7% fat, and a variety of inorganic components. Zymosan administration causes a prolonged inflammatory response and the generation of many inflammatory mediators in experimental animals. When zymosan is administered instead of LPS or CLP, the three-phase inflammatory response is prolonged. It is a suitable paradigm for inquiries that necessitate continuous monitoring. Immediate peritonitis manifests at a dose of 0.8–1.0 mg/g (body weight) and develops into three stages: immediate peritonitis, a period of relative recovery, and a widespread inflammatory response resulting in the failure of numerous organs or death. With the use of this experimental paradigm, scientists may examine the widespread, persistent inflammatory response in the absence of an infection [22, 23].

3. Conclusions

There is currently a great deal of debate on the predictive validity and translational usefulness of many animal models used in medical research, including sepsis, in a number of disease areas and research domains. It is important to understand that no animal model can ever fully replicate every feature of human disease, and that all experimental models have limitations. Any possible advantage from an animal is always compromised by insufficient predictive validity. However, it is vitally important to comprehend the mechanisms behind disease as well as the therapeutic efficacy of innovative pharmacological and genetic therapies. For this reason, animal studies are now carried out.

Though mimicking the clinical profile of shock in animal models is challenging, they are valuable for researching the pathophysiology of shock and gathering data before conducting clinical trials to create new treatment procedures and techniques.

Author details

Alper B. Iskit
Faculty of Medicine, Department of Medical Pharmacology, Hacettepe University, Ankara, Turkey

*Address all correspondence to: alperi@hacettepe.edu.tr

References

[1] Nandi M, Jackson SK, Macrae D, Shankar-Hari M, Tremoleda JL, Lilley E. Rethinking animal models of sepsis - working towards improved clinical translation whilst integrating the 3Rs. Clinical Science (London, England). 2020;**134**(13):1715-1734. DOI: 10.1042/CS20200679

[2] Parker SJ, Watkins PE. Experimental models of gram-negative sepsis. The British Journal of Surgery. 2001;**88**(1):22-30. DOI: 10.1046/j.1365-2168.2001.01632.x

[3] Korneev KV. Mouse models of sepsis and septic shock. Molekuliarnaia Biologiia (Mosk). 2019;**53**(5):799-814. Russian. DOI: 10.1134/S0026898419050100

[4] Remick D, Szabó A, Juffermans N, Osuchowski MF. Basic research in shock and sepsis. Shock. 2023;**59**(3S Suppl. 1):2-5. DOI: 10.1097/SHK.0000000000001953 Epub 2022 Jul 24

[5] Iskit AB, Guc MO. The timing of endothelin and nitric oxide inhibition affects survival in a mice model of septic shock. European Journal of Pharmacology. 2001;**414**(2-3):281-287. DOI: 10.1016/s0014-2999(01)00816-0

[6] Iskit AB, Senel I, Sokmensuer C, Guc MO. Endothelin receptor antagonist bosentan improves survival in a murine caecal ligation and puncture model of septic shock. European Journal of Pharmacology. 2004;**506**(1):83-88. DOI: 10.1016/j.ejphar.2004.10.038

[7] Poli-de-Figueiredo LF, Garrido AG, Nakagawa N, Sannomiya P. Experimental models of sepsis and their clinical relevance. Shock. 2008;**30** (Suppl. 1):53-59. DOI: 10.1097/SHK.0b013e318181a343

[8] Ozer EK, Goktas MT, Kilinc I, Bariskaner H, Ugurluoglu C, Iskit AB. Celecoxib administration reduced mortality, mesenteric hypoperfusion, aortic dysfunction and multiple organ injury in septic rats. Biomedicine & Pharmacotherapy. 2017;**86**:583-589. DOI: 10.1016/j.biopha.2016.11.102 Epub 2016 Dec 23

[9] Kavuklu B, Iskit AB, Guc MO, Ilhan M, Sayek I. Aminoguanidine attenuates endotoxin-induced mesenteric vascular hyporeactivity. The British Journal of Surgery. 2000;**87**(4):448-453. DOI: 10.1046/j.1365-2168.2000.01376.x

[10] Baykal A, Kavuklu B, Iskit AB, Guc MO, Hascelik G, Sayek I. Experimental study of the effect of nitric oxide inhibition on mesenteric blood flow and interleukin-10 levels with a lipopolysaccharide challenge. World Journal of Surgery. 2000;**24**(9):1116-1120. DOI: 10.1007/s002680010181

[11] Ozer EK, Goktas MT, Toker A, Pehlivan S, Bariskaner H, Ugurluoglu C, et al. Thymoquinone protects against the sepsis induced mortality, mesenteric hypoperfusion, aortic dysfunction and multiple organ damage in rats. Pharmacological Reports. 2017;**69**(4):683-690. DOI: 10.1016/j.pharep.2017.02.021 Epub 2017 Mar 24

[12] Özer EK, Kurtgöz S, Göktaş MT, et al. Alterations in hepatic gene expressions of CYP2C11, CYP2C6V, and CYP2D3 enzymes in endotoxemic rats. Yoğun Bakım Dergisi. 2017;**8**:50-53

[13] Ertac-Serdar S, Atilla P, Iskit AB. Effects of PARP Inhibitör 3-Aminobenzamide on impaired mesenteric blood flow and organ injury in CLP-induced septic shock model.

Journal of Critical and Intensive Care. 2022;**13**:32-42

[14] Yang S, Chung CS, Ayala A, Chaudry IH, Wang P. Differential alterations in cardiovascular responses during the progression of polymicrobial sepsis in the mouse. Shock. 2002;**17**(1):55-60. DOI: 10.1097/00024382-200201000-00010

[15] Ulu N, Sokmensuer C, Iskit AB. The effects of inducible nitric oxide synthase blockers on survival and organ injury in a murine Caecal ligation and puncture model of septic shock. Journal of Critical and Intensive Care. 2022;**13**:73-78

[16] Baker CC, Chaudry IH, Gaines HO, Baue AE. Evaluation of factors affecting mortality rate after sepsis in a murine cecal ligation and puncture model. Surgery. 1983;**94**(2):331-335

[17] Ozcelebi E, Iskit AB. Experimental animal models of sepsis and septic shock. Journal of Critical and Intensive Care. 2023;**14**(3):96-100

[18] Agalar F, Iskit AB, Agalar C, Hamaloglu E, Guc MO. The effects of G-CSF treatment and starvation on bacterial translocation in hemorrhagic shock. The Journal of Surgical Research. 1998;**78**(2):143-147. DOI: 10.1006/jsre.1998.5386

[19] Maier S, Traeger T, Entleutner M, Westerholt A, Kleist B, Hüser N, et al. Cecal ligation and puncture versus colon ascendens stent peritonitis: Two distinct animal models for polymicrobial sepsis. Shock. 2004;**21**(6):505-511. DOI: 10.1097/01.shk.0000126906.52367.dd

[20] Scheiermann P, Hoegl S, Revermann M, Ahluwalia D, Zander J, Boost KA, et al. Cecal ligation and incision: An acute onset model of severe sepsis in rats. Journal of Surgical Research. 2008;**151**(1):132-137. DOI: 10.1016/j.jss.2008.02.032

[21] Starr ME, Steele AM, Saito M, Hacker BJ, Evers BM, Saito H. A new Cecal slurry preparation protocol with improved long-term reproducibility for animal models of sepsis. PLoS One. 2014;**9**(12):e115705. DOI: 10.1371/journal.pone.0115705

[22] Volman TJ, Hendriks T, Goris RJ. Zymosan-induced generalized inflammation: Experimental studies into mechanisms leading to multiple organ dysfunction syndrome. Shock. 2005;**23**(4):291-297. DOI: 10.1097/01.shk.0000155350.95435.28

[23] Tanriverdi P, Yuksel BC, Rasa K, Guler G, Iskit AB, Guc MO, et al. The effects of selective nitric oxide synthase blocker on survival, mesenteric blood flow and multiple organ failure induced by zymosan. The Journal of Surgical Research. 2005;**124**(1):67-73. DOI: 10.1016/j.jss.2004.09.004

Chapter 14

Optimizing Initial Resuscitation: Clinical and Perfusion Parameters in Septic Shock

Tetsuya Yumoto

Abstract

Blood lactate assessment is standard for diagnosing suspected sepsis, though its use for guiding therapy is supported by weak, low-quality evidence, as elevated levels do not always indicate tissue hypoperfusion. Trials of early goal-directed therapy focusing on central venous oxygen saturation have shown no benefit over standard care. Alternatives, ranging from physical examination markers like capillary refill time and mottling to objective parameters or biomarkers such as the veno-arterial carbon dioxide gap, near-infrared spectroscopy, and active renin, are emerging. Given the variability in effective perfusion markers, this section will summarize the evidence to better understand the role of lactate levels and identify which other markers are suitable for guiding initial resuscitation in septic shock.

Keywords: blood gas analysis, early goal-directed therapy, lactate, resuscitation, septic shock, tissue hypoperfusion

1. Introduction

Sepsis is characterized as a life-threatening organ dysfunction resulting from a dysregulated host response to infection [1]. Despite advances in understanding and managing sepsis, it continues to cause significant morbidity and mortality worldwide [2]. Prompt treatment and resuscitation are crucial once sepsis is identified. In addition to the administration of antimicrobial agents and source control as needed, fluid resuscitation and vasopressor use are key components of the hemodynamic management of patients with possible impaired tissue perfusion or septic shock [3]. After initial fluid resuscitation, continuous fluid administration is required to restore and maintain organ perfusion. Remarkably, balanced volume resuscitation is crucial to prevent potential adverse outcomes, as excessive resuscitation and fluid overload may lead to positive fluid balance, increasing the risk of pulmonary edema, renal failure, and higher mortality in patients with sepsis [3, 4]. Of note, recent trials comparing restrictive fluid strategy with early vasopressor treatment to more fluid-liberal approaches for septic shock have yielded compatible results [5, 6]. These trials had protocolized strategies of initial resuscitation based on lactate values or knee mottling as tissue perfusion parameters.

Meanwhile, in pragmatic clinical practice, initial resuscitation via fluid administration and vasopressor use is optimized and individualized based on clinical or macro-hemodynamic parameters and/or tissue perfusion or microcirculatory parameters; however, it remains debated which parameters are optimal.

In this chapter, clinical or tissue perfusion parameters to optimize initial resuscitation in adult patients with sepsis or septic shock to improve patients' outcomes are summarized.

2. Parameters for evaluating tissue perfusion and microcirculation

Early resolution of organ injury in part attributed to tissue hypoperfusion is a key aspect of the initial management of sepsis [7, 8]. Vasoactive support alongside fluid resuscitation is an integral step to restore perfusion to end organs at the early stages of sepsis. Although ideal endpoints vary between patients and guidelines for when to ramp down aggressive resuscitation are inconsistent, accomplishing a specific goal such as reversal of shock generally requires hours to days. To avoid irreversible organ damage, numerous studies have been conducted to examine how to optimize or titrate resuscitation, especially focusing on the first several hours after presentation [9–17]. Since the correction of macro-hemodynamic parameters, including blood pressure or cardiac output, is not sufficient to indicate successful resuscitation, the direct identification of organ hypoperfusion using microcirculatory or tissue perfusion parameters is of critical importance [12]. Among the various parameters to guide initial resuscitation, this subsection will focus on tissue hypoperfusion parameters, organized from physical findings to biomarkers (**Figure 1**).

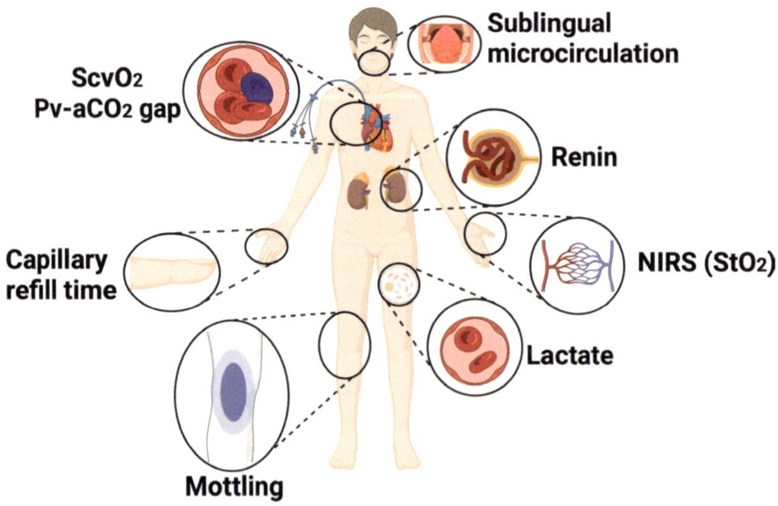

Figure 1.
Parameters for evaluating tissue perfusion and microcirculation. $ScvO_2$: central venous oxygen saturation, Pv-aCO_2 gap: veno-arterial difference in partial pressure of carbon dioxide, NIRS: near-infrared spectroscopy, StO_2: tissue oxygen saturation.

2.1 Capillary refill time

Capillary refill time (CRT), despite being affected by differences in measurement between observers and environmental temperature, is a simple physiological parameter that requires no equipment to measure [18]. To assess CRT, light pressure is applied to blanch the fingernail bed, and the time taken for the color to return after releasing the pressure is recorded.

The ANDROMEDA-SHOCK trial was a significant study comparing CRT-guided therapy with lactate-guided therapy for optimizing the initial resuscitation of septic shock [12]. In this trial, CRT was measured by applying firm pressure with a glass microscope slide to the ventral surface of the right index finger's distal phalanx until the skin blanched, maintaining the pressure for 10 seconds. The time for the skin to return to its normal color was recorded with a chronometer, with a duration of over 3 seconds defined as abnormal. Although the primary outcome of 28-day mortality was not statistically different between the groups (hazard ratio 0.75 (95% confidence intervals 0.55 to 1.02); P = 0.06), patients in the CRT group had significantly lower Sequential Organ Failure Assessment scores at 72 hours and received less fluid within the first 8 hours. A post hoc analysis revealed that patients whose CRT returned to normal following protocolized resuscitation but continued to receive interventions, including fluid resuscitation guided by lactate levels, exhibited higher mortality [19]. These findings indicate that aggressive fluid resuscitation should likely be discontinued once CRT returns to normal, even if lactate levels remain high.

A recent meta-analysis found that CRT has a low predictive value for mortality or adverse events in patients with, or at risk of, acute circulatory failure, though its accuracy improves with high-quality measurement. Despite this, CRT remains a useful parameter for assessing patient severity, comparable to lactate levels, highlighting the need for standardized measurement techniques in clinical practice [20].

Looking ahead, a prototype wearable CRT measurement device has recently been developed, demonstrating moderate or better intra-rater reliability [21]. Additionally, the ANDROMEDA-SHOCK-2 trial is underway, which randomizes septic shock patients to a CRT-targeted resuscitation strategy based on hemodynamic phenotyping or standard care, aiming to provide further insights into the impact of CRT monitoring on patient outcomes [22].

2.2 Skin mottling

Skin mottling in septic shock, characterized by irregular, patchy discoloration primarily around the knees, is a key indicator of cutaneous hypoperfusion due to microcirculation alterations and reduced blood flow. The skin mottling score provides a semi-quantitative evaluation of mottling based on its extension on the legs, ranging from 0 to 5: Score 0, no mottling; Score 1, small mottling area (coin size) localized to the center of the knee; Score 2, mottling area does not exceed the superior edge of the kneecap; Score 3, mottling area does not exceed the middle thigh; Score 4, mottling area does not exceed the fold of the groin; and Score 5, mottling extends beyond the fold of the groin [23]. Studies have shown a significant correlation between mottling and increased mortality, highlighting its importance in assessing the severity of septic shock and guiding treatment [23–25]. A more recent study examined the association of skin mottling with skin temperature measured with infrared thermography around the knee [26]. Although skin temperature was not correlated with the mottling score, the temperature was lower when mottling was present. However, this method did not successfully predict mortality in ICU patients. Another study investigated an Indian ethnic population, who have different skin colors compared to the white-skinned population, and revealed that the incidence of mottling in septic shock was much less in patients of Indian ethnicity with brown skin color than in white-skinned population [27]. In this setting, the occurrence of mottling, rather than delayed CRT, was a better predictor of outcomes. Nonetheless, skin mottling can be easily assessed at the bedside repetitively and is considered effective for evaluating severity and guiding resuscitation.

2.3 Renin

The renin-angiotensin system (RAS) is critical for maintaining circulatory homeostasis. Renin is the primary regulator, released in response to tissue hypoperfusion, sympathetic activation, and hypoxic metabolism. Sepsis induces systemic downregulation of angiotensin I and angiotensin II receptors through proinflammatory cytokines, resulting in systemic hypotension and low aldosterone secretion despite increased plasma renin activity and angiotensin II levels [28]. Several studies have demonstrated that plasma renin serves as a marker of tissue hypoperfusion, and its higher levels are associated with short-term mortality [29–31]. One study even showed that renin outperformed lactate levels [29], suggesting renin as a promising biomarker for tissue hypoperfusion in septic shock.

2.4 Lactate

Blood lactate levels are commonly utilized to indicate impaired tissue perfusion in critically ill patients, especially those with sepsis [32]. Consequently, measuring serum lactate levels is a common practice in managing critical illness, particularly in severe sepsis and septic shock. Serum lactate helps evaluate disease severity, monitor treatment response, and predict prognosis [33, 34]. Measuring blood lactate levels is a standardized first step for patients with suspected sepsis or septic shock, as the Sepsis-3 guidelines recommend including a persistent serum lactate level of more than 2 mmol/L, despite adequate fluid resuscitation, as an essential component in the clinical definition of septic shock [1].

Measuring blood lactate levels in critically ill patients, especially those with septic shock, presents several challenges [35]. Decreased levels may reflect reduced clearance, and factors like increased glycolysis during sepsis can raise lactate levels independently of tissue oxygenation. Lactate serves as an energy substrate, further complicating its role as a perfusion marker. Liver dysfunction, common in sepsis, and certain medications can elevate lactate levels. Persistent hyperlactatemia can result from hypoperfusion and mitochondrial dysfunction. While lactate predicts mortality in sepsis, targeting its reduction without understanding the cause can be ineffective and harmful, necessitating cautious interpretation for accurate clinical decisions [36–39]. Therefore, a weak recommendation with low-quality evidence was issued for lactate-guided therapy during initial resuscitation, since hyperlactatemia does not necessarily indicate tissue hypoperfusion [3]. Nonetheless, despite these challenges, measuring lactate levels and monitoring their trajectory is widely accepted as a method to guide initial resuscitation in septic shock [40].

2.5 $ScvO_2$

Historically, both experimental and clinical studies have revealed that sepsis results in altered tissue oxygen extraction or an imbalance between tissue oxygen demands and supply, which is captured by decreased central venous oxygen saturation ($ScvO_2$) or mixed venous oxygen saturation (SvO_2) [41]. In 2001, a landmark trial by Rivers et al. demonstrated that early goal-directed therapy (EGDT), guided by continuous monitoring of $ScvO_2$, significantly improved ICU mortality compared with standard care [42]. However, three subsequent major trials failed to show a survival advantage with this strategy [43–45]. This discrepancy was partly attributed to the significant difference in initial $ScvO_2$ levels: the mean $ScvO_2$ was 49% at randomization in the original EGDT trial, compared to approximately 71% in the later EGDT trials. It was assumed that half of the patients in these trials had already "achieved the goal" at the time of randomization. While low levels of $ScvO_2$ indicate impaired tissue oxygenation, high levels of $ScvO_2$ are associated with increased mortality, complicating its use due to $ScvO_2$'s U-shaped distribution with respect to cellular oxygen delivery [46, 47]. A recent study indicates that mitochondrial oxidative stress was increased only in the high $ScvO_2$ group [48]. However, serum lactate was also not correlated with mitochondrial oxidative stress in sepsis patients, indicating partial limitation of $ScvO_2$ in guiding resuscitation in septic shock patients.

2.6 Pv-aCO_2 gap

The veno-arterial difference in partial pressure of carbon dioxide (Pv-aCO_2 gap) is gaining recognition as a dependable measure of tissue perfusion and an indicator of poor prognosis in septic shock [49, 50]. The normal Pv-aCO_2 gap ranges between 2 and 6 mmHg, with 6 mmHg or above often indicating an abnormally elevated gap [51, 52]. Elevated Pv-aCO_2 gaps can reflect inadequate cardiac output, impaired tissue perfusion, or issues with CO_2 elimination [53]. While useful, the Pv-aCO_2 gap must be interpreted cautiously due to potential confounding factors such as metabolic shifts, hyperoxia, and measurement inaccuracies. It remains uncertain whether the Pv-aCO_2 gap should be included in resuscitation protocols or if normalizing it improves outcomes in septic shock.

2.7 Sublingual microcirculation

Measuring sublingual microcirculation in septic shock patients allows for the direct assessment of microvascular blood flow, enabling early detection of abnormalities that often precede changes in global hemodynamic parameters [54]. A recent study examined the clinical significance of using handheld, noninvasive sublingual video-microscopes to visualize microcirculation in septic patients. It found a significant reduction in vascular density in small capillaries in septic patients, which correlated with sepsis severity [55]. A recent randomized controlled trial tested whether integrating sublingual microcirculatory perfusion variables into the therapeutic management of ICU patients with shock reduces 30-day mortality. The study concluded that while incorporating these variables led to treatment adjustments, it did not improve survival [56]. Further studies are needed to evaluate the clinical impact of sublingual microcirculation measurements in treating septic shock patients.

2.8 NIRS

Near-infrared spectroscopy (NIRS) for measuring tissue oxygen saturation (StO_2), which can be assessed transcutaneously using several commercially available devices, is proposed as a hemodynamic monitoring tool to evaluate microcirculation [57, 58]. This method assesses the balance between oxygen delivery and consumption in tissues by measuring the ratio of oxygenated to deoxygenated hemoglobin, thus providing an indirect measure of tissue oxygenation. A former study reported that the StO_2 oxygen recovery slope was strongly associated with shock, organ dysfunction, and death in sepsis patients [59]. A recent study found that NIRS-derived StO_2 correlated with organ failure and was linked to outcomes in sepsis. However, it was not highly effective in distinguishing sepsis among emergency department patients with infections [60]. The effectiveness of StO_2 as a diagnostic tool is deemed limited because it does not deviate from normal ranges until shock reaches an advanced stage. To improve its ability to detect tissue hypoperfusion, a dynamic ischemic challenge like the vascular occlusion test could be used [61].

3. Optimal parameters to guide initial resuscitation for septic shock

A recent network meta-analysis included 17 trials that compared various parameters such as lactate, CRT, $ScvO_2$, and the ratio of veno-arterial carbon dioxide tension difference to arterial-venous oxygen content difference ($PvaCO_2/CavO_2$) [62]. The analysis revealed that lactate-guided therapy (risk ratio: 0.59; 95% confidence interval: 0.45–0.76; high certainty) and capillary refill time-guided therapy (risk ratio: 0.53; 95% confidence interval: 0.33–0.86; high certainty) were significantly associated with lower short-term mortality compared to usual care. In contrast, $ScvO_2$-guided therapy (risk ratio: 1.50; 95% confidence interval: 1.16–1.94; moderate certainty) was associated with an increased risk of short-term mortality compared to lactate-guided therapy. Another umbrella review, including 17 systematic reviews and meta-analyses encompassing 15,828 patients, assessed parameters such as mean arterial pressure, $ScvO_2$, systolic or diastolic dysfunction, CO_2 gap, lactate, right ventricular dysfunction, and $PvaCO_2/CavO_2$. Significant correlations with mortality were found for diastolic dysfunction, $PvaCO_2/CavO_2$ ratio, and CO_2 gap, with diastolic dysfunction being the most closely linked to prognosis [63]. However, the clinical applicability of the $PvaCO_2/CavO_2$ ratio and CO_2 gap is limited due to poor evidence quality and low case numbers.

A survey study from the US found that decisions about fluid and vasopressor administration in early sepsis are primarily guided by the fluid volume already received by the patient, rather than other clinical factors such as respiratory status or lactate trend [64]. This study concluded the importance of fluid volume in guiding resuscitation decisions and suggest that future studies should incorporate tools to help personalize care based on fluid management.

4. Biomarkers in sepsis and septic shock

4.1 Procalcitonin

Procalcitonin (PCT) is a valuable biomarker with broad medical applications, especially in sepsis [65]. PCT helps guide antibiotic use in patients with respiratory infections and sepsis by limiting initiation and shortening treatment duration, effectively reducing infection-associated adverse events, 28-day mortality, and hospitalization costs [66, 67]. A recent meta-analysis demonstrated that PCT-guided antibiotic therapy may reduce antibiotic use and 28-day mortality while showing similar ICU and hospital lengths of stay, but it might increase infection recurrence [68]. Further studies are needed to better design PCT-guided antibiotic stewardship in critically ill patients, as PCT alone may be insufficient for diagnosing bacterial infections and assessing their severity, given the complexities in distinguishing between microbial and non-microbial infections.

4.2 Other organ specific biomarkers

Neutrophil gelatinase-associated lipocalin (NGAL) is a biomarker for the early detection of acute kidney injury (AKI), bacterial infection, and systemic inflammation, detectable in plasma and urine before creatinine levels rise [69]. In critically ill patients with sepsis/septic shock, elevated plasma NGAL indicates neutrophil activation even without apparent AKI. Urinary NGAL is a more reliable marker of AKI in septic shock, as its levels remain normal without AKI signs despite high plasma NGAL levels [69]. Regarding the gut, which has long been suspected of playing a crucial role in the development of multiple organ dysfunction [70], intestinal fatty-acid binding protein (I-FABP) has been investigated as a potentially effective biomarker for acute intestinal ischemia [71]. A previous study indicated that I-FABP levels at ICU admission served as a predictor of 28-day mortality and non-occlusive mesenteric ischemia in septic shock patients [72]. Lastly, interleukin-6 (IL-6), which has been extensively investigated, is a cytokine with both pro-inflammatory and anti-inflammatory roles and is significantly elevated in critical illnesses such as sepsis and acute respiratory distress syndrome [73]. The Cochrane review reported that plasma IL-6 concentrations for diagnosing sepsis in critically ill adults reveals significant limitations due to high heterogeneity in evidence regarding diagnosis, setting, threshold, sepsis criteria, and infection origin, highlighting the importance of precision medicine is emphasized, highlighting the need for targeted treatments based on patient-specific profiles [74].

5. Conclusions

Clinical parameters to assess tissue hypoperfusion or microcirculation status in patients with septic shock for initial resuscitation were summarized. Since sepsis is highly heterogeneous and complex, no single reliable parameter exists to adequately guide initial resuscitation. Given the feasibility and real-world clinical settings, an approach combining lactate levels with easily assessed physical findings such as CRT or mottling may be valuable, in addition to dynamic parameters such as systolic blood pressure, cardiac output, or urine output. Despite progress in initial resuscitation strategies, a multifaceted approach that considers both traditional and emerging perfusion markers is essential. Integrating PCT and other organ-specific biomarkers with clinical parameters can improve patient outcomes through more personalized care in septic shock. Future research should refine these tools and develop guidelines to support personalized care, ultimately improving patient outcomes in septic shock.

Conflict of interest

The author declares no conflict of interest.

Author details

Tetsuya Yumoto
Faculty of Medicine, Dentistry, and Pharmaceutical Sciences, Department of Emergency, Critical Care, and Disaster Medicine, Okayama University, Okayama, Japan

*Address all correspondence to: tyumoto@cc.okayama-u.ac.jp

References

[1] Singer M, Deutschman CS, Seymour C, Shankar-Hari M, Annane D, Bauer M, et al. The third international consensus definitions for sepsis and septic shock (sepsis-3). Journal of the American Medical Association. 2016;**315**(8):801-810

[2] Rudd KE, Johnson SC, Agesa KM, Shackelford KA, Tsoi D, Kievlan DR, et al. Global, regional, and national sepsis incidence and mortality, 1990-2017: Analysis for the global burden of disease study. The Lancet. 2020;**395**(10219):200-211

[3] Evans L, Rhodes A, Alhazzani W, Antonelli M, Coopersmith CM, French C, et al. Surviving sepsis campaign: International guidelines for Management of Sepsis and Septic Shock 2021. Critical Care Medicine. 2021;**49**(11):e1063-e1143

[4] Boyd JH, Forbes J, Nakada TA, Walley KR, Russell JA. Fluid resuscitation in septic shock: A positive fluid balance and elevated central venous pressure are associated with increased mortality. Critical Care Medicine. 2011;**39**(2):259-265

[5] Meyhoff TS, Hjortrup PB, Wetterslev J, Sivapalan P, Laake JH, Cronhjort M, et al. Restriction of intravenous fluid in ICU patients with septic shock. New England Journal of Medicine. 2022;**386**(26):2459-2470

[6] National Heart, Lung, and Blood Institute Prevention and Early Treatment of Acute Lung Injury Clinical Trials Network, Shapiro NI, Douglas IS, Brower RG, Brown SM, Exline MC, et al. Early restrictive or liberal fluid management for sepsis-induced hypotension. The New England Journal of Medicine. 2023;**388**(6):499-510

[7] Hotchkiss RS, Moldawer LL, Opal SM, Reinhart K, Turnbull IR, Vincent JL. Sepsis and septic shock. Nature Reviews. Disease Primers. 2016;**2**:16045

[8] Cecconi M, Evans L, Levy M, Rhodes A. Sepsis and septic shock. The Lancet. 2018;**392**(10141):75-87

[9] Hassanein A, Abbas I, Mohammed R. Central blood gases versus lactate level for assessment of initial resuscitation success in patients with sepsis in critical care. Egyptian Journal of Anaesthesia. 2022;**38**(1):439-445

[10] Jansen TC, Van Bommel J, Schoonderbeek FJ, Sleeswijk Visser SJ, Van Der Klooster JM, Lima AP, et al. Early lactate-guided therapy in intensive care unit patients: A multicenter, open-label, randomized controlled trial. American Journal of Respiratory and Critical Care Medicine. 2010;**182**(6):752-761

[11] Zhou X, Liu D, Su L, Yao B, Long Y, Wang X, et al. Use of stepwise lactate kinetics-oriented hemodynamic therapy could improve the clinical outcomes of patients with sepsis-associated hyperlactatemia. Critical Care. 2017;**21**(1):1-10

[12] Hernández G, Ospina-Tascón GA, Damiani LP, Estenssoro E, Dubin A, Hurtado J, et al. Effect of a resuscitation strategy targeting peripheral perfusion status vs serum lactate levels on 28-day mortality among patients with septic shock: The ANDROMEDA-SHOCK randomized clinical trial. Journal of the American Medical Association. 2019;**321**(7):654-664

[13] Jones AE, Shapiro NI, Trzeciak S, Arnold RC, Claremont HA, Kline JA.

Lactate clearance vs central venous oxygen saturation as goals of early sepsis therapy: A randomized clinical trial. Journal of the American Medical Association. 2010;**303**(8):739-746

[14] Zhang Z, Ni H, Qian Z. Effectiveness of treatment based on PiCCO parameters in critically ill patients with septic shock and/or acute respiratory distress syndrome: A randomized controlled trial. Intensive Care Medicine. 2015;**41**(3):444-451

[15] Su L, Tang B, Liu Y, Zhou G, Guo Q, He W, et al. P(v-a)CO_2/C(a-v)O_2-directed resuscitation does not improve prognosis compared with SvO_2 in severe sepsis and septic shock: A prospective multicenter randomized controlled clinical study. Journal of Critical Care. 2018;**48**:314-320

[16] Gattinoni L, Brazzi L, Pelosi P, Latini R, Tognoni G, Pesenti A, et al. A trial of goal-oriented hemodynamic therapy in critically ill patients. SvO_2 collaborative group. The New England Journal of Medicine. 1995;**333**(16):1025-1032

[17] Chen H, Xu J, Wang X, Wang Y, Tong F. Early lactate-guided resuscitation of elderly septic patients. Journal of Intensive Care Medicine. 2022;**37**(5):686-692

[18] Anderson B, Kelly AM, Kerr D, Clooney M, Jolley D. Impact of patient and environmental factors on capillary refill time in adults. The American Journal of Emergency Medicine. 2008;**26**(1):62-65

[19] Kattan E, Hernández G, Ospina-Tascón G, Valenzuela ED, Bakker J, Castro R. A lactate-targeted resuscitation strategy may be associated with higher mortality in patients with septic shock and normal capillary refill time: A post hoc analysis of the ANDROMEDA-SHOCK study. Annals of Intensive Care. 2020;**10**(1):1-9

[20] Jacquet-Lagrèze M, Pernollet A, Kattan E, Ait-Oufella H, Chesnel D, Ruste M, et al. Prognostic value of capillary refill time in adult patients: A systematic review with meta-analysis. Critical Care. 2023;**27**(1):1-13

[21] Shinozaki M, Saito D, Nakada TA, Nomura Y, Nakaguchi T. Feasibility study of wearable capillary refill time measurement device. Artificial Life and Robotics. 2024;**29**(2):334-339

[22] Hernandez G, Carmona P, Ait-Oufella H. Monitoring capillary refill time in septic shock. Intensive Care Medicine. 2024;**50**(4):580-582

[23] Ait-Oufella H, Lemoinne S, Boelle PY, Galbois A, Baudel JL, Lemant J, et al. Mottling score predicts survival in septic shock. Intensive Care Medicine. 2011;**37**(5):801-807

[24] Dumas G, Lavillegrand JR, Joffre J, Bigé N, De-Moura EB, Baudel JL, et al. Mottling score is a strong predictor of 14-day mortality in septic patients whatever vasopressor doses and other tissue perfusion parameters. Critical Care. 2019;**23**(1):1-9

[25] Coudroy R, Jamet A, Frat JP, Veinstein A, Chatellier D, Goudet V, et al. Incidence and impact of skin mottling over the knee and its duration on outcome in critically ill patients. Intensive Care Medicine. 2015;**41**(3):452-459

[26] Ferraris A, Bouisse C, Mottard N, Thiollière F, Anselin S, Piriou V, et al. Mottling score and skin temperature in septic shock: Relation and impact on prognosis in ICU. PLoS One. 2018;**13**(8):1-10

[27] Jog SA, Narasimhan VL, Rajhans PA, Akole PV, Pawar B, Bhurke B, et al. Mottling in septic shock: Ethnicity and skin color matter. Indian Journal of Critical Care Medicine. 2023;**27**(12):902-909

[28] Corrêa TD, Takala J, Jakob SM. Angiotensin II in septic shock. Critical Care. 2015;**19**(1):1-6

[29] Gleeson PJ, Crippa IA, Mongkolpun W, Cavicchi FZ, Van Meerhaeghe T, Brimioulle S, et al. Renin as a marker of tissue-perfusion and prognosis in critically III patients. Critical Care Medicine. 2019;**47**(2):152-158

[30] Leśnik P, Łysenko L, Krzystek-Korpacka M, Woźnica-Niesobska E, Mierzchała-Pasierb M, Janc J. Renin as a marker of tissue perfusion, septic shock and mortality in septic patients: A prospective observational study. International Journal of Molecular Sciences. 2022;**23**(16):9133

[31] Busse LW, Schaich CL, Chappell MC, McCurdy MT, Staples EM, Ten Lohuis CC, et al. Association of active renin content with mortality in critically ill patients: A *post hoc* analysis of the vitamin C, thiamine, and steroids in sepsis (VICTAS) trial∗. Critical Care Medicine. 2024;**52**(3):441-451

[32] Kushimoto S, Akaishi S, Sato T, Nomura R, Fujita M, Kudo D, et al. Lactate, a useful marker for disease mortality and severity but an unreliable marker of tissue hypoxia/hypoperfusion in critically ill patients. Acute Medicine & Surgery. 2016;**3**(4):293-297

[33] Nichol AD, Egi M, Pettila V, Bellomo R, French C, Hart G, et al. Relative hyperlactatemia and hospital mortality in critically ill patients: A retrospective multi-centre study. Critical Care. 2010;**14**(1):1-9

[34] Rishu AH, Khan R, Al-Dorzi HM, Tamim HM, Al-Qahtani S, Al-Ghamdi G, et al. Even mild hyperlactatemia is associated with increased mortality in critically ill patients. Critical Care. 2013;**17**(5):R197

[35] Hernandez G, Bellomo R, Bakker J. The ten pitfalls of lactate clearance in sepsis. Intensive Care Medicine. 2019;**45**(1):82-85

[36] Chertoff J, Chisum M, Garcia B, Lascano J. Lactate kinetics in sepsis and septic shock: A review of the literature and rationale for further research. Journal of Intensive Care. 2015;**3**(1):1-4

[37] Vincent JL, EAQ S, Couto L, Taccone FS. The value of blood lactate kinetics in critically ill patients: A systematic review. Critical Care. 2016;**20**(1):1-14

[38] Filho RR, Rocha LL, Corrêa TD, Souza Pessoa CM, Colombo G, Cesar Assuncao MS. Blood lactate levels cutoff and mortality prediction in sepsis - time for a reappraisal? A retrospective cohort study. Shock. 2016;**46**(5):480-485

[39] Ryoo SM, Lee J, Lee YS, Lee JH, Lim KS, Huh JW, et al. Lactate level versus lactate clearance for predicting mortality in patients with septic shock defined by sepsis-3. Critical Care Medicine. 2018;**46**(6):E489-E495

[40] Lat I, Coopersmith CM, De Backer D, Deutschman CS, Evans L, Ferrer-Roca R, et al. The surviving sepsis campaign: Fluid resuscitation and vasopressor therapy research priorities in adult patients. Intensive Care Medicine Experimental. 2021;**9**(1):623-635

[41] Nguyen HB, Jaehne AK, Jayaprakash N, Semler MW, Hegab S, Yataco AC, et al. Early goal-directed therapy in severe sepsis and septic shock:

Insights and comparisons to ProCESS, ProMISe, and ARISE. Critical Care. 2016;**20**(1):160

[42] Rivers E, Nguyen B, Havstad S, Ressler J, Muzzin A, Knoblich B, et al. Early goal-directed therapy in the treatment of severe sepsis and septic shock. The New England Journal of Medicine. 2001;**345**(19):1368-1377

[43] ProCESS Investigators, Yealy DM, Kellum JA, Huang DT, Barnato AE, Weissfeld LA, et al. A randomized trial of protocol-based care for early septic shock. The New England Journal of Medicine. 2014;**370**(18):1683-1693

[44] The ARISE Investigators and the ANZICS Clinical Trials Group. Goal-directed resuscitation for patients with early septic shock. The New England Journal of Medicine. 2014;**371**(16):1496-1506

[45] Mouncey PR, Osborn TM, Power GS, Harrison DA, Sadique MZ, Grieve RD, et al. Trial of early, goal-directed resuscitation for septic shock. The New England Journal of Medicine. 2015;**372**(14):1301-1311

[46] Vincent JL, De Backer D. Circulatory shock. The New England Journal of Medicine. 2013;**369**(18):1726-1734

[47] Vincent JL, De Backer D. From early goal-directed therapy to late(r) $SCVO_2$ checks. Chest. 2018;**154**(6):1267-1269

[48] Wittayachamnankul B, Apaijai N, Sutham K, Chenthanakij B, Liwsrisakun C, Jaiwongkam T, et al. High central venous oxygen saturation is associated with mitochondrial dysfunction in septic shock: A prospective observational study. Journal of Cellular and Molecular Medicine. 2020;**24**(11):6485-6494

[49] Vallée F, Vallet B, Mathe O, Parraguette J, Mari A, Silva S, et al. Central venous-to-arterial carbon dioxide difference: An additional target for goal-directed therapy in septic shock? Intensive Care Medicine. 2008;**34**(12):2218-2225

[50] Qu YQ, Shen XH, Zhao Q, Guo H, Li XR, Li JG, et al. Central venous-to-arterial carbon dioxide partial pressure difference as a guiding parameter for cardiotonic drug administration in patients with early-stage septic shock. Shock. 2024;**61**(6):836-840

[51] Kriswidyatomo P, Kloping YP, Jaya MG, Nugraha RA, Putri CP, Putra DH, et al. Prognostic value of PCO_2 gap in adult septic shock patients: A systematic review and meta-analysis. Turkish Journal of Anaesthesiology and Reanimation. 2022;**50**(5):324-331

[52] Janotka M, Ostadal P. Biochemical markers for clinical monitoring of tissue perfusion. Molecular and Cellular Biochemistry. 2021;**476**(3):1313-1326

[53] Ltaief Z, Schneider AG, Liaudet L. Pathophysiology and clinical implications of the veno-arterial PCO_2 gap. Critical Care. 2021;**25**(1):1-9

[54] Hernández G, Teboul JL. Is the macrocirculation really dissociated from the microcirculation in septic shock? Intensive Care Medicine. 2016;**42**(10):1621-1624

[55] Rovas A, Sackarnd J, Rossaint J, Kampmeier S, Pavenstädt H, Vink H, et al. Identification of novel sublingual parameters to analyze and diagnose microvascular dysfunction in sepsis: The NOSTRADAMUS study. Critical Care. 2021;**25**(1):1-14

[56] Bruno RR, Wollborn J, Fengler K, Flick M, Wunder C, Allgäuer S, et al.

Direct assessment of microcirculation in shock: A randomized-controlled multicenter study. Intensive Care Medicine. 2023;**49**(6):645-655

[57] Hamaoka T, McCully KK, Quaresima V, Yamamoto K, Chance B. Near-infrared spectroscopy/imaging for monitoring muscle oxygenation and oxidative metabolism in healthy and diseased humans. Journal of Biomedical Optics. 2007;**12**(6):062105

[58] Macdonald SPJ, Brown SGA. Near-infrared spectroscopy in the assessment of suspected sepsis in the emergency department. Emergency Medicine Journal. 2015;**32**(5):404-408

[59] Shapiro NI, Arnold R, Sherwin R, O'Connor J, Najarro G, Singh S, et al. The association of near-infrared spectroscopy-derived tissue oxygenation measurements with sepsis syndromes, organ dysfunction and mortality in emergency department patients with sepsis. Critical Care. 2011;**15**(5):R223

[60] Macdonald SPJ, Kinnear FB, Arendts G, Ho KM, Fatovich DM. Near-infrared spectroscopy to predict organ failure and outcome in sepsis: The assessing risk in sepsis using a tissue oxygen saturation (ARISTOS) study. European Journal of Emergency Medicine. 2019;**26**(3):174-179

[61] Donati A, Damiani E, Domizi R, Scorcella C, Carsetti A, Tondi S, et al. Near-infrared spectroscopy for assessing tissue oxygenation and microvascular reactivity in critically ill patients: A prospective observational study. Critical Care. 2016;**20**(1):1-10

[62] Yumoto T, Kuribara T, Yamada K, Sato T, Koba S, Tetsuhara K, et al. Clinical parameter-guided initial resuscitation in adult patients with septic shock: A systematic review and network meta-analysis. Acute Medicine & Surgery. 2023;**10**(1):1-10

[63] Orso D, Federici N, Lio C, Mearelli F, Bove T. Hemodynamic goals in sepsis and septic shock resuscitation: An umbrella review of systematic reviews and meta-analyses with trial sequential analysis. Australian Critical Care. 2024;**S1036-7314**(24):00059-00056

[64] Munroe ES, Weinstein J, Gershengorn HB, Karlic KJ, Seelye S, Sjoding MW, et al. Understanding how clinicians personalize fluid and vasopressor decisions in early sepsis management. JAMA Network Open. 2024;**7**(4):E247480

[65] Vijayan AL, Ravindran S, Saikant R, Lakshmi S, Kartik R, Manoj G. Procalcitonin: A promising diagnostic marker for sepsis and antibiotic therapy. Journal of Intensive Care. 2017;**5**(1):1-7

[66] Gregoriano C, Heilmann E, Molitor A, Schuetz P. Role of procalcitonin use in the management of sepsis. Journal of Thoracic Disease. 2020;**2**(Suppl. 1):S5-S15

[67] Kyriazopoulou E, Liaskou-Antoniou L, Adamis G, Panagaki A, Melachroinopoulos N, Drakou E, et al. Procalcitonin to reduce long-term infection-associated adverse events in sepsis a randomized trial. American Journal of Respiratory and Critical Care Medicine. 2021;**203**(2):202-210

[68] Papp M, Kiss N, Baka M, Trásy D, Zubek L, Fehérvári P, et al. Procalcitonin-guided antibiotic therapy may shorten length of treatment and may improve survival—A systematic review and meta-analysis. Critical Care. 2023;**27**(1):1-15

[69] Mårtensson J, Bell M, Oldner A, Xu S, Venge P, Martling CR. Neutrophil

gelatinase-associated lipocalin in adult septic patients with and without acute kidney injury. Intensive Care Medicine. 2010;**36**(8):1333-1340

[70] Otani S, Coopersmith CM. Gut integrity in critical illness. Journal of Intensive Care. 2019;**7**(1):17

[71] Sun DL, Cen YY, Li SM, Li WM, Lu QP, Xu PY. Accuracy of the serum intestinal fatty-acid-binding protein for diagnosis of acute intestinal ischemia: A meta-analysis. Scientific Reports. 2016;**6**(September):1-7

[72] Sekino M, Funaoka H, Sato S, Okada K, Inoue H, Yano R, et al. Intestinal fatty acid-binding protein level as a predictor of 28-day mortality and bowel ischemia in patients with septic shock: A preliminary study. Journal of Critical Care. 2017;**42**:92-100

[73] McElvaney OJ, Curley GF, Rose-John S, McElvaney NG. Interleukin-6: Obstacles to targeting a complex cytokine in critical illness. The Lancet Respiratory Medicine. 2021;**9**(6):643-654

[74] Molano Franco D, Arevalo-Rodriguez I, Roqué I, Figuls M, Montero Oleas NG, Nuvials X, et al. Plasma interleukin-6 concentration for the diagnosis of sepsis in critically ill adults. Cochrane Database of Systematic Reviews. 2019;**4**(4):CD011811

Chapter 15

Melatonin-Mediated Protection against Sepsis-Induced Organ Dysfunction

Hilal Üstündağ and Songul Doganay

Abstract

Sepsis-induced organ dysfunction represents a critical challenge in intensive care medicine, characterized by complex pathophysiological mechanisms that can lead to multiple organ failure and death. This review examines the fundamental mechanisms underlying sepsis-induced organ dysfunction and explores the therapeutic potential of melatonin, a multifaceted molecule with potent antioxidant and anti-inflammatory properties. We analyzed the pathophysiological pathways involved in organ damage during sepsis, including inflammatory cascades, oxidative stress, mitochondrial dysfunction, and endothelial injury. Special attention is given to melatonin's protective effects on various organ systems, including cardiac, pulmonary, renal, hepatic, and central nervous system function during sepsis. Recent evidence suggests that melatonin's ability to modulate these pathways, combined with its excellent safety profile, makes it a promising therapeutic agent in sepsis management. Understanding these mechanisms and melatonin's therapeutic applications may provide new strategies for improving outcomes in septic patients.

Keywords: sepsis, organ dysfunction, melatonin, oxidative stress, inflammation, mitochondrial dysfunction, multiple organ failure, therapeutic intervention

1. Introduction

Sepsis remains one of the most challenging conditions in critical care medicine, characterized by a dysregulated host response to infection that leads to life-threatening organ dysfunction [1, 2]. Despite significant advances in understanding its pathophysiology and improvements in therapeutic approaches, sepsis continues to be a leading cause of mortality in intensive care units worldwide [3]. The complex interplay between inflammatory mediators, oxidative stress, and cellular dysfunction creates a devastating cascade that can rapidly progress to multiple organ failure if not properly managed [4].

The pathophysiology of sepsis-induced organ dysfunction involves multiple mechanisms, including excessive inflammation, immune dysregulation, mitochondrial dysfunction, and endothelial damage. These mechanisms create a self-perpetuating cycle of tissue injury that can affect multiple organ systems simultaneously.

Current therapeutic approaches primarily focus on early recognition, source control, and supportive care, yet these interventions often prove insufficient in preventing organ dysfunction and mortality [5].

In recent years, melatonin has emerged as a promising therapeutic agent in sepsis management due to its diverse physiological properties. This endogenous molecule, primarily known for its role in circadian rhythm regulation, demonstrates potent antioxidant, anti-inflammatory, and immunomodulatory effects that may be beneficial in sepsis treatment [6]. Melatonin's ability to cross biological membranes and reach intracellular compartments, combined with its excellent safety profile, makes it an attractive candidate for therapeutic intervention in sepsis [7].

This chapter aims to examine the current understanding of sepsis-induced organ dysfunction and evaluate the potential therapeutic role of melatonin in its management. We explored the pathophysiological mechanisms underlying organ dysfunction in sepsis, with particular focus on the inflammatory cascade, oxidative stress, and mitochondrial dysfunction. Additionally, we assessed the evidence supporting melatonin's protective effects against sepsis-induced organ damage and discuss its potential clinical applications. Understanding these mechanisms and the therapeutic potential of melatonin may provide new strategies for improving outcomes in septic patients.

2. Sepsis-induced organ dysfunction

2.1 Pathophysiological mechanisms

Sepsis-induced organ dysfunction represents a complex pathophysiological condition characterized by dysregulated host response to infection, leading to life-threatening organ dysfunction. The intricate interplay between inflammatory mediators, cellular stress responses, and metabolic alterations creates a devastating cycle that can rapidly progress to multiple organ failure if not properly managed [5].

The inflammatory cascade in sepsis begins with the recognition of pathogenic molecules through specialized cellular receptors. Pattern recognition receptors (PRRs) on immune cells detect both pathogen-associated molecular patterns (PAMPs) and damage-associated molecular patterns (DAMPs), initiating a sophisticated signaling cascade. This recognition process triggers the activation of nuclear factor-κB (NF-κB) and other transcription factors, leading to the production and release of pro-inflammatory cytokines. The resulting "cytokine storm" represents a hallmark of sepsis pathophysiology, where elevated levels of tumor necrosis factor-α (TNF-α), interleukin-1β (IL-1β), and interleukin-6 (IL-6) drive systemic inflammation [1–3].

Recent research has revealed that the inflammatory response in sepsis is far more complex than initially understood. Rather than a simple pro-inflammatory state, sepsis involves simultaneous activation of both pro- and anti-inflammatory pathways. This immunological dysregulation leads to a state of immune paralysis in some patients, characterized by impaired neutrophil function, increased T-cell apoptosis, and reduced antigen presentation capacity. The balance between these competing immune responses significantly influences patient outcomes and presents a major challenge in therapeutic intervention (**Figure 1**) [8].

Oxidative stress emerges as a critical mediator of organ dysfunction in sepsis, extending far beyond simple free radical damage. Multiple cellular sources contribute to the oxidative burden, including activated neutrophils, damaged mitochondria, and compromised antioxidant defense systems. The resulting reactive oxygen species

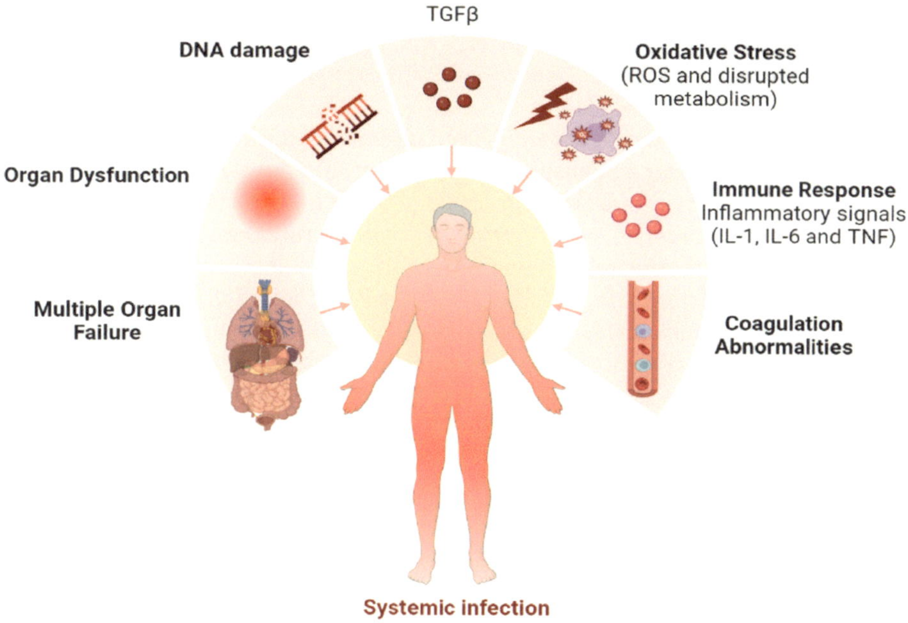

Figure 1.
Pathophysiology of sepsis.

(ROS) and reactive nitrogen species (RNS) induce widespread cellular damage through lipid peroxidation, protein oxidation, and DNA modification. These modifications lead to profound alterations in cellular function, including disrupted membrane integrity, impaired enzyme activity, and altered gene expression patterns [4, 9].

The role of mitochondrial dysfunction in sepsis has gained significant attention as a central mechanism of organ failure. Sepsis induces severe perturbations in mitochondrial function through multiple pathways, leading to what has been termed "cytopathic hypoxia." This phenomenon describes the inability of cells to utilize oxygen effectively despite adequate oxygen delivery, resulting from impaired electron transport chain function and compromised adenosine triphosphate (ATP) synthesis. Research has demonstrated that sepsis disrupts mitochondrial quality control mechanisms, including mitochondrial dynamics, mitophagy, and biogenesis, further compromising cellular energy metabolism [10, 11].

Endothelial dysfunction represents another critical aspect of sepsis pathophysiology, fundamentally altering vascular homeostasis and tissue perfusion. The endothelial response to sepsis involves increased expression of adhesion molecules, enhanced vascular permeability, and altered vasomotor tone. The degradation of the endothelial glycocalyx, a protective layer on the luminal surface of blood vessels, has emerged as a crucial early event in sepsis. This degradation leads to increased vascular permeability, tissue edema, and impaired microcirculatory flow. Recent studies have identified novel mechanisms of endothelial dysfunction in sepsis, including endothelial-to-mesenchymal transition (EndMT) and alterations in mechanotransduction pathways [12, 13].

The complex interplay between these pathophysiological mechanisms creates a self-perpetuating cycle of tissue damage and organ dysfunction. Endothelial activation and dysfunction lead to microcirculatory alterations, which further compromise tissue perfusion and oxygenation. Studies have shown that sepsis-induced microcirculatory dysfunction persists even after normalization of systemic hemodynamic parameters, highlighting the importance of monitoring microvascular function in septic patients (**Figure 2**) [6, 14, 15].

Cellular metabolism undergoes significant alterations during sepsis, characterized by a shift from oxidative phosphorylation to aerobic glycolysis, known as the Warburg effect. This metabolic reprogramming, while initially adaptive, can become maladaptive when prolonged, contributing to organ dysfunction. Recent research has demonstrated that different cell types exhibit distinct metabolic responses to sepsis, with immune cells particularly relying on glycolysis for their effector functions. The altered cellular metabolism affects not only energy production but also influences immune cell function, redox balance, and cell death pathways [16].

The impact of epigenetic modifications in sepsis has emerged as a novel area of research. Sepsis induces significant changes in DNA methylation patterns, histone modifications, and microRNA expression profiles. These epigenetic alterations can persist long after the acute phase of sepsis, potentially explaining the long-term consequences observed in sepsis survivors. Studies have identified specific epigenetic signatures associated with different sepsis phenotypes, suggesting potential therapeutic targets and biomarkers [17, 18].

Autophagy dysregulation represents another crucial mechanism in sepsis-induced organ dysfunction. While autophagy initially serves as a protective mechanism, clearing damaged cellular components and pathogens, prolonged or excessive autophagy can lead to cell death. Research has shown that sepsis induces both excessive and impaired autophagy in different organs and cell types, contributing to organ

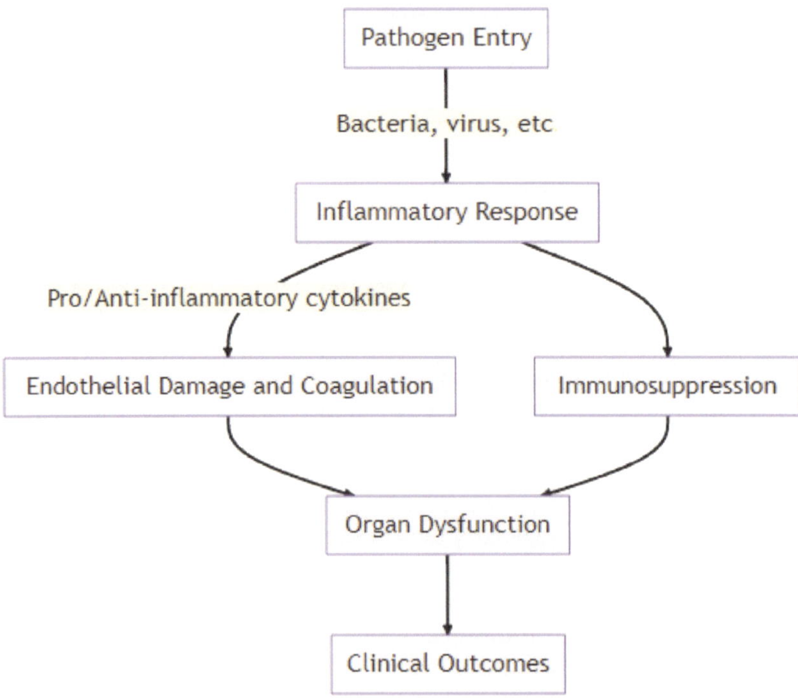

Figure 2.
Pathogenesis of sepsis [6].

dysfunction through various mechanisms, including accumulated cellular damage and compromised pathogen clearance [19].

The role of the coagulation system in sepsis extends beyond simple thrombosis and bleeding complications. Sepsis activates both pro- and anticoagulant pathways, leading to disseminated intravascular coagulation (DIC) in severe cases. The interaction between inflammation and coagulation creates a vicious cycle, where inflammatory mediators activate coagulation, and activated coagulation factors further promote inflammation. Recent studies have highlighted the importance of endothelial protein C receptor and thrombomodulin in regulating this interaction [20, 21].

The neuroendocrine response to sepsis involves complex alterations in hypothalamic-pituitary-adrenal axis function, autonomic nervous system regulation, and hormone signaling. Sepsis induces relative adrenal insufficiency, thyroid hormone alterations, and vasopressin deficiency, contributing to hemodynamic instability and organ dysfunction. The concept of persistent inflammation, immunosuppression, and catabolism syndrome (PICS) has emerged as a framework for understanding chronic critical illness following sepsis [22, 23].

2.2 Major affected organ systems

Sepsis-induced organ dysfunction manifests through a complex pattern of injury affecting multiple organ systems simultaneously. Understanding the specific mechanisms of organ damage is crucial for developing targeted therapeutic strategies. Each organ system demonstrates unique patterns of dysfunction while sharing common pathophysiological pathways.

2.2.1 Cardiovascular system dysfunction

The cardiovascular manifestations of sepsis involve complex interactions between inflammatory mediators, neurohormonal responses, and cellular dysfunction. During the early phase of sepsis, the endothelium undergoes significant functional alterations, characterized by dysregulated production of vasoactive substances such as nitric oxide and prostacyclin. The endothelial activation also leads to enhanced expression of adhesion molecules and increased vascular permeability, contributing to tissue edema and organ dysfunction [24, 25].

A distinguishing feature of septic shock is persistent hypotension despite adequate fluid resuscitation. This cardiovascular collapse results from a complex interplay between myocardial depression, vascular dysfunction, and autonomic dysregulation. The body attempts to compensate through the activation of multiple neurohormonal pathways, particularly the renin-angiotensin-aldosterone system and the sympathetic nervous system. However, these compensatory mechanisms often become maladaptive, contributing to organ dysfunction and poor outcomes [26].

Recent research has revealed that the heart functions not only as a mechanical pump but also as an important endocrine organ during sepsis. Through the production and secretion of specialized proteins known as cardiokines, the heart participates in complex intercellular and interorgan communication networks. These cardiac-derived factors, including natriuretic peptides atrial natriuretic factor (ANF) and brain natriuretic peptide (BNP), growth factors, and various cytokines, play crucial roles in modulating the systemic response to sepsis. Of particular interest is the relationship between cardiac-derived inflammatory mediators and autonomic dysfunction, as evidenced by reduced heart rate variability in septic patients [6, 27].

The endocrine function of the heart during sepsis represents an emerging area of research, with studies identifying numerous cardiokines that influence both local and systemic responses to infection. These factors contribute to the regulation of vascular tone, inflammatory responses, and metabolic adaptation during sepsis [28].

2.2.2 Respiratory system impairment

Acute respiratory distress syndrome (ARDS) represents one of the most severe complications of sepsis. The pathogenesis involves complex interactions between pulmonary endothelial injury, alveolar epithelial damage, and dysregulated inflammation. Recent research has identified novel mechanisms of lung injury in sepsis, including neutrophil extracellular traps (NETs) formation and alterations in surfactant composition and function. The pulmonary endothelium undergoes significant changes during sepsis, leading to increased permeability and pulmonary edema. This process is exacerbated by the release of inflammatory mediators, oxidative stress, and mechanical stress from mechanical ventilation. The concept of "biotrauma" has emerged, highlighting the importance of mechanical ventilation-induced inflammation in perpetuating lung injury [29, 30].

2.2.3 Renal system dysfunction

Sepsis-induced acute kidney injury (S-AKI) represents a distinct entity from other forms of acute kidney injury. Recent evidence suggests that S-AKI involves complex pathophysiological mechanisms beyond simple hypoperfusion. Renal tubular cells undergo significant metabolic reprogramming during sepsis, shifting from oxidative phosphorylation to glycolysis. This metabolic switch, while initially adaptive, can lead to cellular dysfunction and death when prolonged [31].

The role of mitochondrial dysfunction in S-AKI has gained increasing attention. Studies have demonstrated significant alterations in mitochondrial dynamics, including changes in fission and fusion processes, impaired mitophagy, and reduced biogenesis. These changes contribute to persistent tubular dysfunction and may explain the increased risk of chronic kidney disease in sepsis survivors [32].

2.2.4 Hepatic system dysfunction

Sepsis-induced liver dysfunction manifests through multiple pathways, significantly impacting both the metabolic and immunological functions of this vital organ. The liver's unique dual blood supply system and its role as a primary site of immune surveillance make it particularly vulnerable to sepsis-induced injury. Current research has revealed that hepatic dysfunction in sepsis extends beyond traditional markers of liver injury, encompassing complex alterations in metabolic homeostasis, immune function, and protein synthesis [33].

The hepatic microcirculation undergoes significant changes during sepsis, characterized by sinusoidal endothelial cell dysfunction and altered Kupffer cell function. These alterations lead to impaired hepatic blood flow and oxygen delivery, despite maintained systemic perfusion. Recent studies have demonstrated that liver sinusoidal endothelial cells lose their characteristic fenestration during sepsis, contributing to impaired hepatic function and reduced clearance of bacterial products [34].

Metabolic dysfunction in the septic liver manifests through altered glucose homeostasis, impaired protein synthesis, and disrupted lipid metabolism. The liver's capacity to maintain glucose homeostasis becomes compromised, leading to persistent hyperglycemia despite increased insulin levels. This metabolic derangement is further complicated by insulin resistance and altered gluconeogenesis pathways. Additionally, the reduced synthesis of acute-phase proteins and coagulation factors compromises the systemic response to infection and inflammation [33, 35].

2.2.5 Central nervous system dysfunction

Sepsis-associated encephalopathy (SAE) represents a complex manifestation of central nervous system dysfunction that can occur early in the course of sepsis and may persist long after recovery from the acute illness. The pathophysiology of SAE involves multiple mechanisms, including blood-brain barrier disruption, neuroinflammation, and altered neurotransmitter systems. Recent neuroimaging studies have revealed significant structural and functional changes in the brains of septic patients, particularly in regions associated with cognition and emotional processing [36].

The blood-brain barrier undergoes significant alterations during sepsis, leading to increased permeability and allowing the entry of inflammatory mediators and potentially toxic substances into the central nervous system. This process is facilitated by the activation of cerebral endothelial cells and the disruption of tight junction proteins. Moreover, recent research has identified the role of microglial activation and neuroinflammation in perpetuating brain dysfunction during and after sepsis [37, 38].

Long-term cognitive impairment represents a significant concern in sepsis survivors, with studies demonstrating persistent deficits in memory, attention, and executive function. The mechanisms underlying these long-term effects involve both acute injury during the septic episode and ongoing inflammatory processes that persist after recovery from the acute illness. Evidence suggests that sepsis may accelerate neurodegenerative processes and increase the risk of developing cognitive decline and dementia in survivors [38].

2.2.6 Immune system dysregulation

While not traditionally considered an "organ system," the immune system undergoes profound alterations during sepsis that significantly impact multiple organ functions. The concept of sepsis-induced immunosuppression has gained increased recognition, characterized by both innate and adaptive immune dysfunction. This state of immune paralysis increases susceptibility to secondary infections and may contribute to long-term immunological complications in survivors [39].

The bone marrow response to sepsis involves significant alterations in hematopoiesis, with evidence of both enhanced myelopoiesis and impaired lymphopoiesis. These changes result in the production of immature and dysfunctional immune cells, contributing to the compromised immune response. Recent studies have also identified the role of emergency myelopoiesis in altering the phenotype and function of immune cells produced during sepsis [40].

2.2.7 Organ systems crosstalk and clinical implications

The interaction between affected organ systems in sepsis creates a complex network of dysfunction that extends beyond individual organ failure. This "organ crosstalk" phenomenon has emerged as a crucial concept in understanding the progression and persistence of multiple organ dysfunction syndrome (MODS). Research has demonstrated that injury to one organ system can initiate and perpetuate dysfunction in others through various mediators and cellular mechanisms [41].

The lung-kidney axis represents a particularly well-studied example of organ crosstalk in sepsis. Mechanical ventilation strategies required for treating acute respiratory failure can impact renal function through alterations in intrathoracic pressure, neurohormonal activation, and inflammatory mediator release. Conversely, acute kidney injury can exacerbate pulmonary dysfunction through fluid overload, altered acid-base balance, and the accumulation of uremic toxins [42, 43].

3. Melatonin: A multifaceted molecule

Melatonin a lipophilic hormone, primarily secreted by the pineal gland, has garnered significant attention due to its diverse physiological roles beyond its well-known function in regulating circadian rhythms [44]. Additionally, melatonin is produced in various extrapineal tissues, such as the gut, ciliary body, retina, thymus, airway epithelium, bone marrow, immune cells, gonads, placenta, gastrointestinal tract, and skin, and perhaps other organs [45]. This indoleamine molecule, derived from the amino acid tryptophan through a series of enzymatic reactions involving serotonin, is synthesized and released in a rhythmic manner, peaking during the night and declining during the day [44, 46]. While its role in sleep-wake regulation is widely recognized, melatonin's influence extends far beyond circadian rhythm modulation. It is involved in a wide array of biological processes, including sleep regulation, antioxidant defense, immune modulation, anti-inflammatory actions, and even anti-cancer properties [47] Beyond this, it exhibits a multitude of physiological functions, including antioxidant, anti-inflammatory, and mitochondrial-protective properties. Recent studies have highlighted melatonin's potential therapeutic effects, particularly in the context of sepsis—a life-threatening condition characterized by a dysregulated host response to infection.

3.1 Biochemistry and synthesis

Melatonin (N-acetyl-5-methoxytryptamine) is synthesized from the amino acid tryptophan. The biosynthetic pathway involves the conversion of tryptophan to 5-hydroxytryptophan, followed by decarboxylation to serotonin. Serotonin undergoes acetylation by arylalkylamine N-acetyltransferase to form N-acetylserotonin, which is subsequently methylated by hydroxyindole-O-methyltransferase to produce melatonin. This synthesis predominantly occurs in the pineal gland and is tightly regulated by the light-dark cycle, with production peaking during the night (**Figure 3**) [48].

The pineal hormone melatonin plays a crucial role in regulating seasonal reproduction and circadian rhythms through its actions on high-affinity melatonin receptors, primarily located in the pituitary pars tuberalis (PT) and the suprachiasmatic nucleus (SCN) of the hypothalamus. Two subtypes of melatonin receptors, MT1 (Mel1a) and MT2 (Mel1b), have been identified, both belonging to the G protein-coupled receptor (GPCRs) family [49]. ML1-like receptors, including Mel1a and Mel1b, were cloned in various vertebrates [50]. Another ML1-like receptor, Mel1c, is absent in mammals. A third receptor (MT3), GPR50, does not bind melatonin but negatively regulates MT1. The MT1 receptor mediates inhibition of adenylyl cyclase and activation of phospholipase Cβ, while the MT2 receptor inhibits both adenylyl cyclase and the soluble guanylyl cyclase pathway. These receptors are therapeutic targets for sleep

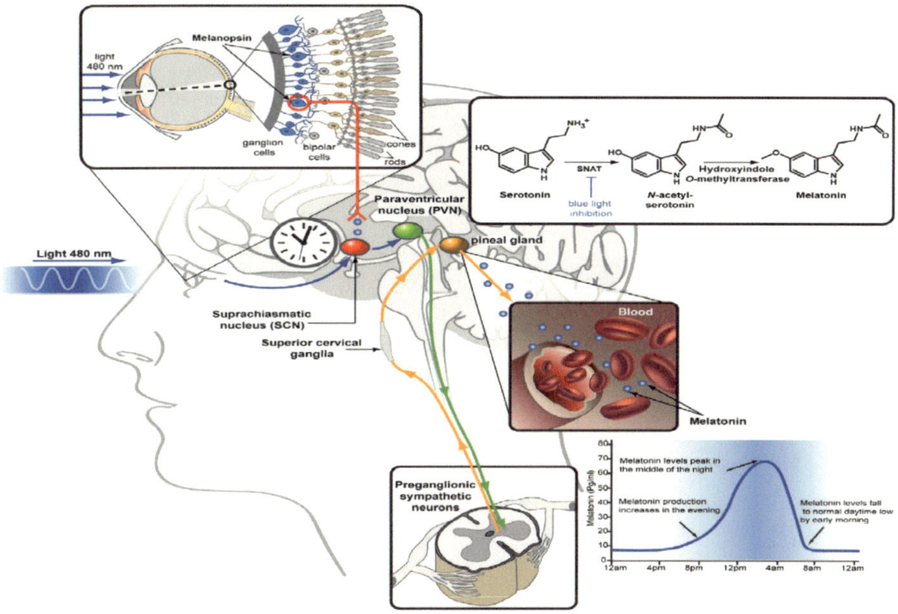

Figure 3.
Melatonin biosynthesis. Serotonin is converted to melatonin in the pineal gland through two enzymatic steps. The first step, N-acetylation, is catalyzed by serotonin N-acetyltransferase (SNAT) and inhibited by blue light signals transmitted via the suprachiasmatic nucleus (SCN), leading to high melatonin production at night and low levels during the day. Melatonin is released into the third ventricle and bloodstream, acting on brain and peripheral tissues via MT1 and MT2 receptors. Its functions include regulating body temperature, blood pressure, and facilitating sleep [48].

disorders, especially given the widespread prevalence of insomnia exacerbated by modern lifestyle factors like light pollution and shift work (**Figure 4**) [46].

Studies using MT1 receptor-deficient mice reveal that the MT1 receptor is essential for melatonin's acute inhibitory effects on SCN activity, though the MT2 receptor can partially compensate for its absence in phase-shifting responses. In the PT, the MT1 receptor is critical for rhythmic expression of the clock gene mPER1 and amplifies cyclic adenosine monophosphate (AMP) signaling at dawn, reinforcing rhythmicity in peripheral tissues. These findings highlight the distinct yet overlapping roles of MT1 and MT2 receptors in regulating circadian and photoperiodic functions, providing insights into the cellular mechanisms of melatonin's actions [50].

Despite structural similarities between melatonin and serotonin receptors, ligand specificity is high, with few dual-acting compounds. Recent advances in structural biology have provided insights into melatonin receptor structures, enabling the rational design of subtype-selective ligands and improved therapeutic agents. Melatonin supplementation and synthetic melatonergics (e.g., ramelteon, agomelatine) are used to address sleep issues and circadian disruptions [52].

3.2 Physiological functions

Melatonin, a hormone primarily secreted by the pineal gland in response to darkness, plays a crucial role in regulating circadian rhythms and promoting sleep. Beyond its involvement in sleep regulation, melatonin exhibits several physiological functions that have significant implications for health. It acts as a potent antioxidant, effectively

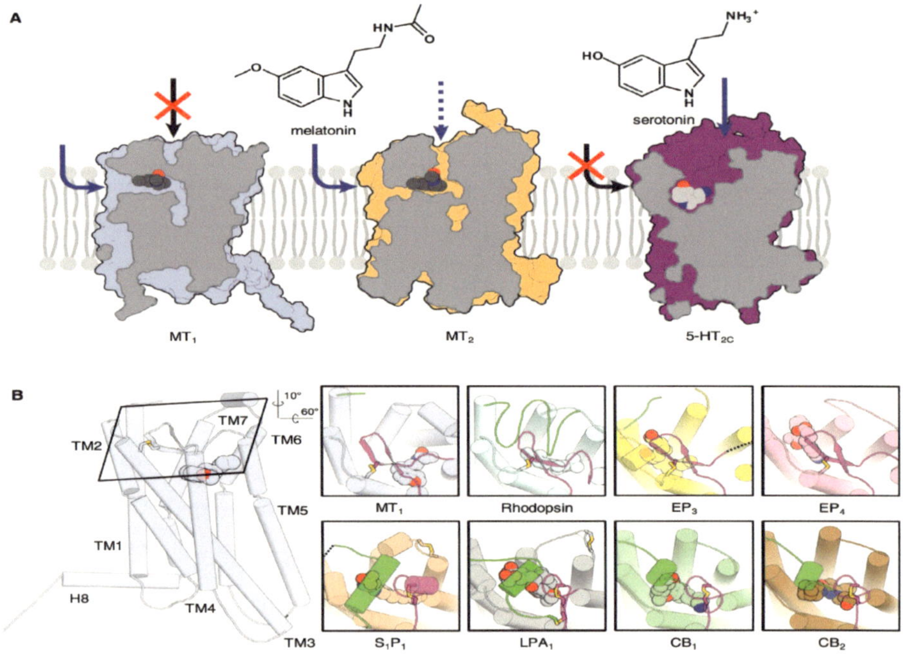

Figure 4.
Comparison of MT receptor binding sites. (A) The surface structure of melatonin receptors MT1 and MT2 is compared to serotonin receptor 5-HT2C (PDB ID: 6bqg), with ligand access routes indicated by blue arrows. The lipid bilayer is shown as a light gray schematic (B) The extracellular conformation of MT1 (PDB ID: 6me2) is compared to rhodopsin (PDB ID: 1u19) and lipid receptors, including prostaglandin (EP3, EP4), sphingosine-1-phosphate (S1P1), lysophosphatidic acid (LPA1), and cannabinoid receptors (CB1, CB2). Structural elements such as the N-terminus (green), extracellular loop 2 (ECL2, magenta), disulfide bonds (yellow), and ligand-binding sites (blue/red spheres) are highlighted, showing differences in ligand accessibility and receptor function [51].

neutralizing free radicals, thereby protecting cellular integrity and reducing oxidative stress. Furthermore, melatonin has been linked to immune function enhancement, showcasing its capacity to modulate immune responses and potentially reduce inflammation [53, 54]. Recent studies suggest that melatonin may also influence endocrine functions, including the regulation of metabolism and reproductive health. The multifaceted roles of melatonin indicate its importance not only in sleep quality and circadian alignment but also as a potential therapeutic agent in managing various health conditions, including sleep disorders, mood disturbances, and even neurodegenerative diseases, highlighting its broader implications for overall well-being. Research indicates that disruptions in melatonin secretion can lead to adverse health outcomes, particularly concerning metabolic disorders and sleep-related issues. For instance, studies suggest that circadian misalignment, such as that experienced during shift work, can impede melatonin production and subsequently affect glucose metabolism and insulin sensitivity [55]. Furthermore, the complex interplay between melatonin and the circadian clock has profound implications for understanding energy balance and risk factors for metabolic diseases [56]. Thus, melatonin emerges as a vital component in maintaining overall physiological health.

3.3 Antioxidant properties and reducing oxidative stress

Melatonin's potent free radical scavenging ability is attributed to its chemical structure, which includes electron-donating indole and methoxy groups that facilitate electron transfer and quench reactive oxygen and nitrogen species (RONS). This action helps reduce oxidative stress by neutralizing free radicals such as H_2O_2, •OH, and O_2•, and mitigates nitrosative stress by inhibiting the formation of peroxynitrite ($ONOO^-$), a highly reactive and cytotoxic molecule. Notably, melatonin's metabolites also exhibit antioxidant capabilities, contributing to a cascade of protective effects against cellular damage [57].

The external melatonin supplementation improves the superoxide dismutase (SOD) and glutathione peroxidase (GPx) activity [58]. This activity is vital not only for preserving cellular integrity but also for modulating immune responses and regulating metabolic processes [59]. Additionally, melatonin plays a crucial role in mitochondrial protection, particularly in conditions like stroke, by enhancing mitochondrial respiration, ATP production, and electron transport chain efficiency. It also prevents mitochondrial permeability transition pore opening and reduces ROS generation, thus maintaining cellular energy homeostasis. Beyond its direct antioxidant effects, melatonin modulates inflammation by reducing the production of pro-inflammatory cytokines, including TNF-α, IL-1β, and IL-6, while inhibiting NF-κB activation. Through these combined mechanisms, melatonin contributes to cellular protection and reduces oxidative and inflammatory damage in various pathological conditions.

Collectively, melatonin's antioxidant functions underscore its significance in maintaining physiological balance and enhancing the body's resilience against oxidative challenges. Additionally, melatonin has demonstrated a capacity to enhance the endogenous antioxidant defenses of cells, further reinforcing its protective role against oxidative stress-related pathologies. Research indicates that melatonin's neuroprotective properties are particularly significant in conditions such as stroke and aging, where its administration has been correlated with reduced cellular damage and improved outcomes [59, 60]. Melatonin's antioxidant properties are crucial in aging, as oxidative stress contributes to neurodegenerative diseases like Alzheimer's and Parkinson's. By scavenging free radicals and reducing oxidative damage, melatonin may help slow cognitive decline. Research indicates that mitochondrial reactive oxygen and nitrogen species (RONS) accelerate cellular aging and age-related deterioration [60]. This suggests that melatonin's antioxidant functions extend beyond mere hormone regulation, positioning it as a promising therapeutic agent in oxidative stress-related disorders.

While melatonin's direct antioxidant effects are well-known, recent research highlights the role of its metabolites in enhancing its antioxidative actions. After metabolism, melatonin undergoes enzymatic reactions that produce metabolites with strong free radical scavenging properties. These metabolites neutralize RONS by donating electrons or hydrogen atoms, contributing to melatonin's overall antioxidant capacity [60]. One of the melatonin metabolite 6-Hydroxymelatonin (6-OHM), formed by cytochrome P450 enzymes, acts as a potent antioxidant by scavenging RONS (H_2O_2, •OH, $ONOO^-$) and reducing oxidative stress. Additionally, it enhances antioxidant enzyme activity and inhibits lipid peroxidation, protecting brain cells from oxidative damage. Another key metabolite, N1-Acetyl-N2-formyl-5-methoxykynuramine (AFMK), is produced *via* cytochrome P450 enzymes, peroxidases, or direct interaction with free radicals. AFMK effectively neutralizes various free radicals, including •OH, $ONOO^-$, and peroxyl radicals (ROO•), contributing to melatonin's overall antioxidative defense [61]. AFMK not only acts as an antioxidant but also has anti-inflammatory properties. Another melatonin metabolite, N1-Acetyl-5-methoxykynuramine (AMK), is produced *via* indoleamine 2,3-dioxygenase (IDO) and functions as a potent free radical scavenger, particularly against peroxyl radicals (ROO•), contributing to melatonin's overall antioxidative defense [62].

Thus, melatonin metabolites maintain their antioxidant appearance by directly scavenging RONS, impairing oxidative stress, and protecting against pathophysiological functions and related organ damage.

3.4 Anti-inflammatory effects

Melatonin's anti-inflammatory effects are mediated through multiple mechanisms. Melatonin's anti-inflammatory effects are well-known and mediated through multiple pathways, including cytokine inhibition, NF-κB suppression, and immune cell modulation. Its therapeutic potential spans a wide range of inflammatory conditions, from acute infections to chronic diseases [63].

Melatonin exerts its anti-inflammatory effects through several pathways to suppress the production and release of pro-inflammatory cytokines. The nuclear factor kappa B (NF-κB) pathway is a major regulator of inflammation and cytokine production. Melatonin inhibits the activation of NF-κB by preventing its translocation to the nucleus, where it would otherwise bind to DNA and promote the transcription of pro-inflammatory genes, including those encoding IL-1β, IL-6, and TNF-α [64]. By blocking NF-κB activation, melatonin reduces the expression of these cytokines at the transcriptional level. Melatonin also influences mitogen-activated protein kinase (MAPK) signaling pathways, such as p38 MAPK and extracellular signal-regulated kinase (ERK), which are involved in cytokine production. By inhibiting these pathways, melatonin further suppresses the synthesis of pro-inflammatory cytokines [65]. Oxidative stress is a key driver of inflammation and cytokine release. Melatonin's potent antioxidant properties help reduce oxidative stress, which in turn decreases the activation of inflammatory pathways and the production of cytokines like IL-1β, IL-6, and TNF-α [47]. Additionally, melatonin modulates the activity of immune cells, such as macrophages, neutrophils, and T-cells, which are primary sources of pro-inflammatory cytokines. For example, it reduces the activation of macrophages, preventing them from releasing excessive amounts of IL-1β and TNF-α [66].

IL-1β is a potent pro-inflammatory cytokine involved in acute and chronic inflammation. Melatonin reduces IL-1β production by inhibiting the inflammasome complex, a multi-protein structure responsible for IL-1β activation. In animal models of sepsis, melatonin administration significantly lowered IL-1β levels, reducing systemic inflammation and improving survival rates [67]. IL-6 is a multifunctional cytokine that promotes inflammation and immune cell recruitment. Melatonin suppresses IL-6 production by inhibiting NF-κB and MAPK pathways in immune cells. Clinical studies have shown that melatonin supplementation reduces IL-6 levels in patients with chronic inflammatory conditions, such as metabolic syndrome and rheumatoid arthritis [68]. TNF-α is a key mediator of inflammation and tissue damage in conditions like rheumatoid arthritis, inflammatory bowel disease, and sepsis. Melatonin reduces TNF-α production by modulating immune cell activity and inhibiting NF-κB signaling. In preclinical models of inflammation, melatonin treatment significantly decreased TNF-α levels, alleviating tissue damage and inflammation [69–71].

4. Protective effects of melatonin in sepsis

Sepsis is a life-threatening condition characterized by a dysregulated immune response to infection, leading to systemic inflammation, organ dysfunction, and, in severe cases, septic shock and death. Melatonin, a hormone with potent anti-inflammatory, antioxidant, and immunomodulatory properties, has shown promise as a therapeutic agent in sepsis [72, 73].

Melatonin plays a protective role in sepsis and inflammation by inhibiting key inflammatory pathways, including NF-κB and NLRP3 inflammasomes, which are crucial in immune response activation. By suppressing these pathways, melatonin reduces excessive inflammation and tissue damage. Melatonin regulates apoptosis and autophagy, two essential cellular processes that help maintain tissue homeostasis and prevent excessive cell death during sepsis [74].

Melatonin exerts its effects in sepsis by suppressing the overproduction of pro-inflammatory cytokines. During sepsis, a "cytokine storm" occurs, characterized by the excessive release of pro-inflammatory cytokines such as interleukin-1β (IL-1β), interleukin-6 (IL-6), INF-γ, and tumor necrosis factor-alpha (TNF-α). Melatonin inhibits the production and release of these cytokines by downregulating the NF-κB and MAPK signaling pathways. NF-κB is a central transcription factor in the inflammatory response, and melatonin prevents its translocation to the nucleus, thereby suppressing the transcription of pro-inflammatory genes [74, 75]. Melatonergic signaling primarily functions through G protein-coupled receptors, leading to cAMP reduction or ERK1/2 activation, a well-documented pathway present in immune cells. While some studies indicate ERK1/2 inhibition, these effects likely result from secondary signaling mechanisms, potentially influenced by epigenetic changes. Melatonin exerts strong anti-inflammatory effects, mainly by inhibiting NF-κB signaling, which reduces the expression of key pro-inflammatory mediators such as iNOS and COX-2. Additionally, melatonin upregulates Nrf2, a crucial regulator of antioxidant and anti-inflammatory responses [65]. Another important pathway involves TLR4 inhibition, which suppresses the production of TNF-α, IL-1β, IL-6, and IL-8, thereby reducing oxidative stress and inflammation. These effects have been observed in various models, including endotoxemia, ischemia/reperfusion injury, and brain inflammation, highlighting the broad anti-inflammatory potential of melatonin. While evidence suggests melatonin may also modulate other toll-like receptors (TLR), further research is needed to confirm its effects on TLR2 and TLR3 [76].

During sepsis, excessive production of ROS and reactive nitrogen species (RNS) leads to oxidative stress. Melatonin, as a potent antioxidant, directly scavenges ROS and RNS. It also upregulates endogenous antioxidant enzymes such as SOD and glutathione peroxidase, thereby reducing oxidative stress [77]. These properties help prevent cellular damage and preserve organ function during sepsis.

Mitochondrial dysfunction is common during sepsis and can lead to organ failure. Melatonin protects mitochondrial integrity by reducing oxidative damage and improving energy production, thereby preserving cellular function [78]. Additionally, melatonin exhibits anti-apoptotic effects. By reducing oxidative stress and inhibiting pro-apoptotic signaling pathways, it prevents cell death and reduces tissue damage [69].

Animal studies have demonstrated the efficacy of melatonin in sepsis. In rodent models, melatonin administration significantly reduced systemic inflammation, oxidative stress, and organ damage [6]. Melatonin has also been shown to protect against sepsis-induced acute lung injury (ALI), liver, testes, and AKI by reducing inflammation and oxidative stress in these organs [67, 72, 79]. Although clinical studies on melatonin in sepsis are limited, preliminary findings are promising. In a small clinical trial, melatonin supplementation in septic patients reduced markers of oxidative stress and inflammation, such as malondialdehyde (MDA) and c-reactive protein (CRP), while improving clinical outcomes [80]. Melatonin has been used as an adjunct therapy in critically ill patients, showing potential to reduce the severity of sepsis and improve recovery [7].

Melatonin's multifaceted actions make it a valuable therapeutic option in sepsis. When used alongside standard treatments such as antibiotics and fluid resuscitation, it can enhance their efficacy and reduce complications. By reducing oxidative stress and inflammation, melatonin helps protect vital organs such as the lungs, kidneys, and liver. Preclinical studies suggest that melatonin improves survival rates in sepsis.

4.1 Organ-specific protection

Sepsis is characterized by an overwhelming inflammatory response, oxidative stress, and subsequent multiple organ dysfunction. Melatonin's multifaceted properties render it a promising candidate for therapeutic intervention in sepsis (**Table 1**).

4.1.1 Cardiac protection

Cardiac dysfunction increases sepsis mortality by 20–50%, resulting from contractile dysfunction, biventricular dilatation, reduced ejection fraction, and

Tissue/organ	Effects of melatonin in sepsis	Mechanisms
Cardiovascular	Improves cardiac function and reduces myocardial injury. Reduces myocardial inflammation, necrosis, and apoptosis. Improves endothelial function and reduces vascular leakage [81].	Reduces mitochondrial dysfunction, oxidative stress, and inflammation, and prevents cardiomyocyte apoptosis. Reduces oxidative stress, inhibits adhesion molecule expression, and enhances NO bioavailability.
Lung	Reduces acute lung injury (ALI), acute respiratory distress syndrome (ARDS), alveolar damage, edema, and inflammatory cell infiltration [82].	Decreases oxidative stress, suppresses pro-inflammatory cytokines (TNF-α, IL-6), and preserves alveolar epithelial integrity.
Kidney	Attenuates acute kidney injury (AKI). Alleviates tubular necrosis, glomerular damage, and interstitial inflammation [83, 84].	Reduces oxidative stress, decreases inflammation, inhibits caspase-dependent apoptosis, and protects tubular epithelial cells
Liver	Protects against hepatic damage and improves liver function. Reduces hepatocyte necrosis, inflammatory cell infiltration, and fatty degeneration [85].	Reduces lipid peroxidation, enhances antioxidant enzymes prevents apoptosis.
Brain	Protects against neuroinflammation and cognitive dysfunction. Reduces neuronal damage, microglial activation, and blood-brain barrier disruption [86].	Reduces blood-brain barrier disruption, oxidative stress, and pro-inflammatory cytokine release, and prevents neuronal apoptosis.
Intestine	Preserves intestinal barrier integrity and reduces bacterial translocation. Prevents villus atrophy, epithelial barrier damage, and inflammatory cell infiltration [87].	Enhances tight junction proteins reduces oxidative stress, and modulates gut microbiota.
Immune System	Modulates immune response and reduces systemic inflammation [66].	Balances pro- and anti-inflammatory cytokines, enhances phagocytic activity, and reduces endotoxin effects.

Table 1.
Effects of melatonin on tissues during sepsis.

hypotension unresponsive to fluids or catecholamines. Key causes include ischemia, direct myocardial suppression, and mitochondrial dysfunction, while endothelial dysfunction in sepsis further impairs microcirculation, exacerbating myocardial ischemia [88, 89].

Melatonin exerts cardioprotective effects in sepsis-induced cardiac dysfunction through multiple molecular mechanisms. It reduces oxidative stress by scavenging reactive oxygen and nitrogen species (RONS), including superoxide ($O_2\bullet^-$), hydroxyl radicals (•OH), and peroxynitrite ($ONOO^-$), while enhancing the activity of antioxidant enzymes such as SOD, glutathione peroxidase (GPx), and catalase (CAT), thereby minimizing oxidative damage in myocardial cells. Additionally, melatonin preserves mitochondrial function by preventing mitochondrial permeability transition pore opening, improving electron transport chain efficiency, and increasing ATP production, ensuring cardiac energy metabolism [81]. It also inhibits inflammatory pathways by suppressing NF-κB activation and downregulating NLRP3 inflammasome activation, leading to a reduction in pro-inflammatory cytokines such as TNF-α, IL-1β, and IL-6. Furthermore, melatonin modulates apoptosis and autophagy by upregulating Bcl-2 expression while suppressing Bax and caspase-3 activity, thereby preventing cardiomyocyte death and maintaining cellular homeostasis *via* the AMP-activated protein kinase (AMPK) pathway [90, 91]. In addition, melatonin enhances NO bioavailability by reducing its oxidative degradation and stimulating endothelial nitric oxide synthase activity, which supports coronary blood flow and overall cardiac function. Through these mechanisms, melatonin effectively mitigates oxidative and inflammatory damage, preserves myocardial contractility, and enhances cardiac resilience in sepsis [92].

4.1.2 Pulmonary protection

Sepsis patients develop acute lung injury (ALI) involves pulmonary endothelial dysfunction, alveolar damage, vascular leakage, and fibrosis, leading to respiratory distress. Inflammatory cell recruitment increases epithelial permeability, with elevated IL-6, IL-1β, TNF-α, and IFN-γ levels contributing to lung inflammation [93]. Macrophage overactivation drives excessive cytokine production, exacerbating lung damage, while neutrophil accumulation in pulmonary capillaries obstructs blood flow, impairing gas exchange [94]. Reactive oxygen species generated in the lungs further damage mitochondria and alveolar walls, increasing vascular permeability. Destruction of alveolar epithelial cells compromises fluid clearance, promoting pulmonary edema. In severe cases, sepsis-induced ALI can progress to acute respiratory distress syndrome (ARDS), a critical condition characterized by hypoxemia and pulmonary infiltrates, leading to severe lung failure [95].

Melatonin has demonstrated protective effects against sepsis-induced ALI through various mechanisms. Although clinical data on melatonin remains limited, several animal studies have demonstrated its potential to alleviate sepsis-induced acute lung injury (ALI) and improve survival rates. Melatonin exerts anti-inflammatory, antioxidant, and mitochondrial-protective effects, reducing pro-inflammatory cytokines (IL-6, IL-1β, TNF-α) and inhibiting NF-κB activation, which helps mitigate lung inflammation [96, 97]. Additionally, melatonin protects alveolar fluid clearance by upregulating epithelial sodium channel (ENaC) expression *via* the SIRT1/SGK1/Nedd4-2 pathway, maintaining alveolar-capillary barrier integrity and reducing pulmonary edema. Its strong antioxidant capacity also helps scavenge reactive oxygen species (ROS) and preserve mitochondrial function, preventing further oxidative damage in lung tissues [98]. Moreover, melatonin is safe with no clinically significant side effects, making it a promising therapeutic agent for sepsis-induced ALI [99].

4.1.3 Renal protection

Acute kidney injury (AKI) is a common and severe complication in sepsis, leading to high morbidity and mortality. Sepsis is a major cause of acute kidney injury (AKI), accounting for 26–50% of AKI cases in the U.S., compared to 7–10% of primary kidney disease. In children, AKI affects 5% of inpatients and 30–50% of Intensive Care Unit (ICU) patients, highlighting its high incidence and critical impact, especially in intensive care settings [100]. Currently, there is no specific treatment for sepsis-induced AKI (SAKI), with only symptomatic management available. Therefore, identifying effective therapeutic targets and strategies remains a critical priority for improving SAKI outcomes [101].

Sepsis-induced AKI results from multiple factors, including ischemia-reperfusion injury, nephron inflammation, hypoxia, oxidative stress, and cytokine-induced tubular damage. Sepsis-induced AKI multiple pathological factors, including ROS, endoplasmic reticulum stress, and epithelial-mesenchymal transition. Under normal conditions, ROS levels are balanced, but during sepsis, disrupted renal microcirculation leads to ROS overproduction, causing fibrosis, hypoxemia, and renal dysfunction. Excess ROS further reduces ATP levels, increases inflammatory mediators, and disrupts calcium homeostasis in cells and mitochondria. Given the harmful effects of ROS on the kidneys, developing new therapeutic strategies is urgently needed [83]. Thus, RONS clearance is considered a potential strategy for AKI treatment. Various antioxidants have been investigated for their protective effects, with melatonin being one of the most extensively studied compounds [102].

Melatonin has demonstrated protective effects against sepsis-induced AKI through several mechanisms. One key pathway involves the activation of SIRT, a mitochondrial deacetylase that plays a crucial role in maintaining mitochondrial function. By promoting SIRT3-mediated deacetylation of transcription factor A, mitochondrial (TFAM), melatonin enhances mitophagy, the process of clearing damaged mitochondria, thereby preserving renal tubular epithelial cell integrity and function [101, 103]. Additionally, melatonin exhibits potent antioxidant properties, reducing oxidative stress by scavenging reactive oxygen species and upregulating antioxidant enzymes. This reduction in oxidative damage contributes to improved renal function in sepsis conditions. Furthermore, melatonin's anti-inflammatory effects play a significant role in renal protection. By inhibiting pro-inflammatory cytokine production and suppressing inflammatory pathways, melatonin mitigates inflammation-induced renal damage during sepsis [104]. A study demonstrated that early melatonin administration (25 μg/ml) reduces oxidative stress in CLP-induced sepsis by inhibiting Nox4, lowering ROS levels, and downregulating inflammatory factors (IL-1α, IL-1β, MCP-1, TGF-β), which helps mitigate tubular and glomerular injury, inflammation, and fibrosis [83]. Another research, found that melatonin inhibits kinase 1, reducing mitochondrial autophagy and suppressing NLRP3 inflammasome activation, preventing cell death [105]. Collectively, these findings suggest that melatonin's modulation of mitochondrial function, oxidative stress, and inflammation contributes to its renoprotective effects in sepsis-induced AKI.

4.1.4 Hepatic protection

Sepsis, a systemic inflammatory response to infection, can lead to significant liver injury through various molecular mechanisms. Despite its strong regenerative capacity and resilience, the incidence of sepsis-induced liver injury (SLI) is lower compared to other organs. However, SLI-associated mortality ranges from 54 to 68%, surpassing the mortality rates of pulmonary dysfunction or failure, which are more commonly affected in sepsis [88]. One primary factor is the disruption of hepatic microcirculation due to systemic inflammation, resulting in reduced blood flow and oxygen delivery to liver tissues. This ischemia-reperfusion injury causes hepatocyte damage and necrosis. Inflammatory mediators, such as TNF-α, IL-1β, and IL-6, are released during sepsis and play crucial roles in liver injury. These cytokines activate Kupffer cells, the liver's resident macrophages, which in turn produce ROS and NO, leading to oxidative stress and further hepatocyte damage [33]. Additionally, neutrophil extracellular traps (NETs) can exacerbate hepatic injury by promoting inflammation and thrombosis within the liver's microvasculature [106]. Activation of molecular pathways such as NF-κB and MAPK leads to increased transcription of pro-inflammatory genes, amplifying the inflammatory response and contributing to hepatocyte apoptosis [107].

Melatonin's structure has remained unchanged across species for billions of years. Studies show that melatonin reduces neutrophil infiltration, lowers alanine aminotransferase (ALT) and aspartate aminotransferase (AST) levels, and suppresses pro-inflammatory cytokines in sepsis-induced liver injury. Additionally, serum melatonin levels correlate with sepsis severity and mortality. Melatonin therapy has significantly improved survival rates in polymicrobial sepsis models [73, 108]. In septic conditions, the hepatic SIRT1/STAT3 pathway is often inhibited, leading to liver dysfunction and disrupted glucose metabolism. Melatonin administration has been shown to promote SIRT1 expression and STAT3 phosphorylation, thereby attenuating liver injury and normalizing glucose levels [109].

5. Conclusion

Melatonin's multifaceted properties, including its potent antioxidant, anti-inflammatory, and immunomodulatory effects, provide comprehensive protection against sepsis-induced organ damage. The evidence supports melatonin's protective effects across multiple organ systems, from preserving cardiac function and maintaining alveolar-capillary barriers to preventing acute kidney injury and hepatic dysfunction. Its ability to cross biological membranes, combined with an excellent safety profile and cost-effectiveness, positions melatonin as an attractive therapeutic agent in sepsis management. However, several aspects require further investigation through large-scale clinical trials, including optimal dosing regimens, timing of administration, and potential interactions with standard sepsis treatments. Future research should focus on identifying specific patient populations who might benefit most from melatonin intervention and investigating potential synergistic effects with other therapeutic agents. While additional clinical evidence is needed to optimize its application in sepsis treatment, the current understanding of melatonin's protective mechanisms strongly supports its continued investigation as an adjunctive therapy in sepsis care. The integration of melatonin into sepsis treatment protocols could potentially improve patient outcomes and reduce the burden of sepsis-induced organ dysfunction in critical care settings.

Acknowledgements

The Figure 1 was created by BioRender.com.

Conflict of interest

The authors declare no conflict of interest.

Author details

Hilal Üstündağ[1*] and Songul Doganay[2]

1 Department of Physiology, Faculty of Medicine, Erzincan Binali Yıldırım University, Erzincan, Türkiye

2 Department of Physiology, Faculty of Medicine, Sakarya University, Sakarya, Türkiye

*Address all correspondence to: hilal.ustundag@ebyu.edu.tr

References

[1] van der Poll T et al. The immunopathology of sepsis and potential therapeutic targets. Nature Reviews Immunology. 2017;**17**(7):407-420

[2] Üstündağ H. The role of antioxidants in sepsis management: A review of therapeutic applications. Eurasian Journal of Molecular and Biochemical Sciences. 2023;**2**(2):38-48

[3] Timmermans K et al. Danger in the intensive care unit: Damps in critically ill patients. Shock. 2016;**45**(2):108-116

[4] Mantzarlis K, Tsolaki V, Zakynthinos E. Role of oxidative stress and mitochondrial dysfunction in sepsis and potential therapies. Oxidative Medicine and Cellular Longevity. 2017;**2017**(1):5985209

[5] Cecconi M et al. Sepsis and septic shock. The Lancet. 2018;**392**(10141):75-87

[6] Üstündağ H et al. A new treatment approach: Melatonin and ascorbic acid synergy shields against sepsis-induced heart and kidney damage in male rats. Life Sciences. 2023;**329**:121875

[7] Srinivasan V et al. Melatonin in septic shock: Some recent concepts. Journal of Critical Care. 2010;**25**(4):656.e1-656.e6

[8] Hotchkiss RS, Monneret G, Payen D. Sepsis-induced immunosuppression: From cellular dysfunctions to immunotherapy. Nature Reviews Immunology. 2013;**13**(12):862-874

[9] Galley HF. Oxidative stress and mitochondrial dysfunction in sepsis. British Journal of Anaesthesia. 2011;**107**(1):57-64

[10] Singer M. The role of mitochondrial dysfunction in sepsis-induced multi-organ failure. Virulence. 2014;**5**(1):66-72

[11] Arulkumaran N et al. Mitochondrial function in sepsis. Shock. 2016;**45**(3): 271-281

[12] Ince C et al. The endothelium in sepsis. Shock. 2016;**45**(3):259-270

[13] Opal S, Van Der Poll T. Endothelial barrier dysfunction in septic shock. Journal of Internal Medicine. 2015;**277**(3):277-293

[14] De Backer D et al. Pathophysiology of microcirculatory dysfunction and the pathogenesis of septic shock. Virulence. 2014;**5**(1):73-79

[15] Damiani E et al. Microcirculation-guided resuscitation in sepsis: The next frontier? Frontiers in Medicine. 2023;**10**:1212321

[16] Cheng S-C et al. Broad defects in the energy metabolism of leukocytes underlie immunoparalysis in sepsis. Nature Immunology. 2016;**17**(4):406-413

[17] Cross D et al. Epigenetics in sepsis: Understanding its role in endothelial dysfunction, immunosuppression, and potential therapeutics. Frontiers in Immunology. 2019;**10**:1363

[18] Wu D et al. Epigenetic mechanisms of immune remodeling in sepsis: Targeting histone modification. Cell Death and Disease. 2023;**14**(2):112

[19] Yin X et al. The role of autophagy in sepsis: Protection and injury to organs. Frontiers in Physiology. 2019;**10**:1071

[20] Conway Morris A et al. Cell-surface signatures of immune dysfunction

risk-stratify critically ill patients: INFECT study. Intensive Care Medicine. 2018;**44**:627-635

[21] Levi M, van der Poll T. Coagulation and sepsis. Thrombosis Research. 2017;**149**:38-44

[22] Mehdi SF et al. Endocrine and metabolic alterations in response to systemic inflammation and sepsis: A review article. Molecular Medicine. 2025;**31**:16

[23] Hiser SL et al. Post-intensive care syndrome (PICS): Recent updates. Journal of Intensive Care. 2023;**11**(1):23

[24] Martin L et al. The septic heart: Current understanding of molecular mechanisms and clinical implications. Chest. 2019;**155**(2):427-437

[25] Song J et al. Sepsis-induced cardiac dysfunction and pathogenetic mechanisms. Molecular Medicine Reports. 2023;**28**(6):1-12

[26] Poveda-Jaramillo R. Heart dysfunction in sepsis. Journal of Cardiothoracic and Vascular Anesthesia. 2021;**35**(1):298-309

[27] Lv X, Wang H. Pathophysiology of sepsis-induced myocardial dysfunction. Military Medical Research. 2016;**3**:1-9

[28] Brierre S, Deboisblanc BP, Kumari R. The endocrine system during sepsis. The American Journal of the Medical Sciences. 2004;**328**(4):238-247

[29] Matthay MA et al. Acute respiratory distress syndrome. Nature Reviews Disease Primers. 2019;**5**(1):18

[30] Kim W-Y, Hong S-B. Sepsis and acute respiratory distress syndrome: Recent update. Tuberculosis and Respiratory Diseases. 2016;**79**(2):53-57

[31] Gomez H et al. A unified theory of sepsis-induced acute kidney injury: Inflammation, microcirculatory dysfunction, bioenergetics, and the tubular cell adaptation to injury. Shock. 2014;**41**(1):3-11

[32] Parikh SM et al. Mitochondrial function and disturbances in the septic kidney. In: Seminars in Nephrology. WB Saunders; 2015. p. 108-119

[33] Beyer D et al. The liver in sepsis: Molecular mechanism of liver failure and their potential for clinical translation. Molecular Medicine. 2022;**28**(1):84

[34] Yan J, Li S, Li S. The role of the liver in sepsis. International Reviews of Immunology. 2014;**33**(6):498-510

[35] Zhu L et al. The mechanisms of sepsis induced coagulation dysfunction and its treatment. Journal of Inflammation Research. 2025;**18**:1479-1495

[36] Tauber SC et al. Sepsis-associated encephalopathy and septic encephalitis: An update. Expert Review of Anti-Infective Therapy. 2021;**19**(2):215-231

[37] Xin Y et al. The key drivers of brain injury by systemic inflammatory responses after sepsis: Microglia and neuroinflammation. Molecular Neurobiology. 2023;**60**(3):1369-1390

[38] Ji M-H et al. Acute and long-term cognitive impairment following sepsis: Mechanism and prevention. Expert Review of Neurotherapeutics. 2023;**23**(10):931-943

[39] Liu D et al. Sepsis-induced immunosuppression: Mechanisms, diagnosis and current treatment options. Military Medical Research. 2022;**9**(1):56

[40] Rincon JC, Efron PA, Moldawer LL. Immunopathology of chronic critical

illness in sepsis survivors: Role of abnormal myelopoiesis. Journal of Leukocyte Biology. 2022;**112**(6):1525-1534

[41] Borges A, Bento L. Organ crosstalk and dysfunction in sepsis. Annals of Intensive Care. 2024;**14**(1):147

[42] Husain-Syed F, Slutsky AS, Ronco C. Lung–kidney cross-talk in the critically ill patient. American Journal of Respiratory and Critical Care Medicine. 2016;**194**(4):402-414

[43] Koyner JL, Murray PT. Mechanical ventilation and lung–kidney interactions. Clinical Journal of the American Society of Nephrology. 2008;**3**(2):562-570

[44] Claustrat B, Leston J. Melatonin: Physiological effects in humans. Neurochirurgie. 2015;**61**(2-3):77-84

[45] Slominski AT et al. Melatoninergic System in the Skin. Springer; 2012

[46] Zisapel N. New perspectives on the role of melatonin in human sleep, circadian rhythms and their regulation. British Journal of Pharmacology. 2018;**175**(16):3190-3199

[47] Reiter RJ et al. Melatonin as a mitochondria-targeted antioxidant: One of evolution's best ideas. Cellular and Molecular Life Sciences. 2017;**74**:3863-3881

[48] Barrenetxe J, Delagrange P, Martinez J. Physiological and metabolic functions of melatonin. Journal of Physiology and Biochemistry. 2004;**60**(1):61-72

[49] Skubis-Sikora A et al. Regulation of adipose-derived stem cell activity by melatonin receptors in terms of viability and osteogenic differentiation. Pharmaceuticals. 2023;**16**(9):1236

[50] Dubocovich ML et al. Molecular pharmacology, regulation and function of mammalian melatonin receptors. Frontiers in Bioscience. 2003;**8**(10):1093-1108

[51] Stauch B, Johansson LC, Cherezov V. Structural insights into melatonin receptors. The FEBS Journal. 2020;**287**(8):1496-1510

[52] Cardinali DP et al. Melatonin and its analogs in insomnia and depression. Journal of Pineal Research. 2012;**52**(4):365-375

[53] Meléndez-Fernández OH, Liu JA, Nelson RJ. Circadian rhythms disrupted by light at night and mistimed food intake alter hormonal rhythms and metabolism. International Journal of Molecular Sciences. 2023;**24**(4):3392

[54] Megha K et al. Significance of melatonin in the regulation of circadian rhythms and disease management. Molecular Neurobiology. 2024:1-31

[55] Arble DM et al. Impact of sleep and circadian disruption on energy balance and diabetes: A summary of workshop discussions. Sleep. 2015;**38**(12):1849-1860

[56] Plano SA et al. Circadian and metabolic effects of light: Implications in weight homeostasis and health. Frontiers in Neurology. 2017;**8**:558

[57] Ahmad SB et al. Melatonin and health: Insights of melatonin action, biological functions, and associated disorders. Cellular and Molecular Neurobiology. 2023;**43**(6):2437-2458

[58] Mayo J et al. Melatonin regulation of antioxidant enzyme gene expression. Cellular and Molecular Life Sciences CMLS. 2002;**59**:1706-1713

[59] Carlomagno G et al. From implantation to birth: Insight into molecular melatonin functions. International Journal of Molecular Sciences. 2018;**19**(9):2802

[60] Carretero VJ et al. Non-excitatory amino acids, melatonin, and free radicals: Examining the role in stroke and aging. Antioxidants. 2023;**12**(10):1844

[61] Galano A, Tan DX, Reiter RJ. On the free radical scavenging activities of melatonin's metabolites, AFMK and AMK. Journal of Pineal Research. 2013;**54**(3):245-257

[62] Bocheva G et al. The vital role of melatonin and its metabolites in the Neuroprotection and retardation of brain aging. International Journal of Molecular Sciences. 2024;**25**(10):5122

[63] Sayan M, Karabulut D, Özdamar S. Assessment of the protective and therapeutic effect of melatonin against thioacetamide-induced acute liver damage. Journal of Biochemical and Molecular Toxicology. 2020;**34**(4):e22450

[64] Zhao Q et al. Melatonin inhibits the endoplasmic reticulum stress-induced, C/EBP homologous protein-mediated pathway in acute pancreatitis. Molecular Medicine Reports. 2020;**22**(2):1647-1655

[65] Hardeland R. Melatonin and inflammation—Story of a double-edged blade. Journal of Pineal Research. 2018;**65**(4):e12525

[66] Carrillo-Vico A et al. Melatonin: Buffering the immune system. International Journal of Molecular Sciences. 2013;**14**(4):8638-8683

[67] Üstündağ H et al. Protective effect of melatonin and ascorbic acid combination on sepsis-induced lung injury: An experimental study. Clinical and Experimental Pharmacology and Physiology. 2023;**50**(8):634-646

[68] Ali M, Aziz T. The combination of zinc and melatonin enhanced neuroprotection and attenuated neuropathy in oxaliplatin-induced neurotoxicity. Drug Design, Development and Therapy. 2022:3447-3463

[69] Maestroni GJ. The immunotherapeutic potential of melatonin. Expert Opinion on Investigational Drugs. 2001;**10**(3):467-476

[70] Vaghari-Tabari M et al. Melatonin and inflammatory bowel disease: From basic mechanisms to clinical application. Biochimie. 2023;**209**:20-36

[71] de Carvalho JF, Skare TL. Melatonin supplementation improves rheumatological disease activity: A systematic review. Clinical Nutrition ESPEN. 2023;**55**:414-419

[72] Doganay S et al. Protective role of melatonin against testicular damage caused by polymicrobial sepsis in adult rats. Turkish Journal of Trauma and Emergency Surgery. 2022;**28**(6):723

[73] Çokluk E et al. Investigation of the effect of melatonin administration on inflammatory mediators; MMP-2, TGF-β and VEGF levels in rats with sepsis. International Journal of Clinical Practice. 2021;**75**(11):e14832

[74] Xu L et al. Protective effect of melatonin against polymicrobial sepsis is mediated by the anti-bacterial effect of neutrophils. Frontiers in Immunology. 2019;**10**:1371

[75] Hu W et al. Utilizing melatonin to combat bacterial infections and septic injury. British Journal of Pharmacology. 2017;**174**(9):754-768

[76] Chuffa LGA et al. Melatonin attenuates the TLR4-mediated

inflammatory response through MyD88- and TRIF-dependent signaling pathways in an in vivo model of ovarian cancer. BMC Cancer. 2015;**15**:1-13

[77] Reiter RJ et al. Melatonin as an antioxidant: Under promises but over delivers. Journal of Pineal Research. 2016;**61**(3):253-278

[78] López LC et al. Melatonin restores the mitochondrial production of ATP in septic mice. Neuroendocrinology Letters. 2006;**27**(5):623-630

[79] Doganay S et al. Antioxidant and anti-inflammatory effects of nicotinamide adenine dinucleotide (NAD+) against acute Hepatorenal oxidative injury in an experimental sepsis model deneysel sepsis modelinde nikotinamid adenin dinükleotidin (NAD+) akut hepatorenal oksidatif hasara Karşı antioksidan ve anti-inflamatuar etkileri. Kafkas Universitesi Veteriner Fakultesi Dergisi. 2022;**28**(1):121-130

[80] Gitto E et al. Melatonin reduces oxidative stress in surgical neonates. Journal of Pediatric Surgery. 2004;**39**(2):184-189

[81] Taha AM et al. Melatonin as a potential treatment for septic cardiomyopathy. Biomedicine and Pharmacotherapy. 2023;**166**:115305

[82] Tordjman S et al. Melatonin: Pharmacology, functions and therapeutic benefits. Current Neuropharmacology. 2017;**15**(3):434-443

[83] Chen L et al. Melatonin alleviates renal injury in mouse model of sepsis. Frontiers in Pharmacology. 2021;**12**:697643

[84] Berberoglu AS et al. Melatonin relieves kidney damage caused by polymicrobial sepsis with its antioxidant and anti-inflammatory effect. Acta Physiologica. 2023;**240**:84-85

[85] Hu B et al. Melatonin promotes mitochondrial biogenesis and mitochondrial degradation in hepatocytes during sepsis. Alternative Therapies in Health and Medicine. 2023;**29**:284-289

[86] Sieminski M et al. Antioxidant and anti-inflammatory properties of melatonin in secondary traumatic brain injury. Antioxidants. 2024;**14**(1):25

[87] Srinivasan V, Mohamed M, Kato H. Melatonin in bacterial and viral infections with focus on sepsis: A review. Recent Patents on Endocrine, Metabolic and Immune Drug Discovery. 2012;**6**(1):30-39

[88] Hollenberg SM, Singer M. Pathophysiology of sepsis-induced cardiomyopathy. Nature Reviews Cardiology. 2021;**18**(6):424-434

[89] Lochner A, Marais E, Huisamen B. Melatonin and cardioprotection against ischaemia/reperfusion injury: What's new? A review. Journal of Pineal Research. 2018;**65**(1):e12490

[90] Yang C-S et al. The AMPK-PPARGC1A pathway is required for antimicrobial host defense through activation of autophagy. Autophagy. 2014;**10**(5):785-802

[91] Liu Q et al. Identification of PIK3CG as a hub in septic myocardial injury using network pharmacology and weighted gene co-expression network analysis. Bioengineering and Translational Medicine. 2023;**8**(1):e10384

[92] Chen L et al. Melatonin alleviates cardiac function in sepsis-caused myocarditis via maintenance of

mitochondrial function. Frontiers in Nutrition. 2021;**8**:754235

[93] Zhou Y et al. Exosomes from endothelial progenitor cells improve the outcome of a murine model of sepsis. Molecular Therapy. 2018;**26**(5):1375-1384

[94] Qiao X et al. Endothelial cell dynamics in sepsis-induced acute lung injury and acute respiratory distress syndrome: Pathogenesis and therapeutic implications. Cell Communication and Signaling. 2024;**22**(1):241

[95] Rawal G, Yadav S, Kumar R. Acute respiratory distress syndrome: An update and review. Journal of Translational Internal Medicine. 2018;**6**(2):74-77

[96] Ling J et al. Melatonin attenuates sepsis-induced acute lung injury via inhibiting excessive mitophagy. Drug Design, Development and Therapy. 2023:2775-2786

[97] Wang W, Gao J. Effects of melatonin on protecting against lung injury. Experimental and Therapeutic Medicine. 2021;**21**(3):1-1

[98] Li J et al. Melatonin attenuates sepsis-induced acute lung injury through improvement of epithelial sodium channel-mediated alveolar fluid clearance via activation of SIRT1/SGK1/Nedd4-2 signaling pathway. Frontiers in Pharmacology. 2020;**11**:590652

[99] Barlow KM et al. Efficacy of melatonin in children with postconcussive symptoms: A randomized clinical trial. Pediatrics. 2020;**145**(4)

[100] Ismy J et al. The effect of superoxide dismutase on inhibition of acute kidney injury induced by sepsis based on kidney tissue histology and murine sepsis score. The Scientific World Journal. 2021;**2021**(1):1827296

[101] Deng Z et al. Melatonin attenuates sepsis-induced acute kidney injury by promoting mitophagy through SIRT3-mediated TFAM deacetylation. Autophagy. 2024;**20**(1):151-165

[102] Yang J et al. Effects of melatonin against acute kidney injury: A systematic review and meta-analysis. International Immunopharmacology. 2023;**120**:110372

[103] Bai X-Z et al. Melatonin prevents acute kidney injury in severely burned rats via the activation of SIRT1. Scientific Reports. 2016;**6**(1):32199

[104] Liu R et al. Melatonin: A window into the organ-protective effects of sepsis. Biomedicine and Pharmacotherapy. 2022;**154**:113556

[105] Dai W et al. Melatonin prevents sepsis-induced renal injury via the PINK1/Parkin1 signaling pathway. International Journal of Molecular Medicine. 2019;**44**(4):1197-1204

[106] Looney MR. Platelets Induce Neutrophil Extracellular Traps in Transfusion-Related Acute Lung Injury. Washington, DC: American Society of Hematology; 2014

[107] Chen J-W et al. Sepsis-associated liver injury: Mechanisms and potential therapeutic targets. World Journal of Gastroenterology. 2024;**30**(42):4518

[108] Peng Z et al. Melatonin attenuates airway inflammation via SIRT1 dependent inhibition of NLRP3 inflammasome and IL-1β in rats with COPD. International Immunopharmacology. 2018;**62**:23-28

[109] Yang X-R et al. Role of sirtuins in sepsis and sepsis-induced organ dysfunction: A review. International Journal of Biological Macromolecules. 2024:134853